men's
health

men's
health

Edited by

Roger S Kirby MA MD FRCS (Urol) FEBU
Consultant Urologist, St. George's Hospital, London, UK

Michael G Kirby MB BS LRCP MRCS MRCP
Family Practitioner, The Surgery, Nevells Road, Letchworth, Hertfordshire, UK

Riad N Farah MD FACS
Vice-Chairman, Urology, Henry Ford Hospital, Detroit, MI, USA

Foreword by
Professor Sir Donald Acheson

I S I S
MEDICAL
MEDIA

© 1999 Isis Medical Media Ltd
59 St Aldates
Oxford OX1 1ST, UK

First published 1999
Reprinted 1999

British Library Cataloguing in Publication Data
A catalogue record for this title is available from the British Library.

ISBN 1 899066 92 6

Kirby, R. S. (Roger)
Men's Health
Roger S. Kirby, Michael G. Kirby and Riad N. Farah (eds)

Always refer to the manufacturer's Prescribing Information
before prescribing drugs cited in this book.

Isis Medical Media Staff
Commissioning Editor: John Harrison
Senior Editorial Controllers:
Catherine Rickards, Sarah Carlson
Production Controller: Geoff Holdsworth

Typeset by
Creative Associates,
115 Magdalen Road, Oxford OX4 1RS, UK

Medical illustration by
Dee McLean

Printed and bound by
Craft Print Pte Ltd., Singapore

Distributed in the USA by
Books International Inc.,
P.O. Box 605, Herndon, VA 20172, USA

Distributed in the rest of the world by
Plymbridge Distributors Ltd.,
Estover Road, Plymouth, PL6 7PY, UK

Contents

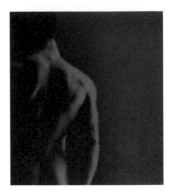

Contributors vii

Foreword ix

Preface xi

Dedication xiii

1. Men's health: closing the gender gap 1
   R. S. Kirby and M. G. Kirby

2. Anatomy and physiology of male sexual function 5
   S. D. Shetty and R. N. Farah

3. Impact of prostatic disease on men's health 11
   R. S. Kirby and M. G. Kirby

4. Testicular cancer 25
   W. F. Hendry

5. Duodenal and gastric ulcer disease 33
   S. E. Patchett and M. J. G. Farthing

6. Groin hernias 43
   H. B. Devlin

7. Colorectal cancer 51
   J. Northover

8. Tobacco smoking, cancer and premature death in men 63
   P. Boyle

9. Lumps, lesions and skin cancer 77
   G. R. Mikhail, S. D. Shetty and R. N. Farah

10a. Heart disease: lipids and hypertension 89
   A. F. Winder and I. James

10b. Heart disease: interventional cardiology 101
   A. E. Abdelmeguid

11. Diet, fat and cancer of the prostate 117
   M. J. Hill

12a. Male sexual dysfunction: diagnosis and treatment of erectile dysfunction 125
   C. C. Carson

12b.   Male sexual dysfunction: the male menopause   137
       W. D. Dunsmuir

13.   Infertility in men   147
       L. S. Ross

14.   Men as risk takers   155
       S. Griffiths

15.   Sexually transmitted diseases and men   161
       J. F. Jovanovich

16.   Men and suicide: assessment and management in a primary care setting   185
       D. P. Sugrue

17.   Office treatment and prevention of common sports injuries   197
       J. B. Ryan

18.   Osteoporosis in men   211
       A. C. Scane

19.   Disorders of the head and neck   221
       M. S. Benninger and G. M. Gardner

20.   Setting up a Well Man clinic in primary care   231
       M. G. Kirby

       Index   245

Contributors

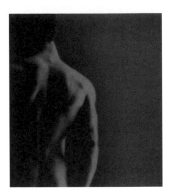

Alaa E. Abdelmeguid
Consultant Interventional Cardiologist, Heart Care Centers of Illinois, Kankakee, Illinois, USA

Michael S. Benninger
Chairman, Department of Otolaryngology – Head and Neck Surgery, Henry Ford Hospital, Detroit, MI, USA

Peter Boyle
Director, Division of Epidemiology and Biostatistics, European Institute of Oncology, Milan, Italy

Culley C. Carson III
Professor, Division of Urology, UNC School of Medicine, North Carolina, USA

H. Brendan Devlin (deceased)
Honorary Consultant Surgeon, North Tees General Hospital, Stockton on Tees, UK

William D. Dunsmuir
Senior Surgical Registrar in Urology, South West Thames Region, UK

Riad N. Farah
Vice Chairman, Department of Urology, Henry Ford Hospital, Detroit, MI, USA

Michael J. G. Farthing
Professor of Gastroenterology, Digestive Disease Research Centre, St Bartholomew's and Royal London School of Medicine and Dentistry, London, UK

Glendon M. Gardner
Department of Otolaryngology – Head and Neck Surgery, Henry Ford Hospital, Detroit, MI, USA

Siân Griffiths
Director of Public Health and Health Policy, Oxfordshire Health Authority, Oxford, UK

William F. Hendry
Genito-Urinary Surgeon, St Bartholomew's and Royal Marsden Hospitals, London, UK

Michael J. Hill
Chairman, European Cancer Prevention Organisation, Lady Sobell Gastrointestinal Unit, Wexham Park Hospital, Slough, UK

Ian James (deceased)
Reader and Consultant Physician, Academic Department of Medicine, Royal Free and University College Medical School, London, UK

John F. Jovanovich
Division of Infectious Diseases and Hospital Epidemiology, Henry Ford Hospital, Detroit, MI, USA

Michael G. Kirby
General Practitioner, The Surgery, Letchworth, Hospital Practitioner in Cardiology, Lister Hospital, Stevenage and Director of HertNet Primary Care Research Group, Hertfordshire, UK

Roger S. Kirby
Consultant Urologist, 149 Harley Street, London, UK and St. George's Hospital, London, UK

George R. Mikhail
Department of Mohs Surgery, Henry Ford Health Sysytem, Detroit, MI, USA

John Northover
Consultant Surgeon and Honorary Director, ICRF, Colorectal Cancer Unit, St Mark's Hospital, Harrow, Middlesex, UK

Stephen E. Patchett
Senior Lecturer/Honorary Consultant Gastroenterologist, Digestive Disease Research Centre, St Bartholomew's and Royal London School of Medicine and Dentistry, London, UK

Lawrence S. Ross
Clarence C. Saelhof Professor, Department of Urology, University of Illinois at Chicago College of Medicine, Chicago, Illinois, USA

John B. Ryan
St John Macomb Orthopedics and Sports Medicine, Warren, MI, USA

Andrew C. Scane
Consultant Physician, North Tees General Hospital, Stockton on Tees, UK

Sugandh D. Shetty
Senior Staff Urologist, Henry Ford Hospital, Detroit, MI, USA

Dennis P. Sugrue
Associate Division Head, Outpatient Psychiatry, Henry Ford Health System, West Bloomfield, MI, USA

Anthony F. Winder
Professor, Department of Molecular Pathology and Clinical Biochemistry, Royal Free and University College Medical School, London, UK

Foreword

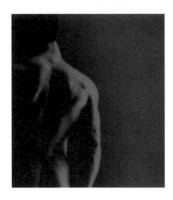

It is sometimes said that doctors tend to write too much, and that it might be better if we stuck more closely to our clinical work. With these thoughts in mind, I consulted the librarian of one of the largest collections of medical books in England. The results were remarkable. Even when 114 books and reports on obstetrics and gynaecology were excluded, there remained 90 further books on women's health. For children, setting aside 274 books and reports on paediatrics, there were 258 more dealing with child health. In contrast there were only five entries in the index dealing specifically with the health of men.

I therefore conclude with some confidence that a comprehensive, up-to-the-minute text such as this dealing with the main afflictions prevalent among men will be welcomed, and that its publication should prove to be a major literary event.

One of the ironies about the prevailing lack of attention to the health of men is that at all stages of life from the foetus to old age, the mortality of males is higher than that of females and taken overall expectation of life in Britain is five years longer in women than in men. In early life most of the male excess is associated with trauma due presumably to our hormone-derived rash and venturesome nature (Chapter 14 deals with men as risk takers). Later in life, excesses in mortality from cardiovascular disease and a number of cancers are added and come to dominate the picture.

But it is when one looks at the health of men and women in the context of the various degrees of socio-economic disadvantage that the starkest contrast between the sexes is revealed. This is illustrated by the fact that women living in the least favourable circumstances have a substantially better mortality experience than men living in the most favourable conditions [1]. To reduce these differences there will need to be new health policies directed at the problems of men.

As might be expected, *Men's Health* deals comprehensively with male sexual function in all its aspects including anatomy, physiology, sexual dysfunction and the male menopause, with additional chapters on sexually transmitted diseases in men and on infertility. Many doctors doubtless will turn to this book to seek clinical advice on the only too prevalent problems of erectile dysfunction (which affects 1 in 10 of all men at some stage). The text combines authority with a sensitive approach in dealing with this devastating issue.

However, the problems of men's health extend far beyond their sexual function. The book is touchingly dedicated to Roger and Michael Kirby's father, Professor Kenneth Kirby, who died of coronary heart disease in the prime of life in 1967. There are admirable chapters on heart disease and hypertension and a number of other conditions commonly occurring in men are also dealt with.

I was glad to see that *Men's Health* recognises the importance of suicide as a serious and increasing problem in young men. In Britain there is a phenomenal differential in suicide according to social circumstances with rates four times higher among the unskilled and socially excluded than the best off [1]. If I may add a personal impression on the basis of work in the prison system, many of these young men suffer from the depressing combination of a lack of marketable skills and of any expectation of a settled role in family life.

Fittingly, *Men's Health* concludes with a chapter on setting up 'Well Man' clinics in primary care. The chapter is drafted within the framework of the national strategy for health and emphasises the need for health promotion to be based on proven effectiveness and audit. Many who read this excellent book will join me in the view that, subject to regular evaluation as the idea develops, 'Well Man' clinics are likely soon to achieve an accepted place alongside 'Well Woman' and 'Mother and Baby' clinics throughout our primary care system.

Professor Sir Donald Acheson

1. Acheson, D. Independent Inquiry into Inequalities in Health Report, London: TSO, 1998;78–81,102

Preface

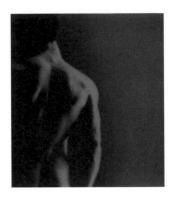

Men die on average five years younger than women, and many well before their sixty-fifth birthday. This difference between men and women has been termed the 'gender gap', and the means of closing it constitute the subject of this book. Poor health impacts not only on the sufferer, but also on his entire family. The premature death of the father figure and main income generator leaves the family bereft, as two of the authors of this book know first hand (see Dedication), and can have a profound effect on the next generation.

Although the prevention of premature death constitutes the headline story, avoidance of preventable chronic ill health provides an important backdrop to the subject. In the UK alone, for example, 187 million working days are lost through sickness. And this is only the tip of the iceberg, since the retirement years of very many men are blighted by preventable ill health.

Men's Health focuses on these issues and stresses the central role of health education. It is no good a man waiting until he is ill and then stating, "If I had known I would live this long I would have taken more care of myself." Men and the doctors who care for them must learn to think in preventative terms.

Contributions from some of the world's experts on men's diseases cover cardiac, pulmonary, urological and many other illnesses. The role of primary prevention is discussed for each. In the final chapter practical recommendations for setting up and running a men's health clinic are outlined.

The editors and Isis Medical Media acknowledge with grateful thanks the role of Sir Christopher Lewinton, Chairman of TI Group plc, and his Board of Directors in supporting work in this area of health and in encouraging the development and production of this book. Sir Christopher's and TI Group's belief in the importance of sharing experience and knowledge between businesses and between nations has been a significant element in the successful growth of TI Group. This belief, applied to the sharing of medical knowledge between the US and the UK has been a valuable guiding principle for the editors.

We are grateful, as well, for the outstanding contributions from all our authors, the tireless editing of Christine McKillop and Ben Jeapes, and the beautifully lucid artwork of Dee McLean. We very much hope this book will help men all over the world to live happier, healthier and longer lives.

Roger S. Kirby, Michael G. Kirby and Riad N. Farah

Dedication

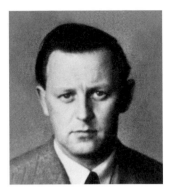

This book is dedicated to Professor Kenneth Kirby who died prematurely of heart disease at the age of 49, having sustained his first infarction at the age of 46. Professor Sir Alexander Haddow contributed the following obituary in The Times (13 November 1967):

'Cancer research, chemistry and science in general have sustained a grievous loss in the death on November 10th 1967, of Professor Kenneth Kirby, after severe ill-health lasting for several years. Aged 49, in spite of his affliction he was at the height of his knowledge and powers.

'Kenneth Kirby graduated B.Sc. with first-class honours at the University of Manchester in 1940. He took his Ph.D. at the University of Leeds in 1949, where he specialised in the chemistry of textiles and leather — an experience which was to stand him in great stead, and which largely fashioned his contributions to biological chemistry in later years. He proceeded to D.Sc. of the University of Manchester in 1962. After his first graduation, Kirby worked successively in the water pollution research laboratories, and in the Wellcome laboratories of tropical medicine (on the chemotherapy of amoebiasis). Later, he became attached to the Forestal, Land, Timber and Railways Co. Ltd., where he developed an expert knowledge of the complex chemistry of the tannins which he was later to apply to our understanding of the carcinogenic potentiality of these substances.

'In 1953 Kirby was appointed to the Chester Beatty Research Institute (of the Institute of Cancer Research: Royal Cancer Hospital) as a Fellow of the British Empire Cancer Campaign, and soon became a member of the permanent scientific staff working in the Institute's research station at Pollards Wood, Chalfont St Giles, Buckinghamshire. Very rapidly he established his own school actively engaged in exploration of natural products in normal and abnormal cells both animal and human. He was named Reader in Chemistry in the University of London in 1965 and was granted the title of Professor of Cell Chemistry in February of the present year. His main contribution lay in the field of nucleic acids, in their fractionation, isolation, characterization and functions, in studies of the enzymes controlling nucleic acid synthesis, of protein synthesis itself, and one of the nucleic acid:protein association. He introduced highly novel methods and techniques for the isolation of the nucleic acids by the use of phenolic solvents — techniques which were soon accepted throughout the world and which made a substantial impact upon the development of this sphere of chemistry. Kirby thus acquired international acclaim soon reflected in the large number of students from many lands who came to work with him and to seek his guidance. His great contributions to technique and methodology must not be allowed to obscure his clear views on the future of nucleic acid chemistry. He regarded these technical improvements as a mere if essential prelude, and had he been spared, we would certainly have seen the ultimate flowering. Even so, Kirby's work has already added materially to our knowledge of cancer and the adjacent field of virology, and to that of cell growth, cell transformation and differentiation. As a person, Kirby was in my own experience unique in his humanity and sympathy. Most of us have our ridiculous faults and foibles, antipathies and animosities, but Kirby had none of these. Outstanding were his gaiety and humour — maintained to the end — often Rabelaisian and earthy but never unkind, and which made him the joy of any gathering. I have rarely met a man so much liked and respected, or more universally and affectionately accepted as a leader. Death came to him as a friend. If we are bereft, yet do we hold strong and grateful memories which must bring succour also to his loving wife and family to whom our hearts extend.'

© Alexander Haddow/The Times, London 1967

CHAPTER 1

Men's health: closing the gender gap

R. S. Kirby and M. G. Kirby

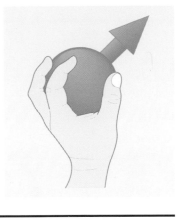

Introduction

Men live, on average, for 5 years less than women. Currently, the average expectation of life in the UK is 73.9 years for men compared with 79.2 for women. For many years, this phenomenon has been attributed to some intrinsic difference in overall disease susceptibility between the sexes. Of late, however, it has become apparent that at least some of the difference in life expectancy between the sexes reflects the fact that men look after themselves very much less well than do women. This general lack of health awareness among males has been termed the 'gender gap'.

Despite these disturbing health differences between men and women, a Men's Health Matters Gallup Survey carried out in 1997 found that only half of the men surveyed were worried about developing heart disease [1]. Only 16% of men said that they would consult their doctor immediately if they had a mildly irritating health problem; 31% said they would wait until the problem worsened. Also, 32% of men over 65 had experienced problems urinating (a potential indicator of prostate problems), but only 11% had been diagnosed as having a prostate problem.

Nevertheless, it may be an oversimplification to state that women consistently report higher levels of ill-health than men. It appears that the difference in reporting of ill-health between men and women may vary according to the particular symptom or condition and the patient's phase of life [2]. Mid-life in men is often a peak time for work and family responsibilities. Stresses due to the fulfilment of these responsibilities, finances, relationships with children and the loss of parents commonly occur in mid-life, with a consequent negative effect on the man's health. In addition, reaching the midpoint in the life span implies a recognition of declining energy, memory, physical fitness and health. In the late 1990s, being a mid-

dle-aged man also means facing up to the current changes in society, such as the changing traditional male roles in response to women's changing roles and the possible prospect of redundancy and early retirement. Work is an important central role for many men and its loss can have devastating effects.

Cardiovascular disease

Cardiovascular problems are the main cause of male deaths in the UK, closely followed by cancer (Table 1.1) [3]. One in five men dies prematurely before the age of 75 from cardiovascular disease [3]. Men's greater susceptibility to heart disease has generally been ascribed to a lack of the protective effects of oestrogen. However, most of the preventable risk factors for myocardial infarction or stroke — such as smoking, central obesity and hypertension — are considerably more common in men than women. Of UK males, 10% have high blood pressure but are not receiving treatment [3]; a further 13% of men are

Table 1.1. *Relative causes of male deaths in the UK [3]*

Disease	Percentage of male deaths
Coronary heart disease	27
Stroke	6
Other cardiovascular diseases	7
Lung cancer	10
Prostate cancer	4
Colorectal cancer	3
Other cancers	15
Respiratory disease	9
Injuries and poisoning	7
All other causes	12

currently being treated for high blood pressure but, because of inadequate therapy, half of these still have significant hypertension.

Cancer

In 1990, over 136 000 men in the UK had cancer diagnosed; in 1994, over 82 000 men died of the disease [4]. Prostate cancer is the second most common male cancer, and a leading cause of cancer death, with over 15 000 new cases and around 10 000 deaths per year in the UK (Table 1.2) [4].

Reduced awareness among men of the malignant diseases to which their bodies are prone may also be a factor in the gender gap. Lung cancer can largely be prevented by abstinence from smoking, a habit more commonly and more heavily indulged in by men. Colon cancer, particularly in those with a positive family history, can be detected early and cured with little morbidity by the use of faecal occult blood testing and flexible colonoscopy. Prostate cancer, which may have a familial link in up to 9% of cases, can be detected early by means of prostate-specific antigen (PSA) testing and digital rectal examination (DRE), and cured by radiotherapy

or surgery. In a recent study of stored serum, PSA testing was strongly predictive of the subsequent development of clinical prostate cancer [5]. In spite of this, there have been no concerted efforts yet in the UK to reduce the rising death toll of the malignancies most prevalent among men. This is in contrast to the £60 million or more spent annually on screening for breast and cervical cancer in women.

Lifestyle factors

Many premature deaths are linked to unhealthy dietary and lifestyle habits, as well as risk-taking behaviour. Studies show that 44% of men in England are overweight, with an additional 15% classed as obese [3]. A total of 28% of men still smoke, even though lifelong male smokers have only a 42% chance of reaching the age of 73 compared with a 78% chance for men who have never smoked [6]; furthermore, 27% of men drink more than the recommended limit of 3–4 units per day [3]. High blood cholesterol (> 6.5 mmol/l) is present in 28% of men and only 31% of men take part in physical activity that will afford them some protection against coronary heart disease [3].

Although trauma is far less common as a cause of death than either cardiovascular disease or malignancy, mortality from trauma — as a result of accidents, violence or suicide — contributes significantly to the total loss of anticipated life years because such incidents so often involve young people. Here again, men are very much more susceptible than women: risk-taking behaviour is predominantly the province of young men and could potentially be reduced by focused education.

Psychological problems

The major causes of mortality among young men in England and Wales are injury and poisoning, included in which are homicide, suicide and accidents. During 1992, deaths from injury and poisoning accounted for 52% of all deaths in the 15–39 age group in men [7]; the predominant portion of deaths due to injury and poisoning can be attributable to men rather than to women. Emphasis needs to be placed on discussing and managing specific problems with young men, particularly homelessness, drugs and unemployment.

Table 1.2. *Male cancers: incidence and causes of death*

The 10 most common sites of cancer in men	The 10 most common sites of cancer causing death in men
Lung	Lung
Prostate	Prostate
Skin (non-melanoma)	Bowel
Bowel	Stomach
Bladder	Oesophagus
Non-Hodgkin's lymphoma	Pancreas
Pancreas	Leukaemia
Stomach	Bladder
Oesophagus	Non-Hodgkin's lymphoma
Leukaemia	Brain

Social inequalities

The English Green Paper on public health, *Our Healthier Nation — a Contract for Health*, recognizes that ill-health is not spread evenly across our society. Statistics show the following:

- More people die of lung cancer in the north of England than in the south;
- Children in the lowest social class are five times more likely to die as the result of an accident than are those in the top social class;
- In nearly every case, the highest incidence of illness is experienced by the worst-off people.

Differences in health between groups of men are of concern. The inverse social gradient for mortality is unlikely to be due solely to social class differences in individual lifestyles. Research shows that men of lower social status suffer more financial problems, more stressful life events, less adequate social support and more feelings of disempowerment within the workplace.

In the UK, Asian men have higher rates of heart disease than their White counterparts [8]. Also, Afro-Caribbean men are more likely to suffer from severe mental illness and to be admitted to secure wards [9]. It has been suggested that improving the health of men from the ethnic minorities will require a reduction in stress due to unemployment, poor housing and other forms of racism. One of the key aims of the Green Paper is to improve the health of the worst-off in society and to narrow the health gap.

Male-specific problems

Almost half of the 22.5 million men aged over 16 are suffering from a specific male complaint. Benign prostatic hyperplasia (BPH) affects an estimated 2 million men in the UK [10], while 14% of men in their 40s and 40% of men in their 70s have clinical symptoms of BPH [11]. Autopsy studies indicate that the disease affects almost 80% of males over 80 years of age.

Erectile dysfunction is a common complaint in men, with an estimated 10% of men over the age of 16 suffering from the condition at some time in their life [12]. Although in many cases the erectile dysfunction can be treated, many men do not seek help because of embarrassment or the belief that nothing can be done to help. It

has also been estimated that 1% of men suffer from Peyronie's disease; the curvature that occurs on erection can be severe, resulting in painful erection and excluding the possibility of sexual intercourse. Surveys have suggested that premature ejaculation is another common problem: eight out of 10 men are thought to ejaculate within 1–5 minutes of penetration, with two of these eight doing so within a minute [13].

Testicular pain can be due to infection or torsion of the testes, but many men fear it, thinking that it is a sign of testicular cancer. The longer the patient delays seeing a doctor about a torsion, the worse the prognosis. However, testicular cancer is usually detected by the presence of a lump and not the presence of pain. The reluctance among men for self-examination often means that patients with testicular cancer present late and have a poorer chance of cure and greater morbidity.

What can be done

What steps should be taken to improve the health of menfolk worldwide? A campaign of public information seems appropriate, since the answer to these problems lies largely in the hands of individuals themselves, rather than the endeavours of bureaucrats. Men should be actively encouraged to adopt a healthier lifestyle, in terms of both diet and exercise, and exhorted to give up smoking. A visit to a Well Man Clinic could include a health check for cardiovascular disease, and enquiry should be made about rectal bleeding as well as symptoms of prostatism. A focused examination based on family and clinical history should be conducted. In addition, an examination of the testes or information on self-examination seems appropriate, especially since the incidence of testicular cancer has doubled over the last 20 years. It seems appropriate to counsel men over 45 years of age (especially those with a family history of prostate cancer) about PSA testing, as well as to perform a dipstick examination of the urine. Transitional cell carcinoma more commonly occurs in men, especially those who are heavy smokers, and may present as microscopic haematuria. Erectile dysfunction, although not in itself life threatening, is associated with reduced quality of life; it can now be safely and effectively treated and should be discussed.

Regular health checks not only allow the detection of diseases, at a stage when they can be treated effectively, but also provide an opportunity for men to be educated about the way to stay fit, as well as to discuss their health concerns. Men have a much greater tendency than women to bury their heads in the sand on health matters, often hiding behind the excuse that they do not want to bother the doctor [14]. The result is that they often present with disease that has progressed beyond the stage of cure. Education should be targeted in the workplace — by, for example, campaigns to give up smoking and the importance of diet and regular exercise — to raise general and specific health awareness among men.

Conclusions

Much remains to be done to prove in prospective randomized controlled studies that preventative strategies are effective; however, while more men are dying prematurely every year, there seems no better time than the present to encourage men of all ages to live healthier, happier and *longer* lives.

References

1. Men's health matters in the nineties: a report of the Men's Health Matters Gallup Survey 1997; Gallup: London
2. MacIntyre S, Hunt K, Sweeting H. Gender differences in health: are things really as simple as they seem? *Soc Sci Med*, 1996; 42: 617–624
3. Coronary Heart Disease Statistics. British Heart Foundation, 1997: 1–25
4. Imperial Cancer Research Fund Cancer Statistics Fact Sheet, London: ICRF, June 1997
5. Parkes C, Wald N, Murphy P *et al*. Prospective observational study to assess the value of prostate specific antigen as a screening test for prostate cancer. *Br Med J* 1995; 311: 1338–1343
6. Philips AN, Wannamether SG, Walter M *et al*. Life expectancy in men who have never smoked and those who have smoked continuously: 15 year follow up of large cohort of middle aged British men. *Br Med J* 1996; 313: 907–908
7. Charlton J, Kelly S, Dunnell K, Evans B. Trends in suicide deaths in England and Wales. *Pop Trends* 1992; 69: 10–16
8. Gupta S, de Belder A, O'Hughes L. Avoiding premature coronary deaths in Asians in Britain. *Br Med J* 1995; 311: 1035–1036
9. Griffiths S. Men's health: unhealthy lifestyles and an unwillingness to seek medical help. *Br Med J* 1996; 312: 69–70
10. Kirby RS. Costs and options in BPH. Medicom Excel: London, 1996: 1–8
11. Garraway WM, Collins GN, Lee RJ. High prevalence of benign prostatic hyperplasia in the community. *Lancet* 1991; 338: 469–471
12. Men's Health Trust Factsheet 2. The penis: 1–17
13. Bradford N. Men's health matters: the complete A to Z of male health. Vermilion: London, 1995, 380
14. Carroll S. The Which Guide to Men's Health. Penguin, London 1995: 173–230

CHAPTER 2

Anatomy and physiology of male sexual function

S. D. Shetty and R. N. Farah

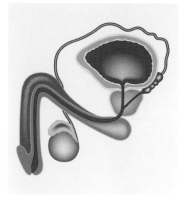

Penile anatomy

The penile erectile apparatus consists of paired vascular spongy organs, the corpora cavernosa, which are closely attached to each other except in the proximal third. Ventral to the penile shaft is the corpus spongiosum, through which the urethra passes; it expands distally to form the glans penis. The penile skin is continuous with that of the lower abdominal wall and continues over the glans penis to form the prepuce and then folds on itself to reattach at the coronal sulcus. The penile skin envelops the shaft and can be moved freely over the erect organ. The underlying fascial layer or the dartos fascia (Colles' fascia) is continuous with Scarpa's fascia of the lower abdominal wall. It continues inferiorly as the dartos fascia of the scrotum and Colles' fascia of the perineum and attaches to the posterior border of the perineal membrane. The superficial dorsal vein lies in this layer of the fascia. Buck's fascia is the deep layer of the penile fascia that covers both the corpora cavernosa and the corpus spongiosum in separate fascial compartments (Fig. 2.1). Proximally, Buck's fascia is attached to the perineal membrane; distally, it is tightly attached to the base of

the glans penis at the coronal sulcus, where it fuses with the ends of the corpora. The ischiocavernosus and the bulbospongiosus muscles lie beneath Colles' fascia but superficial to Buck's fascia, to which their intrinsic fascia is loosely attached. Buck's fascia has a dense structure composed of longitudinally running fibres and is firmly attached to the underlying tunica albuginea. It encloses the deep dorsal vein, the dorsal arteries and the dorsal nerves (Fig. 2.2).

The fundiform ligament is a thickening of the superficial penile fascia, deep within which is the suspensory ligament, which is in continuity with Buck's fascia. The attachment of this ligament to the pubic symphysis maintains the penile position during erection; consequently, its severance will lead to a lower angulation of the penile shaft during erection.

The tunica albuginea forms a thick fibrous coat over the spongy tissue of the corpora cavernosa and corpus spongiosum. It consists of two layers — the outer longitudinal and the inner

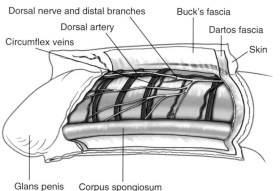

Figure 2.1. *Fascial layers of the penile shaft.*

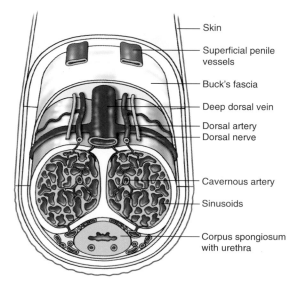

Figure 2.2. *Cross-section of the mid-penile shaft.*

circular. The tunica albuginea provides a tough uniform backing for the engorged sinusoidal spaces. It is thinner in the region of the corpus spongiosum and contains smooth muscle that aids ejaculation. The glans penis is devoid of tunica albuginea. The corpora are separated centrally by an intercavernous septum, which is perforated on its dorsal margin by vertical openings that provide communication between the corpora. Along the inner aspect of the tunica albuginea, numerous flattened columns or sinusoidal trabeculae — composed of fibrous tissue, elastin fibres and smooth muscle — surround the endothelial-lined sinusoids or cavernous spaces.

Muscles of erectile function

The ischiocavernosus is a paired muscle that increases penile turgor during erection beyond that attainable by arterial pressure alone. It is innervated by the perineal branch of the pudendal nerve (S3–4).

The bulbospongiosus muscle invests the bulb of the urethra and the distal corpus spongiosum. It is supplied by a deep branch of the perineal nerve. This muscle helps to empty the last few drops of urine and to ejaculate semen.

Arterial blood supply to the penis

The arterial supply to the erectile apparatus originates from superficial and deep arterial systems. The superficial arterial system arises as two symmetrically arranged vessels from the inferior external pudendal artery — a branch of the femoral artery. Each vessel divides into a dorsolateral and ventrolateral branch, supplying the skin of the penile shaft and the prepuce. There is communication between the superficial and deep arterial systems at the coronal sulcus. The deep arterial system arises from the internal pudendal artery, which is the final branch of the anterior trunk of the internal iliac artery. The internal pudendal artery divides into the perineal and penile arteries (Fig. 2.3). The penile artery divides into three branches — the bulbo-urethral artery, the urethral artery and the cavernous artery or deep artery of the penis; it terminates as the deep dorsal artery of the penis. An accessory internal pudendal may arise from the obturator, the inferior vesical or the superior vesical arteries; this may be damaged during radical prostatectomy in as many as 50% of patients. The dorsal artery may arise from the accessory internal pudendal artery within the pelvis, endangering it during radical pelvic surgery. On its way to the glans penis, it gives off the circumflex arteries which supply the corpus spongiosum.

Intracorporal circulation

Arterial blood is conveyed to the erectile tissue in the deep arterial system by means of the dorsal, cavernous and bulbo-urethral arteries. The cavernous artery gives off multiple helicine arteries among the cavernous spaces within the centre of the erectile tissue. Most of these open directly into the sinusoids bounded by trabeculae; a few helicine arteries terminate in capillaries which supply the trabeculae. The emissary veins at the periphery collect the blood from the sinusoids through the subalbugineal venular plexuses and empty it into the circumflex veins, which drain into the deep dorsal vein. With erection, the arteriolar and sinusoidal walls relax and the cavernous spaces dilate, enlarging the corporal bodies and stretching the tunica albuginea. The veins are compressed and trapped between the trabeculae, preventing outflow of blood. The direction of blood flow can be summarized as follows: cavernous artery → helicine arteries → sinusoids → post-cavernous venules → subalbugineal venous plexus → emissary vein.

Venous drainage

The venous drainage system consists of three distinct groups of veins — superficial, intermediate and deep. The superficial drainage system consists of venous drainage from the penile skin and prepuce into the superficial dorsal vein, which joins the saphenous vein via the external pudendal vein. The intermediate system consists of the deep dorsal and circumflex veins, which drain via the prostatic plexus into the deep dorsal vein. The deep drainage system consists of the cavernous veins, the bulbar vein and the crural veins. Blood from the sinusoids in the proximal one-third of the penis drains directly

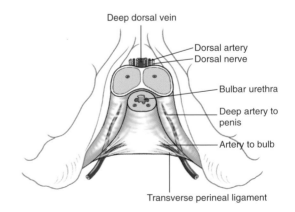

Figure 2.3. *Arterial and venous supply of the penis at the level of the perineal membrane.*

into cavernous veins. The two cavernous veins join to form the main cavernous vein, which drains into the internal pudendal vein to form the main venous drainage of the corpora cavernosa. Crural veins arise from the dorsolateral surface of each crus and unite to drain into the internal pudendal vein. The bulb is drained by the bulbar vein, which drains into the prostatic plexus.

Lymphatic drainage

The lymphatics from the penile skin and prepuce run proximally towards the presymphyseal plexus and then divide into right and left trunks; these join the lymphatics from the scrotum and the perineum. Some drainage occurs through the femoral canal into Cloquet's node. The lymphatics from the glans penis and the penile urethra drain into the deep inguinal nodes and presymphyseal nodes, and occasionally into external iliac nodes.

Nerves

Somatic innervation arises from sacral spinal segments S2–4 via the pudendal nerve. The perineal branch of the pudendal nerve supplies the posterior part of the scrotum and the rectal nerve to the inferior rectal area. The pudendal nerve continues as the dorsal nerve of the penis. In epispadias and bladder exstrophy, the dorsal nerves are displaced laterally in the middle and distal portion of the penile shaft. Cutaneous nerves to the penis and the scrotum arise from the dorsal and posterior branches of the pudendal nerve. The anterior part of the scrotum and proximal penis is supplied by the ilio-inguinal nerve after it leaves the superficial inguinal ring. The pudendal nerve supplies the ischiocavernosus and bulbocavernosus muscles; it branches into the inferior rectal nerve and the scrotal nerve and continues as the dorsal nerve of the penis.

The autonomic nerves consist of sympathetics which arise from lumbar segments L1 and L2 and parasympathetics from S2–4 (nervi erigentes or pelvic nerve). Lumbar splanchnic nerves join the superior hypogastric plexus and, from here, right and left hypogastric nerves travel to the inferior hypogastric plexus. The pelvic plexus adjacent to the base of the bladder, prostate, seminal vesicles and rectum also contains parasympathetic fibres. Nerves from the inferior pelvic plexus supply the prostate, the seminal vesicles, the epididymis, the membranous and penile urethra, and the bulbourethral gland.

Cavernous nerves/Neurovascular bundle

The cavernous nerves arise from the pelvic plexus from the lateral surface of the rectum. The branches from the cavernous nerve accompany the branches of the prostatovesicular artery and provide a macroscopic landmark for nerve-sparing radical prostatectomy. The cavernous nerve supplies each corpus cavernosum, the corpus spongiosum and the penile urethra, and ends as a delicate network around the erectile tissue.

Testes, spermatic cord and scrotum

The testes are the primary reproductive organs in males and hang in the scrotum by the spermatic cord, which contains the vas deferens, the testicular and vasal arteries, the pampiniform plexus and the lymphatics. The testes measure approximately $5 \times 3 \times 2$ cm and weigh 10–14 g each. The testes are covered by the tunica albuginea, within which are the seminiferous tubules. These tubules are lined by Sertoli cells and spermatogonia. Interspersed between the tubules are the Leydig cells, which produce testosterone. Spermatozoa are produced in the tubules and travel through the vasa efferentia into the epididymis; the vas deferens, a thick muscular tube 2–3 mm in diameter, serves as a conduit. The terminal portion of the vas deferens is dilated to form the ampulla and opens on the verumontanum.

The seminal vesicles are pyramidal, paired, glandular organs that lie behind the prostate and the bladder neck. The secretions from seminal vesicles contribute 70% of the ejaculate and form a seminal coagulum. Spermatozoa mature in the epididymis and the ampulla of the vas deferens. Seminal vesicles have both cholinergic and adrenergic innervation, and contract during ejaculation.

Accessory male sexual organs

Prostate

The prostate is a chestnut-shaped fibromuscular gland situated at the base of the bladder neck and through which runs the prostatic urethra. Secretions from the prostrate form 13–32% of the ejaculate volume and empty into the prostatic urethra via the ejaculatory duct.

Cowper's glands

Cowper's glands are paired organs located in the urogenital diaphragm lateral to the membranous urethra. Ducts from the glands pierce the perineal membrane and enter the bulbar urethra. They secrete a milky white or yellowish fluid into the urethra during sexual excitement.

Glands of Littré

Glands of Littré line the penile urethra and secrete a clear mucus on sexual arousal, which lubricates the urethra.

Physiology of male sexual function

The normal male sexual function is the result of an interaction between the hypothalamus, the pituitary gland and the testes (Fig. 2.4) [1]. The hypothalamus has the central role of integrating the signals that modulate the release of luteinizing hormone (LH) and follicle-stimulating hormone (FSH). Gonadotrophin-releasing hormone (GnRH) is released from the hypothalamus in response to adrenergically and humorally mediated stimuli. GnRH stimulates the release of LH and FSH from the basophils of the anterior pituitary, which regulate testosterone synthesis and spermatogenesis. LH controls testosterone synthesis and release from the Leydig cells; the release of LH is controlled by a negative feedback system based on the levels of testosterone and oestradiol. FSH stimulates spermatogenesis by increasing the local production of androgen-binding protein, resulting in greater intracellular binding of testosterone. Sertoli cells release inhibin, which modulates the FSH secretion. Prolactin is also secreted by the anterior pituitary under the regulation of prolactin inhibitory factor. Hyperprolactinaemia can cause impotence and is usually associated with decreased levels of circulating testosterone.

Testosterone plays an important part in the initiation of spermatogenesis, meiosis and spermatid maturation. It is converted in the target organs to dihydrotestosterone (DHT) by the enzyme 5-alpha-reductase. The effects of testosterone are (a) regulatory, (b) trophic and (c) maintenance of libido. As noted previously, testosterone regulates the release of GnRH and LH by a negative feedback mechanism. The target organs for testosterone include the prostate, the seminal vesicles and Cowper's and Littré's glands. Each of these accessory organs contributes to the ejaculatory volume, a decrease in which is a sign of androgen insufficiency.

Testosterone is necessary for maintenance of sexual desire or libido. Hypogonadal men have impaired sexual function through diminished desire (libido) rather than a failure of erectile function. The level of testosterone required for adequate sexual desire is not known, although higher levels do not increase libido or erectile function.

Mechanism of erection

Central and peripheral sexual stimulation lead to increased impulses in the pelvic nerves and subsequently to increased blood flow through the pudendal arteries and the corpora cavernosa. On initiation of erection, the sinusoidal smooth muscle relaxes, causing an increase in the diameter of the sinusoids and in blood content, resulting in elongation of the corpora. The intracorporal pressure remains fairly constant during the initial phase and the corporal diameter increases before any change in rigidity. With further filling, the intracavernosal pressure rises and rigidity increases. A fully rigid penis requires 80–115 ml of blood for a 7.5 cm increase in penile length; pressure increases to 90–100 mmHg in the corpora cavernosa and 40–50 mm in the glans penis. Animal and penile cast studies have demonstrated that, in the flaccid state, the arterioles are constricted and the sinusoidal trabeculae are contracted, offering maximal resistance for arterial inflow. In

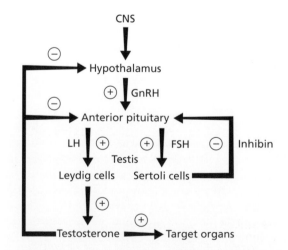

Figure 2.4. *The hypothalamus–pituitary–testis axis in a male: CNS, central nervous system; GnRH, gonadotrophin-releasing hormone; LH, luteinizing hormone; FSH, follicle-stimulating hormone.*

addition, the venules interspersed between the sinusoids are dilated. The maintenance of erection is brought about by the compression of the subalbugineal venous plexus against the tough tunica albuginea and compression of the emissary veins (Fig. 2.5). This leads to decreased venous outflow from, and engorgement of, the corpora. Contraction of the ischiocavernosus muscles raises the corporal pressure further to 350 mmHg, to produce a rigid erection.

Neurotransmitters

Nitric oxide (NO) has recently been identified as an important neurotransmitter in the erectile process [2]. It is derived from L-arginine by the action of the enzyme nitric oxide synthase (NOS). NO activates guanyl cyclase, which converts guanosine triphosphate (GTP) to cyclic guanosine monophosphate (cGMP) — an important second messenger (Fig. 2.6).

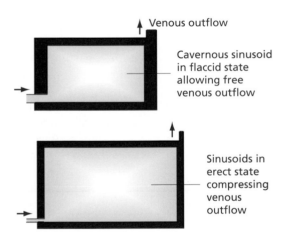

Figure 2.5. *A diagrammatic representation of the mechanism of erection.*

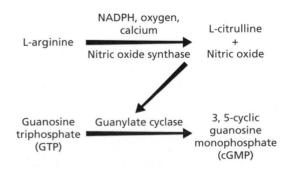

Figure 2.6. *The nitric oxide pathway in the erectile process: NADPH, reduced nicotinamide–adenine dinucleotide phosphate.*

Studies in vitro of bovine penis and of rat and mouse anococcygeus muscle provide the first evidence that NO produces genital smooth muscle relaxation. In studies in vitro on cavernous tissue specimens from human penis, direct application of NO or its substrate L-arginine caused tissue relaxation, which was blocked by infusion of tetrodotoxin. This was a non-adrenergic, non-cholinergic (NANC) reaction, since cholinergic and adrenergic blockade did not affect the relaxation. Electrically induced erections can be blocked by intravenous or intracavernous administration of inhibitors of NOS, and these effects are reversed by administration of NO or NO substrates. Further evidence comes from intracavernous injection of NO-releasing substances (sodium nitroprusside and S-nitroso N-acetylpenicillamine), cGMP or specific cGMP phosphodiesterase inhibitors, which leads to penile tumescence in the dog, cat and monkey.

Immunohistochemical studies have shown that NOS is localized to neuronal elements supplying the penis, including the pelvic plexus, cavernous nerves and their terminal endings. Bilateral cavernous nerve transection abolished the immunostaining in NOS-containing neurons but not in the vascular endothelium. These studies strongly indicate that NO is produced in nerves and acts as a postganglionic neurotransmitter of NANC-mediated penile erection. Local diffusion of NO to the vascular and trabecular smooth muscle in the penis results in vasodilatation. NO is also produced by the trabecular and vascular endothelium. The major stimulus for vascular endothelial NO is acetylcholine released by the parasympathetic nerve terminals that contact the endothelium.

Detumescence occurs when the erection signals cease, the trabecular smooth muscles contract and the venules dilate. Failure of detumescence leads to persistent erection (priapism).

Emission, ejaculation and orgasm

Emission is the deposition of semen in the posterior urethra and is mediated by the sympathetic contraction of the seminal vesicles, terminal vas deferens and prostate. Ejaculation is the expulsion of seminal fluid from the urethra. During ejaculation the bladder neck is closed and a forward propulsion occurs as a result of rhythmic contraction of the bulbospongiosus and pelvic musculature at 0.8-second intervals, as well as intermittent relaxation of the external sphincter. Loss of the bladder-neck closure mechanism following transurethral resection of the prostate or retroperitoneal lymph-node dissection may lead to retrograde ejaculation.

Orgasm consists of pleasurable sensations associated with emission and ejaculation. It results from cerebral processing of afferent stimuli via the pudendal nerve and is associated with reversal of the generalized physiological changes occurring with the build-up of sexual excitement [3].

References

1. Klein EA. The anatomy and physiology of normal male sexual function. In: Montague DK (ed) Disorders of male sexual function. Chicago: Year Book Medical, 1988: 2–19
2. Burnett AL. Nitric oxide control of lower genito-urinary tract functions: a review. *Urology* 1995; 45: 1071–1083
3. Carson C, Kirby RS, Goldstein I. Textbook of erectile dysfunction. Isis Medical Media, Oxford, 1999

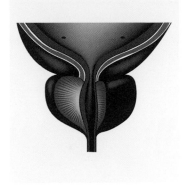

CHAPTER 3

Impact of prostatic disease on men's health

R. S. Kirby and M. G. Kirby

Introduction

The prostate, although relatively small in size compared with other organs such as the liver or heart, looms large as a source of disease, especially in men beyond middle age. Lower urinary tract symptoms (LUTS) due to benign prostatic hyperplasia (BPH) have been estimated to affect 43% of men over 65 [1]. Prostate cancer is the second-commonest cause of cancer death in men after lung neoplasms, and prostatitis is one of the commonest causes of recurrent inflammatory disease in younger and middle-aged men. As a consequence, disorders of the prostate, together with cardiovascular disease, feature prominently as a cause of ill-health among men and may significantly impair quality of life.

For many years prostatic disorders have been something of a 'Cinderella' subject. With the greying of the 'baby boomers', however, these diseases have recently begun to receive the attention that they undoubtedly deserve. The current state of the art with regard to causes, diagnosis and management of these three highly prevalent causes of ill-health in men form the subject of this chapter.

Anatomy and physiology

In the human male, in contradistinction to all other species (with the exception of the dog), the prostate surrounds the urethra, guarding the exit to the bladder (Fig. 3.1). On the positive side, the antibacterial properties of the prostate in this strategic location makes urinary tract infections in young men unusual. Less helpful, however, is the toll taken, in terms of symptom burden and reduced quality of life, by BPH, prostate cancer and prostatitis, not least because any disease affecting the prostate is liable to affect both filling and emptying phases of bladder function.

The prostate has been divided into distinct anatomical zones [2]. The central and peripheral zones have phylogenetic links with the axial and caudal prostates in lower species; between the two, there is the so-called transition zone (Fig. 3.2). These separate zones have different disease susceptibilities: the peripheral zone is the common site of development of prostate cancer; in contrast, the transition zone is where the characteristic adenomyomatous nodule formation of BPH is initiated.

The anatomy of the prostatic ducts also has an impact on predisposition of the peripheral zone towards acute and chronic prostatitis. Peripheral zone ducts enter the prostatic urethra almost at right angles, making them liable to intraprostatic urinary reflux. In contrast, central zone ducts enter obliquely, ensuring that the central zone is seldom affected by this inflammatory disorder.

The major function of the prostate is to add its secretions to semen, which is made in the testes and stored in the seminal vesicles. In this location, semen is bound together in a coagulum

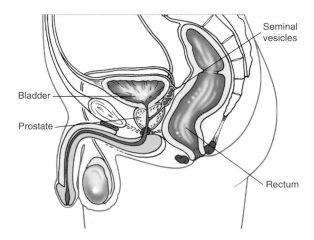

Figure 3.1. *Diagram showing the location of the prostate surrounding the urethra as it exits the bladder.*

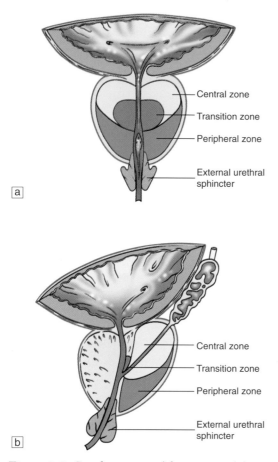

Figure 3.2 labels:
- Central zone
- Transition zone
- Peripheral zone
- External urethral sphincter

[a]

- Central zone
- Transition zone
- Peripheral zone
- External urethral sphincter

[b]

Figure 3.2. *Zonal anatomy of the prostate: (a) antero-posterior view; (b) sagittal view.*

formed by proteins such as seminogelin, which facilitate the ejaculatory process. Prostatic secretions, by contrast, are liquid and contain high concentrations of the glycoprotein prostate-specific antigen (PSA). This powerful protease liquifies semen after ejaculation by degrading seminogelin, thus freeing spermatozoa to migrate within the female genital tract.

Although most PSA is secreted from the columnar epithelium lining into the lumen of the prostatic acini, a very small proportion is absorbed across the basal cell layer and basement membrane into the bloodstream. Here it occurs either as free PSA or complexed to antichymotrypsin in concentrations usually less than 4.0 ng/ml. In normal healthy males, the ratio of free to complexed PSA is usually greater than 18%. In diseases of the prostate, however, especially prostate cancer, there is disruption of the normal barriers to PSA absorption. The consequence is a rise in serum PSA levels and a reduction in the ratio of free to complexed PSA [3].

BPH

BPH is the most prevalent disorder to afflict the prostate. In most men beyond the age of 40, the transition zone of the gland begins to show signs of hyperplasia (Fig. 3.3). The stimulus for this hyperplasia affects both stromal and glandular elements and results in the formation of characteristic nodules, which compress the prostatic urethra, making voiding progressively more difficult. Androgens certainly have a permissive role: testosterone, secreted from the Leydig cells of the testis, enters prostatic cells by simple diffusion and is converted to dihydrotestosterone (DHT) by the enzyme 5 alpha-reductase. DHT is roughly five times more potent as an androgen in the prostate than testosterone itself. DHT binds to androgen receptors (ARs) located within the nuclei of prostatic stromal and epithelial cells. The act of DHT binding induces a conformational change and dimerization of the ARs, and the release of heat-shock protein (hsp). The result of these molecular interactions is the transcription of several large segments of DNA. These segments encode, among other things, a number of growth factors, such as epidermal growth factor (EGF) and fibroblast growth factor (FGF). Both EGF and FGF molecules bind to specific growth- factor receptors located on the cell membrane of stromal and epithelial cells, producing the stimulus for hyperplasia (Fig. 3.4).

BPH develops as the result not only of positive signals for cell division but also of a lack of the normal programmed cell death, or apoptosis pathways, that function to maintain organ size. In this respect, transforming growth factor beta (TGFβ) is important. Reduced levels of TGFβ, which normally acts through the *bc1–2* and *bax* apoptosis genes, will result in abnormally pro-

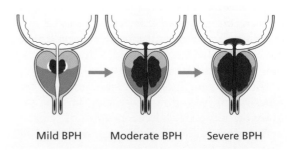

Mild BPH   Moderate BPH   Severe BPH

Figure 3.3. *Progressive enlargement of the transition zone of the prostate characteristic of benign prostatic hyperplasia.*

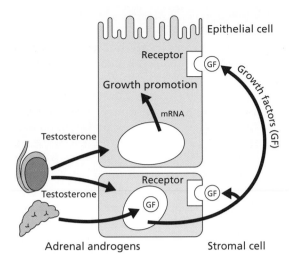

Figure 3.4. *Testosterone secreted from the testes enters prostate cells by simple diffusion and is converted by 5 alpha-reductase to dihydrotestosterone. This molecule stimulates the androgen response area of the genome to transcribe the regions that encode a number of growth factors, including epidermal growth factor.*

longed cell survival. The normal balance between cell division and cell death is disturbed and BPH results.

Risk factors for BPH

BPH is so prevalent among men beyond middle age that it has been difficult to identify specific risk factors. Age is certainly the strongest, and the presence of functioning testes is a prerequisite. Recently, a familial trait towards BPH has been identified, with almost all the males in some families being affected by early onset of obstruction and LUTS, often requiring surgery.

Effects of obstruction

As bladder outflow obstruction due to prostatic enlargement progresses, a number of secondary effects develop. From the patient's point of view, the most important of these is the development of LUTS. These symptoms have been divided into two groups: these are (1) the irritative symptoms of frequency, nocturia, urgency and urge incontinence, and (2) the obstructive symptoms of hesitancy, poor flow and incomplete bladder emptying.

As might be imagined, the irritative symptoms are most bothersome to patients, while the obstructive symptoms correlate more strongly with the eventual necessity for prostatic surgery [4]. Taken together, this cluster of symptoms has

a significant impact on the sufferer's quality of life. The activities of daily living that are affected by BPH are listed in Table 3.1.

Left untreated, symptomatic BPH tends to progress slowly: symptoms worsen, the impact on quality of life increases and, eventually, urinary retention develops. Acute urinary retention (AUR) is, in fact, more common than is often appreciated. The Olmsted County Study examined the natural history of AUR in 2113 men and found that the rate of this complication of BPH increased with age [5]. The cumulative incidence of AUR at 5 years in men aged 40–49 years was 1.6%, rising to 10% in men aged 70–79 years. A number of other risk factors for AUR have been identified (Table 3.2).

For prostate volumes greater than 30 ml, the risk of AUR increased threefold. The study also found that prostate size increased with age at approximate rates of 0.4 ml/year and 1.2 ml/year in men aged 40–50 and 60–79, respectively. In addition, symptom severity increased and urinary flow rate decreased with age: a linear decrease in uroflow was noted, starting at age 40 and progressing to age 80.

Diagnosis of BPH

The diagnosis of bladder outflow obstruction due to BPH depends on a careful history, a

---

Table 3.1. *Impact of BPH on activities of daily living*

- Limits outdoor sporting activities (e.g. golf)
- Unable to drive for more than 1 hour without stopping
- Limits visits to the cinema, theatre, etc.
- Restricts fluid intake during evenings

Table 3.2. *Risk factors for acute urinary retention (AUR)*

- Severe symptoms
- Enlarged prostate
- Previous history of AUR
- Very reduced flow rate
- Large post-void residual urine volume

physical examination and specific investigations.

History

LUTS associated with BPH can be quantified simply by means of the well-validated International Prostate Symptom Score (IPSS) [6]. As a case-finding exercise, most clinicians prefer a truncated approach and simply ask the so-called 'three questions': (1) do you wake up at night to pass urine; (2) is your urinary flow reduced and (3) are you bothered by your bladder symptoms? If answers to any of these are positive, the severity of the problem may be quantified by a self-administered IPSS questionnaire.

Other important points in the history include previous episodes of AUR, haematuria or prostatic surgery, co-morbid conditions, such as cardiovascular disease or erectile dysfunction, and enquiry about concomitant medications. A number of drugs used for other conditions, especially antidepressants and anticholinergic agents, may have a deleterious effect on bladder function.

Examination

Digital rectal examination (DRE) constitutes the cornerstone of the physical examination of patients suffering from LUTS as a result of BPH. The normal prostate has the same springy consistency as the tip of the nose and is about the size of a chestnut. A median sulcus is usually palpable. In BPH, the gland is diffusely enlarged, and can be palpated projecting dorsally into the rectum. The abdomen should also be examined to exclude chronic retention or other intra-abdominal pathology. A general physical examination is necessary to exclude other important co-morbidity, such as neurological or cardiovascular pathology, especially hypertension which coexists with BPH in around one-third of all patients.

Special investigations

Routine investigations include urine culture; measurements of electrolytes, urea and creatinine; and a blood sugar test if diabetes is suspected. In patients with excessive frequency and dysuria, urine cytology should be performed to identify possible carcinoma in situ of the bladder. The degree of obstruction caused by prostatic enlargement can be conveniently assessed non-invasively by a combination of ultrasound imaging and uroflowmetry. The more severe the obstruction, the more reduced is the uroflow and the greater is the post-void residual urine (PVR). Complications of BPH, such as bladder stone, diverticulum formation and upper tract dilatation, can also be excluded by these means.

In more complex cases — where previous prostatic surgery has been performed, for example — pressure/flow urodynamic studies may be necessary. If there is a history of haematuria or suspicion of carcinoma in situ of the bladder, cysto-urethroscopy is mandatory to exclude more sinister bladder pathology.

Treatment options for BPH

Traditionally, treatment for obstructive BPH has been surgical, usually by transurethral resection of the prostate (TURP). TURP remains the gold standard therapy for all patients with any of the complications of BPH listed in Table 3.3. For uncomplicated cases, however, increasingly safe and effective medical treatment options are often employed as first-line therapy, with surgery being reserved for non-responders or those who progress despite therapy.

Medical therapy for BPH

Although plant extracts continue to be prescribed for BPH, there is very little firm evidence from randomized controlled trials of genuine efficacy. By contrast, two classes of drugs have withstood scrutiny in large placebo-controlled studies, namely, 5 alpha-reductase inhibitors and alpha-1-adrenoceptor antagonists.

5-alpha-reductase inhibitors act by blocking the conversion of testosterone to DHT. As a result of reduced androgen drive, the prostatic epithelium undergoes apoptosis and the prostate shrinks by 20–30%. The reduction of prostate volume is accompanied by a modest improvement in symptom score, and an enhanced uroflow [7]. Recent studies have also demonstrated that finasteride reduces the risk of AUR or surgery by around 50% compared with placebo [8]. Finasteride works better in men with larger glands.

Table 3.3. *Complications of benign prostatic hyperplasia*

- Acute or chronic urinary retention
- Bladder stone(s)
- Diverticulum formation
- Upper tract dilatation
- Recurrent urinary tract infections
- Haematuria

Alpha-1-adrenoceptor blockers act mainly by relaxing prostatic smooth muscle, producing rapid relief of symptoms and increased uroflow. By reducing adrenoceptor-stimulated smooth muscle contraction they also lower blood pressure (BP) in hypertensive men, but have little impact on BP in normotensives. Recently, three subtypes have been identified — alpha-1A, alpha-1B and alpha-1D. The alpha-1A subtype seems to be functionally predominant in the prostate, but it is not clear whether the marginal selectivity of tamsulosin for alpha-1A over alpha-1B in fact confers clinical benefit in terms of safety compared with non-selective compounds such as doxazosin [9]. More alpha-1A selective compounds are under development.

Compounds such as doxazosin have other non-prostatic effects that could be construed as beneficial, such as reducing low-density lipoprotein and serum triglycerides. There are also emerging data that doxazosin may improve erectile function, possibly by reducing adrenergic vasoconstriction tone in the corpora cavernosa. Finally, it has been suggested that doxazosin may induce apoptosis in prostatic smooth muscle by blocking the trophic effect of noradrenaline within the gland. To date, however, no actual prostatic shrinkage has been observed in patients with BPH treated with alpha-blockers.

Surgical therapy for BPH

The bothersome symptoms of BPH stem from the obstructive effect of the adenoma on the prostatic urethra [10]. It is, therefore, not surprising that surgical resection of the hyperplastic transition zone tissue results in a dramatic improvement in symptoms and restoration of normal uroflow patterns (Fig. 3.5); bladder emptying is also enhanced. These benefits are achieved at the price of complications in around 18% of cases and a small but significant mortality [11].

More than half of all patients undergoing TURP suffer retrograde ejaculation afterwards, but only a small percentage develop erectile dysfunction. These drawbacks of surgery suggest that operative intervention should mainly be confined to those with absolute indications for surgery due to BPH complications (e.g. bladder stone or recurrent haematuria) or those in whom medical therapy has failed.

Recently, a range of less-invasive options to TURP have been developed in an attempt to maintain the advantages of reducing tissue bulk while also lessening complications such as bleeding: these include hyperthermia using microwave generators, laser ablation and, most recently,

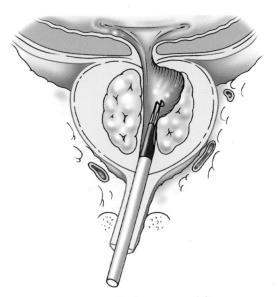

Figure 3.5. *Transurethral resection of the prostate involving endoscopic removal of obstructing transition zone tissue.*

electrovaporization. At the time of writing it is not clear whether these newer methods will be sufficiently robust in terms of durability of effect eventually to supplant TURP.

Prostate cancer

Prostate cancer has recently become the most frequently diagnosed cancer in the USA and the second most common cause of cancer death. In the UK, almost 10 000 men die annually from the disease and, because of the 'greying' of society, the death rate seems set to rise still further.

Adenocarcinoma of the prostate develops as a result of neoplastic changes affecting the epithelial lining of prostatic acini. Bostwick has identified a premalignant transformation of these cells and termed it prostatic intra-epithelial neoplasia (PIN) [12]. Observational studies have confirmed that more than 50% of men whose prostatic biopsies reveal a focus (or foci) of high-grade PIN will eventually develop frank adenocarcinoma of the prostate.

The molecular events resulting in prostate cancer have yet to be elucidated. There is evidence that cancer induction, in common with other adenocarcinomata, is a stepwise process. Sequential deletion of tumour suppressor genes and the activation of oncogenes is accompanied by the loss of metastasis suppressor genes such as E-cadherin. The result is a cancer that develops the ability to invade the basal cell layer and base-

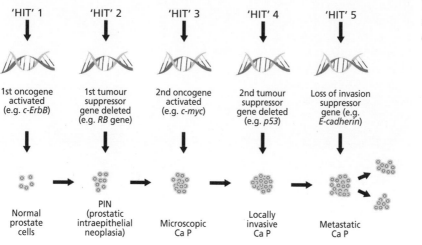

Figure 3.6. *Stepwise induction of prostate cancer.*

ment membrane and to metastasize to lymph nodes and bone through lymphatic and vascular channels (Fig. 3.6).

Risk factors for prostate cancer

Like BPH, one of the strongest risk factors for prostate cancer is age. Of all the solid tumours, adenocarcinoma of the prostate correlates most strongly with age (Fig. 3.7). Recently, it has also become clear that prostate cancer runs in certain families. Linkage analysis performed by Smith and colleagues has localized a genetic abnormality to the short arm of chromosome 1q, but the actual tumour suppressor gene or oncogene involved has yet to be identified [13]. Prostate cancer is also more common in African-American men; moreover the tumours that they develop are more aggressive and occur at a younger age than those in White males.

Diagnosis of prostate cancer

Prostate cancer develops as a microscopic focus of malignancy and progresses to become a tumorous nodule. Because over 70% of tumours develop in the peripheral zone, many such nodules are palpable on DRE. Unfortunately, by the time that such a lesion becomes palpable, invasion of the prostatic capsule may have occurred and the tumour is often incurable, at least by surgical means.

As mentioned previously, prostatic malignancy is associated with an elevation of serum PSA values and a decline in the ratio of free to complexed PSA. A PSA value of between 4 and 10 ng/ml carries a 22% probability of prostate cancer, while a PSA value of 10 ng/ml increases the chances of cancer to more than 60% [14]. Similarly, the lower the ratio of free to complexed PSA, the more likely is that individual to have prostate cancer.

Screening for prostate cancer has been advocated by some. The arguments for this relate to the observation that PSA-detected prostate cancer is much more frequently found to be gland confined than is the case in men presenting clinically. In the USA, where PSA testing is widely utilized, prostate cancer mortality has fallen by almost 3% per annum for the past 3 years; elsewhere in the world, prostate cancer deaths continue to rise. Randomized studies of screening are now underway, but it will be some years before the results are available. Until then, it is unlikely that population-based screening programmes will be introduced. Informed individuals, however, are

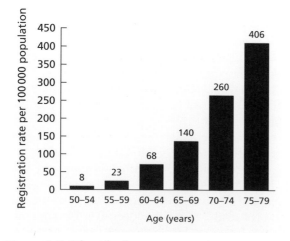

Figure 3.7. *The risk of prostate cancer in men substantially rises with age.*

likely to continue to demand that their PSA be measured. It will always be hard to refuse these requests, but individuals should be informed about the possible consequences of PSA testing and of the current uncertainties about optimal treatment modalities before blood is drawn for this purpose.

Confirmation of the diagnosis requires histological evidence of cancer. This is accomplished by sextant transrectal ultrasound (TRUS)-guided biopsy under antibiotic cover. Information about the local stage of the tumour can be derived from computed tomography (CT) or magnetic resonance imaging, but both these imaging modalities carry a low sensitivity and specificity for identifying spread through the capsule or to the lymph nodes. The degree of PSA elevation also provides some information about the local tumour stage. Men with PSA values above 20 ng/ml very seldom have cancer still confined to the prostate [15].

In men with PSA values greater than 10–20 ng/ml, a radionuclide bone scan should be performed to rule out bone metastases [16]. A chest radiograph should also be ordered, although pulmonary metastases are uncommon from this primary source.

Treatment options

Treatment of prostate cancer is best considered in terms of (a) local disease and (b) advanced disease. Largely because of the increased utilization of PSA testing, a downward shift has occurred in terms of stage of diagnosis in most developed societies. More patients are now seen with localized, potentially curable disease and fewer with disseminated disease.

Localized disease

A number of treatment options are available for men with localized prostate cancer. In those with low-volume, well-differentiated lesions, a policy of watchful waiting with PSA monitoring may be appropriate. Even when more extensive and/or aggressive disease is present, watchful waiting may still be a valid option in men whose life expectancy is less than 10 years. In younger, fitter men with lesions of Gleason sum greater than 4, active intervention is usually considered appropriate. In many countries, the favoured option is usually radical prostatectomy, by either the retropubic or the perineal route. When the nerve-sparing technique of Walsh (Fig. 3.8) is employed, incontinence rates should be less than 3% and more than 70% of patients should have a PSA value that falls below 0.5 ng/ml postoperatively. Even with a nerve-spar-

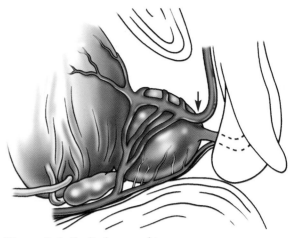

Figure 3.8. *Radical retropubic prostatectomy: an important step in this procedure is to secure the dorsal venous complex (arrowed).*

ing technique, many patients will suffer erectile dysfunction after surgery. This problem can often be resolved, however, with modern therapies such as intracavernosal or intra-urethral prostaglandin E_1 or the selective phosphodiesterase type 5 inhibitor sildenafil.

An alternative treatment option is external beam radiotherapy, with or without conformal targeting and hormonal cytoreduction therapy. This therapy is less demanding of patients, does not involve hospitalization and carries lower risks of inducing erectile dysfunction; on the other hand, it does not reliably eradicate all cancer in every patient, nor does it suppress PSA levels as effectively as surgery in the longer term. In patients with locally advanced disease, however, it is often the treatment of choice, especially when combined with androgen ablation therapy to achieve pretreatment tumour downsizing [17]. An alternative means of delivering radiotherapy to the prostate is to implant radioactive pellets of palladium or iodine under ultrasound control [18]. This technique is known as brachytherapy and initial results appear promising [19]; however, long-term data on its safety and effectiveness are awaited and, as yet, there are no randomized studies comparing brachytherapy with standard therapies.

Unfortunately, no results are yet available of randomized trials comparing radical surgery with radiotherapy or watchful waiting, although the relevant studies are now under way. In the absence of these data it is imperative that all treatment options are carefully discussed with patients, so that an informed decision about management can be reached.

Metastatic disease

Despite rising awareness about prostate cancer, many patients still present with metastatic disease, or develop it after unsuccessful attempts at cure of localized disease. In such cases, first-line therapy is usually androgen ablation, since most patients will respond dramatically to such intervention. Debate about the timing of the initiation of androgen withdrawal continues, but the results of the Medical Research Council (MRC) study of early versus delayed therapy have suggested that patients in the early treatment arm fare better overall [20].

By what means should androgen ablation be achieved? Bilateral orchiectomy is now much less popular as a means of depriving prostate cancer cells of testosterone, because of the psychological effects of surgical castration. Three-monthly depot injections of either goserelin or leuprolide achieve results equivalent to orchiectomy, but leave the testes in place. Since both these luteinizing hormone-releasing hormone (LHRH) analogues stimulate the hypothalamus before blocking LHRH production, it is essential that an anti-androgen such as bicalutamide or flutamide be administered immediately before, and for 6 weeks after, commencing LHRH analogue therapy. Failure to do so risks stimulation of metastases, causing the so-called 'tumour flare', and has been reported to result in spinal cord compression.

More controversial is the claim that the 5% or so of adrenal androgens still secreted after LHRH analogue therapy need to be counteracted by continuing anti-androgen therapy in the longer term [21]. Although several studies have reported a small survival advantage in those treated with combination therapy [22,23], others have shown no difference. A recent meta-analysis of all studies failed to confirm a survival advantage of dual therapy, which does carry disadvantages in terms of cost as well as the potential for added side effects such as diarrhoea.

Unfortunately, in almost all cases, despite the initial dramatic response to androgen ablation, eventually prostate cancer cells acquire the ability to grow and divide in spite of the absence of androgens. This is known as 'hormonal escape' (Fig. 3.9). When this occurs, anti-androgens should be stopped, as anti-androgen withdrawal has been reported to result in a remission in a proportion of cases. Unfortunately, current second-line therapies are seldom very effective and most patients are still managed palliatively at this stage. A number of new agents are in development, however, and the prospects for more effec-

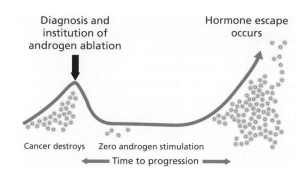

Figure 3.9. *Hormone escape of prostate cancer. A clone of androgen-independent cancer cells allows the tumour to progress in spite of androgen ablation.*

tive second-line therapy are now beginning to look more promising.

Prostatitis

Prostatitis literally means inflammation of the prostate. However, by no means all patients who are labelled as suffering from prostatitis in fact have genuine inflammation of the gland. Although prostatitis is less common than the other two major afflictions of the prostate (BPH and prostate cancer), it is estimated that prostatitis accounts for up to one-quarter of all visits to urologists and for a substantial number to family practitioners [24]. Moreover, since the disease affects younger and middle-aged men predominantly, the disorder often has a significant economic impact, not only on the sufferer but also on his dependants, as well as considerably reducing quality of life [25].

Even though prostatitis affects many hundreds of thousands of men worldwide, there have been few scientific studies to elucidate its aetiology and even less to confirm the sensitivity and specificity of investigations or objectively to evaluate the response to therapy. Because of the difficulty in eradicating symptoms completely and preventing recurrence, frustration and anxiety often develop, not only among the patients themselves and their families, but also in the clinicians caring for them. As a result, a careful stepwise approach to diagnosis and a clear sympathetic explanation of the diagnosis and prognosis is paramount in this disease. Treatment often needs to be prolonged and careful follow-up arranged.

Pathogenesis of prostatitis
Infective aetiology

The male urethra, being longer than its female counterpart, affords considerably greater protection against ascending infection. None the less, pathogens such as *Escherichia coli*, *Pseudomonas aeruginosa* and *Enterococcus* spp. can either ascend the urethra or enter by intraprostatic reflux and subsequently initiate an inflammatory process within the prostate. Risk factors for prostatic infection include indwelling intra-urethral catheters, external urinary appliances and unprotected anorectal intercourse, as well as active lower urinary tract infection. Haematogenous spread of organisms to the prostate may also occur.

Of the many serotypes of *E.coli*, those most frequently implicated in lower urinary tract infections are 04, 08, 025, 050 and 075. Using filamentous adhesions (fimbriae), *E. coli* attach to carbohydrate structures on uroepithelial surfaces. *E. coli* have been subdivided into those with type 1 fimbriae and those with type P fimbriae. It is the former variety that are mainly involved in lower urinary tract infections, including prostatitis.

The adhesive mechanisms of Gram-positive bacteria such as *Enterococcus* spp. are less clearly defined, although several mechanisms of adhesion have been detected. An adhesion molecule called 'aggregation substance' mediates attachment to epithelial cells and can be visualized as hair-like structures under electron microscopy.

Several urogenital pathogens, including *Proteus* spp. and *Ureaplasma urealyticum*, produce human immunoglobulin A1-specific proteases. These induce local paralysis of immune defence mechanisms, facilitating bacterial colonization and penetration through the mucosal barrier. Attachment and invasion of bacteria is followed by epithelial inflammation induced by lipid A, cytotoxic haemolysin and cytotoxic necrotizing factors. This induces immigration of inflammatory cells from the vessels of the prostatic stroma. The epithelium of the prostatic acini becomes infiltrated with neutrophil granulocytes, with local destruction and desquamation. The lumen of the acini becomes filled with an exudate of inflammatory cells. In the stroma there is a lesser infiltration of plasma cells, lymphocytes and neutrophils. Important in terms of the pathogenesis of chronic bacterial prostatitis is the formation of a glycocalix, which encloses and protects bacterial microcolonies within prostatic ducts and acini. The immune system therefore does not recognize the causative bacteria because they are embedded within this protective coat.

Non-infective, inflammatory causes of prostatic inflammation

Intraprostatic urinary reflux Since the prostate empties the contents of its glandular secretions into the prostatic urethra, there is clearly the opportunity for urine, at the time of micturition, to reflux into the prostate and set up an inflammatory response. As mentioned previously, the horizontal direction of the peripheral zone ducts on entering the urethra may make them especially susceptible to such reflux.

There is no question that intraprostatic reflux of urine can occur. It is not uncommonly visualized on voiding cysto-urethrography. Moreover, in a series of men who were undergoing prostatectomy for BPH, carbon particles (Indian ink) were placed in the bladder and they were asked to void: in eight of nine cases, carbon particles were visualized in the prostatic ducts of these men [26].

In an ancilliary study, men with chronic nonbacterial prostatitis also underwent placement of carbon particles in the bladder and were asked to void. Subsequent microscopic analysis of expressed prostatic secretions revealed macrophages that had ingested carbon particles in all patients studied, again confirming the existence of this phenomenon. As yet unanswered, however, is why some patients should develop intraprostatic urinary reflux, whereas others do not. Urodynamic factors may be important: lack of distal sphincter relaxation or a urethral stricture can both cause a rise in pressure within the prostatic urethra during voiding.

Prostatic calculi The prostate ducts are prone to become obstructed by multiple prostatic calculi, which on occasion may become quite large. Stones are commonly visualized protruding from the ducts entering the urethra at the verumontanum. Prostatic calculi are therefore a further risk factor for prostatitis: not only can they cause obstruction and set up an inflammatory response around themselves, they may also harbour bacteria and make them difficult to eradicate with antibiotics, which penetrate these structures poorly, if at all.

Classification of prostatitis

Prostatitis syndromes are most usefully divided into acute and the more commonly encountered chronic variants (Table 3.4). Although acute prostatitis is nearly always caused by a bacterial infection, chronic prostatitis is most commonly non-bacterial in origin. Patients who have neither infection nor inflammation of the prostate,

Table 3.4. *Classification of common prostatic syndromes*

- Acute bacterial prostatitis
- Chronic bacterial prostatitis
- Chronic non-bacterial prostatitis
- Prostatodynia

Table 3.5. *Unusual forms of prostatitis*

- Gonococcal prostatitis
- Tuberculous prostatitis
- Mycotic prostatitis
- Granulomatous prostatitis

yet complain of symptoms relating to the gland, are best described as suffering from prostatodynia.

Rarer causes of prostatitis are listed in Table 3.5 but are not considered further here.

Acute bacterial prostatitis

Patients suffering from acute bacterial prostatitis typically experience sudden chills, fever, low back and perineal pain, and acute onset of LUTS. Generalized malaise and myalgia may develop. DRE is extremely painful and, when performed, reveals a swollen, tender prostate. A midstream urine (MSU) may demonstrate many leucocytes and macrophages and, if there is an associated urine tract infection, bacteria and a positive culture. Histology of the gland reveals an acute inflammatory response.

E. coli is the organism most commonly implicated (in about 80% of cases). Less commonly, *Pseudomonas* spp. or *Enterococcus faecalis* are involved. The organisms that commonly cause acute bacterial prostatitis are listed in Table 3.6.

Prostatic abscess

Acute prostatitis may, unusually, progress to abscess formation. *E. coli* is most commonly implicated, with occasionally *Staphylococcus aureus* or *Pseudomonas* spp. involved. Men with diabetes and chronic renal failure, as well as immunosuppressed patients, are especially at risk of this complication. Abscess formation is best imaged by CT scanning, as TRUS is usually too painful to be tolerated.

Treatment

High doses of the appropriate antibiotic constitute the most effective treatment (Table 3.7). If an abscess has formed, aspiration under ultrasound control is important to identify the causative pathogen. Although some prostatic abscesses have been cured by the insertion of a percutaneous catheter, in general the most effective drainage is accomplished by transurethral incision into the prostatic urethra using a resectoscope. Any pus drained at the time should be sent for culture and determination of antibiotic sensitivities.

Chronic bacterial prostatitis

It surprises many to know that only 5% of men with chronic prostatitis syndrome in fact have bacterial infection of the prostate gland. In spite of

Table 3.6. *Pathogens involved in bacterial prostatitis*

Gram negative

- *Escherichia coli*
- *Proteus* spp.
- *Klebsiella* spp.
- *Enterobacter* spp.
- *Pseudomonas* spp.

Gram positive

- *Enterococcus faecalis*
- *Staphylococcus aureus*

Table 3.7. *Antibiotics useful in bacterial prostatitis*

Acute bacterial prostatitis

- Gentamicin: 80 mg i.v., 8-hourly
- Ampicillin: 500 mg i.v. 6-hourly

Chronic bacterial prostatitis

- Ciprofloxacin: 500 mg orally, twice daily
- Ofloxacin: 400 mg orally, once daily
- Trimethoprim: 200 mg orally, twice daily
- Doxycycline: 100 mg orally, once daily
- Cephalexin: 500 mg orally, four times daily

Table 3.8. *Risk factors for chronic bacterial prostatitis*

- Urethral inoculation by pathogenic vaginal bacteria

- Unprotected insertive anorectal intercourse

- Indwelling urethral catheter or external condom drainage systems

- Untreated infected urine after transurethral resection of the prostate

this, many men with symptoms suggestive of chronic prostatitis are treated empirically with antibiotics — often with predictably modest results. However, chronic bacterial prostatitis is the underlying cause of recurrent urinary tract infection in men in a significant number of cases. The risk factors for this disorder are listed in Table 3.8.

Diagnosis

Relapsing urinary tract infection in men is a common clinical feature of chronic bacterial prostatitis, although other men complain of perineal discomfort and either irritative or obstructive voiding symptoms. Rectal examination is non-specific, the prostate feeling variably normal, indurated, tender or boggy. The diagnosis cannot be made on physical examination or by simply requesting an MSU, as this will often be sterile; a lower-tract localization test is required to elucidate the problem (Fig. 3.10) [27]. Transrectal colour Doppler ultrasound imaging often confirms hypervascularity associated with the inflammatory response. Urodynamic studies may reveal bladder outflow obstruction, either at the level of the bladder neck or due to the prostate itself.

Treatment

The treatment course is often protracted and unsatisfactory for both the patient and his doctor. In the absence of the intense inflammation in acute prostatitis, the penetration of antibiotics into the prostate is low. Drugs that are lipid soluble, non-ionized and weakly bound to plasma proteins are better able to achieve adequate concentrations in prostatic fluid. The 4-quinolones, such as ciprofloxacin or norfloxacin, are usually the most efficacious, while other useful drugs include doxycycline and cephalexin.

The optimum duration of treatment is uncertain, but at least 6 weeks of therapy is usually recommended. Surgical treatment by TURP is seldom effective because the peripheral zone of the prostate, which is the main site of the inflammatory process, is not effectively removed by this

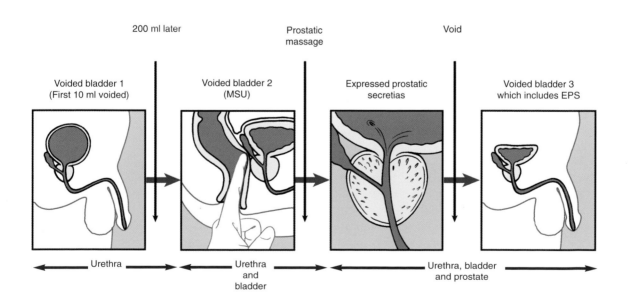

Figure 3.10. *Lower-tract localization test. Secretions expressed from the prostate result in positive cultures in patients with bacterial prostatitis.*

procedure. In spite of some reports to the contrary [28], microwave therapy to the prostate is also usually ineffective, at least in these authors' experience.

Chronic non-bacterial prostatitis

Although chronic non-bacterial prostatitis (CNBP) is estimated to be eight or nine times more frequent than the bacterial form of the disorder, it remains a condition of uncertain aetiology. Occasionally, *Chlamydia trachomatis*, *Ureaplasma urealyticum* and *Mycoplasma hominis* are cultured; however, the failure to document an immune response to these organisms raises serious questions about their genuine causative role.

The proposal mentioned earlier, that the chronic inflammatory process could be the result of intraprostatic reflux of urine, has recently been corroborated by Persson and Ronquist [29], who additionally suggest that CNBP may be a chemical inflammatory response to the intraprostatic reflux of urinary urate.

Diagnosis

Diagnosis rests on a characteristic history of perineal pain and variable urinary and sexual dysfunction. There is no history of recurrent bladder infections. The presence of prostatic inflammation is confirmed by the finding of raised counts of leucocytes and lipid-laden macrophages on microscopy of expressed prostatic secretions. Further evidence of an inflammatory response comes from colour Doppler imaging of the gland by TRUS.

Treatment

Because the exact cause of chronic non-bacterial prostatitis is unknown, treatment is often difficult. Some patients improve with antibiotics, so a trial of an oral 4-quinolone is often employed. If *C. trachomatis* or *U. urealyticum* are present on culture of expressed prostatic secretions, patients should be treated, usually with doxycycline. Patients responding to antimicrobials should be treated for at least 6 weeks. Anti-inflammatory agents may also be helpful. Non-steroidal agents, such as ibuprofen, may be used singly or in combination with antibiotics. The outcome, however, is often less than ideal, and there is a marked tendency towards relapse of symptoms and further presentation.

Prostatodynia

Prostatodynia is the term given to the pelvic pain disorder and associated urinary symptoms troubling patients in whom investigations reveal neither evidence of inflammation nor infection affecting the prostate. Culture of prostatic secretions reveal neither an excess of white cells nor bacterial growth. TRUS colour Doppler studies are normal. Prostatic calculi may sometimes be present, but these often occur in patients who have no symptoms related to the prostate.

Treatment

Increased tension and spasm of smooth muscle in the bladder neck has been reported to result in an increased pressure in the prostatic urethra. Patients may therefore sometimes respond to alpha-blockers, such as doxazosin, alfuzosin or tamsulosin. If effective, these compounds may need to be continued indefinitely. Patients with tension myalgia of the pelvic floor may occasionally respond to diazepam, although caution should be used when advising long-term usage of this anxiolytic drug.

Symptomatic therapy, using hot baths and biofeedback, sometimes brings relief. Prostatic massage is reported to help those with a congested prostate caused by infrequent sexual activity [30]. A select group of patients has been reported to respond to zinc supplements. Others are claimed to benefit from microwave therapy [27], but there are no controlled studies of these therapies and a placebo effect cannot be excluded.

Conclusions

Prostatic diseases continue to take a considerable toll on the health of men beyond middle age. As the proportion of the population over the age of 60 expands, this burden is likely to increase. Recent advances in diagnosis and management are enabling treatment to be offered to the very many sufferers of these various disorders, with less-invasive therapies that have fewer side effects. Nevertheless, much remains to be done to improve staging and to provide a sound evidence base for therapy, as well as to raise awareness of the risks of prostatic disease, almost all of which may be managed more safely and effectively when diagnosed at an earlier, less advanced stage.

References

1. Garraway WM, Collins GN, Lee RJ. High prevalence of benign prostatic hypertrophy in the community. *Lancet* 1991; 338: 469–471

2. McNeal JE. Regional morphology and pathology of the prostate. *Am J Clin Pathol* 1968; 49: 347–357

3. Oesterling JE, Jacobsen SJ, Lee GG *et al.* Free, complexed and total serum prostate specific antigen: the establishment of appropriate reference ranges for their concentrations and ratios. *J Urol* 1995; 154: 1090–1095

4. Arrhigi HM, Guess HA, Metter EJ, Fozard JL. Symptoms and signs of prostatism as risk factors for prostatectomy. *Prostate* 1990; 16: 253–261

5. Jacobson SJ, Jacobson DJ, Girman C. Natural history of prostatism: risk factors for acute urinary retention. *J Urol* 1997; 158: 481–487

6. Barry MJ, Fowler FJ, O'Leary MP *et al.* The American Urological Association symptom index for benign prostatic hyperplasia. *J Urol* 1992; 148: 1549–1557

7. Gormley GJ, Stoner E, Bruskewitz RC *et al.* The effect of finasteride in men with benign prostatic hyperplasia. *N Engl J Med* 1992; 327: 1185–1191

8. McConnell JD, Bruskewitz RC, Walsh PC *et al.* The effect of finasteride on the risk of acute urinary retention and the need for surgical treatment among men with benign prostatic hyperplasia. *N Engl J Med* 1998; 338: 557–563

9. Kirby RS, Pool JL. Alpha-adrenoceptor blockade in the treatment of benign prostatic hyperplasia: past, present and future. *Br J Urol* 1997; 80: 521–532

10. Garraway WM, Kirby RS. Benign prostatic hyperplasia: effects on quality of life and impact on treatment decisions. *Urology* 1994; 44: 629–636

11. Mebust WK, Holtgrewe HL, Cockett ATK. Transurethral prostatectomy: immediate and postoperative complications. A cooperative study of 13 participating institutions evaluating 3885 patients. *J Urol* 1989; 41: 243–247

12. Bostwick DG, Brawer MK. Prostatic intraepithelial neoplasia and early invasion in prostate cancer. *Cancer* 1987; 59: 778–794

13. Smith JR, Freije D, Carpten JD *et al.* Major susceptibility locus for prostate cancer on chromosome 1 suggested by genome-wide search. *Science* 1997; 274: 1371–1376

14. Catalona WJ, Richie JP, Ahmann FR *et al.* A multicentre examination of PSA and digital rectal examination for early detection of prostate cancer in 6,374 volunteers. *J Urol* 1993; 194: 412A

15. Partin A, Kattan MW, Subong MS *et al.* Combination of prostate-specific antigen, clinical stage and Gleason score to predict pathological stage of localised prostate cancer. *JAMA* 1997; 277: 1445–1451

16. Oesterling JE. Using prostate-specific antigen to eliminate the staging radionuclide bone scan: significant economic implications. *Urol Clin North Am* 1993; 20: 705–712

17. Bolla M, Gonzalez D, Warde P *et al.* Improved survival in patients with locally advanced prostate cancer treated with radiotherapy and goserelin. *N Engl J Med* 1997; 337: 295–300

18. Blasko JC, Fowler FJ, Grimm PD, Ragde H. Prostate-specific antigen based disease control following ultrasound guided 125 iodine implantation for stage T1/T2 prostatic carcinoma. *J Urol* 1995; 154: 1096–1099

19. Grimm PD, Blasko JC, Ragde H. Ultrasound-guided transperineal implantation of iodine 125 and palladium 103 for the treatment of early stage prostate cancer. *Atlas Urol Clin North Am* 1994; 2: 113–125

20. Kirk D. Medical Research Council immediate versus deferred treatment study: how important is local progression in advanced prostate cancer? *Br J Urol* 1998; 81: 30S

21. Labrie F, Dupont A, Belanger A *et al.* New approaches in the treatment of prostate cancer: complete instead of partial withdrawal of androgens. *Prostate* 1983; 4: 579–594

22. Crawford ED, Eisenberger MA, McLeod DG. A controlled trial of leuprolide with or without flutamide in prostate cancer. *N Engl J Med* 1989; 321: 419–424

23. Janknegt RA. International Anandron Study Group: Efficacy and tolerance of a total androgen blockade with anandron and orchiectomy. A double-blind, placebo-controlled multicentre study. *J Urol* 1991; 145: 425A

24. Roberts RO, Lieber MM, Bostwick D, Jacobsen SJ. A review of clinical and pathological prostatitis syndromes. *Urology* 1997; 49: 809–821

25. Wenninger K, Heinman TR, Rothman I *et al.* Sickness impact of chronic non-bacterial prostatitis and its correlates. *J Urol* 1996; 155: 956–968

26. Kirby RS, Lowe D, Bultitude MI, Shuttleworth KED. Intraprostatic urinary reflux: an aetiological factor in abacterial prostatitis. *Br J Urol* 1992; 54: 729–734

27. Meares EM, Stamey TA. The diagnosis and management of bacterial prostatitis. *Br J Urol* 1972; 44: 175–179

28. Nickel JC, Sorenson R. Transurethral microwave thermotherapy of non-bacterial prostatitis and prostatodynia: initial experience. *Urology* 1994; 44: 458–460

29. Persson BE, Ronquist G. Evidence for the mechanistic association between abacterial prostatitis and the levels of urate and creatinine in expressed prostatic secretions. *J Urol* 1996; 155: 968–960

30. Hennenfent BR, Feliciano AE. Changes in white blood cell counts in men undergoing thrice-weekly prostatic massage, microbial diagnosis and anti-microbial therapy for genitourinary complaints. *Br J Urol* 1998; 81: 370–376

CHAPTER 4

Testicular cancer

W. F. Hendry

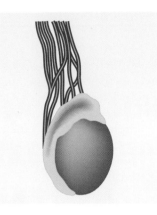

Introduction

Recent developments in the management of testicular cancer make it a rarity for patients to die of this disease, provided that they are treated adequately. Cure is dependent upon early diagnosis, prompt treatment of the primary lesion, careful staging and correct initial treatment. Mistakes in management that allow metastases to become bulky will reduce the chance of cure [1]. Vigilant follow-up is also essential in order to allow early detection of relapse and to deal with any residual disease left after chemotherapy. One study on 449 men with non-seminomatous tumours showed that the risk of dying was more than doubled if the patient was not managed in a specialist testicular tumour unit [2].

The size of the problem

The incidence of testicular cancer has risen during the 20th century and it is now the most common neoplasm in men aged 25–34; one man in 500 can expect to develop this disease by the age of 50. However, the tumour is rare in men of African descent [3]. Death rates are highest amongst professional, administrative and clerical workers, and lowest among manual workers [4].

Aetiology

Men with a history of cryptorchism have an increased chance of developing testicular malignancy compared with the normal population. Approximately 10% of testicular tumours occur in testes that are or have been maldescended [5]; the risk is six times greater for intra-abdominal testes than for lower-lying testes. Consequently, it is recommended that such testes should always be removed if they cannot be placed in the scrotum. Of patients with bilateral maldescent who develop a tumour in one testis, 25% will go on to develop a contralateral tumour. When one testis is maldescended, 20% of the tumours that develop will occur in the contralateral, normally situated testicle [6]. Although some reports have observed no tumours in boys who had undergone orchiopexy before the age of 6 [7], a review of 69 testicular tumour patients at the Royal Marsden Hospital who had a history of cryptorchism indicated that age of treatment had no effect on the risk of cancer [5].

Testicular tumours are more likely to occur in testes that are atrophic, whether following orchiopexy [8], torsion [9] or trauma [10]. The incidence of these abnormalities, and hence perhaps the risk of testicular tumours, is higher in males exposed prenatally to exogenous hormones such as diethylstilboestrol [11], or to radiation [12].

Diagnosis

Diagnosis of testicular cancer may be problematic for a number of reasons. Although the tumour usually presents as a painless enlargement, it can be mistaken for epididymitis when the swollen testis is tender. In fact, about 10% of men with a testicular tumour complain of pain from the outset [13]. Many of these testes show evidence of haemorrhage on pathological examination. A small bleed into or adjacent to the tumour not only causes pain and sudden swelling but also its subsequent resorption may account for subsidence of the swelling. This may coincide with antibiotic therapy, thus reinforcing the wrong diagnosis of infection. Pain on presentation can also lead to the condition being treated incorrectly as an inflammation [14].

A history of trauma, recent or remote, is recorded in about 20% of cases and this 'red herring' should not be allowed to distract attention from the true underlying condition. Previous surgery to the testis or inguinal canal may make the findings more difficult to interpret, and may alter the pattern of lymphatic spread. Orchiopexy, for example, may deflect metastases to the inguinal or iliac lymph nodes; sometimes, the resulting lymphoedema may lead to a swollen leg as the presenting feature.

The patient who has already had a testicular tumour represents a particular problem. Of 769 men attending the Royal Marsden Hospital (RMH) between 1952 and 1976, 21 (2.7%) developed a tumour in the contralateral testis: in two instances, this occurred synchronously; in the remainder, development was at intervals from 4 months to 15 years [15]. All patients are instructed to examine the remaining testicle at regular intervals, as a result of which tumours as small as 0.5 cm in diameter have been self-diagnosed. In addition, biopsy is offered to all patients with infertility, a history of maldescent or an atrophic testis, in order to monitor for carcinoma in situ [16].

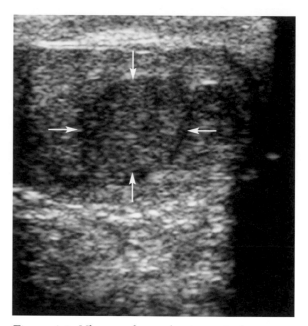

Figure 4.1. *Ultrasound scan showing testicular tumour, indicated by arrows.*

Clinical examination

Careful clinical examination of the testis remains the best method of detecting a tumour. It is worth starting the physical examination of the testes with the patient standing. A tumour will cause the testis to lie lower than normal, whereas inflammatory lesions or torsion tend to raise the testis. Once the patient is lying down, the entire outline of the body of the testis can be assessed for consistency and localization of any induration. A tumour is first identifiable as a firm or hard swelling in the body of the testis, and then as an enlargement of the testicle, which may feel relatively heavy. It also causes the testicle to lose its normal sensation on gentle squeezing. Abnormal firmness in the body of the testis is the most reliable finding; however, difficulty may arise when the tumour lies in the groove between the testis and epididymis. Scrotal ultrasound will help to confirm the diagnosis in such cases (Fig. 4.1) [17,18].

If diagnosis is still inconclusive, then surgical exploration of the testicle is advised. The differential diagnosis includes epididymitis, torsion, tuberculosis, gumma and granulomatous orchitis. Evidence supports the view that all non-transilluminable testicular swellings should be explored unless the swelling is strictly confined to the epididymis or there are pus cells in the urine to confirm the diagnosis of epididymitis.

Occasionally, patients present with metastatic germ-cell malignancy and no primary tumour can be palpated in either testis. Many have advanced disease, presenting with abdominal pain and systemic symptoms [19]. Biopsy of enlarged abdominal or cervical lymph nodes or of the lung can establish the diagnosis, as well as the finding of high serum marker levels, which should always be checked in such patients. Certain patients have a history of testicular atrophy and histological examination may reveal evidence of a microscopic primary tumour. Although the primary tumour can disappear, leaving only a scar [20], biopsy is likely to show the presence of carcinoma in situ [21].

Tumour markers

Three-quarters of non-seminomatous germ-cell tumours (NSGCT) produce either alpha-fetoprotein (AFP) or beta-human chorionic gonadotrophin (β-hCG) [22]. Blood should always be taken for estimation of AFP and β-hCG before the testicle is explored. These measurements are repeated at twice-weekly intervals following removal of the testis until they have become normal, and at each follow-up visit.

Histological classification

The histological classification of testicular tumours is shown in Table 4.1. Of 3196 tumours

Table 4.1. *Histological classification of testicular tumours described by the Testicular Tumour Panel of Great Britain**

Seminoma

Teratoma (non-seminomatous germ cell tumours)[†]

- TD: teratoma differentiated (teratoma)

- MTI: malignant teratoma intermediate (teratocarcinoma)

- MTU: malignant teratoma undifferentiated (embryonal carcinoma)

- MTT: malignant teratoma trophoblastic (choriocarcinoma)

Combined tumour: a malignant tumour, that is a combination of seminoma and teratoma

*See ref. 36.
[†]Corresponding American terminology in parentheses.

Table 4.2. *Royal Marsden Hospital staging for testicular cancer [38]*

Stage	Definition
I	No evidence of metastases
M	Rising serum markers with no other evidence of metastases
II	Abdominal node metastases
A	< 2 cm diameter
B	2–5 cm diameter
C	> 5 cm diameter
III	Supradiaphragmatic nodal metastases
M	Mediastinal
N	Supraclavicular, cervical or axillary
O	No abdominal disease
IV	Extralymphatic metastases
L1	< 3 lung metastases
L2	> 3 lung metastases all < 2 cm in diameter
L3	> 3 lung metastases, one or more > 2 cm in diameter
H+	Liver metastases
Br+	Brain metastases
Bo+	Bone metastases

analysed by the Testicular Tumour Panel of Great Britain between 1958 and 1973, 39.5% were seminomas, 31.7% teratomas (NSGCT) and 13.5% combined tumours [23].

Staging classification

Patients are staged as precisely as possible using non-invasive imaging methods. Computed tomography (CT) scanning gives an accurate assessment of the size and upper limit of para-aortic nodal masses, and can detect lung and mediastinal metastases that are not visible on conventional radio-graphy [24]. Because the volume of metastases exerts an influence on therapeutic response, this measurement is included in the RMH clinical staging system, with formation of subgroups (Table 4.2). The distribution and volume of metastases is of critical importance in planning a treatment strategy [25].

Treatment

The most important variables affecting the outcome of treatment for testicular tumours are tumour volume and serum marker levels at presentation. In one study, 91% of patients with

small-volume metastases and low levels of serum markers were alive at 3 years compared with 47% of those with very bulky disease and high serum marker level [26]. Fortunately, the latter group accounted for only 16% of patients with metastases.

Delay in diagnosis has been found to correlate with clinical stage of disease. In one study, the median patient-plus-physician delay for stage I tumours was 75 days; for stage II it was 101 days and, for stage III, 134 days [27]. In another study, there was a significant delay in presentation, the correct diagnosis being established at the first consultation in only 43% of 526 cases [28].

The importance of early diagnosis relates to the adverse prognostic influence of bulky metastatic disease and high serum concentrations of AFP and/or β-hCG, as well as to the possibility of avoiding chemotherapy if tumour is confined to the testis. In order to achieve cure in patients with bulky metastases and high markers, more intensive chemotherapy is required than is the case for patients with a small tumour burden [29]. The avoidance of chemotherapy altogether in stage I disease and of very toxic chemotherapy in patients with metastatic disease is particularly desirable in patients with decades of life ahead of them, in whom treatment-related morbidity, including recovery of fertility and the fathering of normal children, is of importance. The essence of the modern treatment of testicular tumours is maximizing benefit with minimum toxicity.

Surgical exploration and orchiectomy
Ideally, the surgical approach to a testicular tumour should be through an inguinal incision, although scrotal incision is used if a hydrocele obscuring the testis is present. If a tumour is evident, a second incision can easily be made in the groin to remove the testis and cord. A slightly more liberal approach to scrotal orchiectomy is acceptable in this era of effective chemotherapy, but electively a groin approach is preferable. Once the results of histopathological examination of the testicle are available, the tumour can be classified and further treatment planned.

Seminoma
Seminomas tend to present with early-stage disease and consequently high success rates can be achieved with radiotherapy. Between 1964 and 1983 at the RMH, no death from stage I seminoma was reported and relapse rate was only 2% [30]. In a review of 16 series totalling more than 2600 patients, the recurrence rate was 4.4% and the cause-specific mortality only 2.1% [31]. Recurrences were equally distributed within supradiaphragmatic nodes and lung fields; relapse at other sites was rare. The great majority of recurrences were salvaged with chemotherapy. The morbidity of radiotherapy is low but not negligible: peptic ulcer has been recorded in 6% of patients following treatment [30].

The results of radiotherapy in stage II seminoma are influenced by tumour volume. Relapse rates in stages IIA, IIB and IIC disease of 10, 18 and 38%, respectively, have been reported in 63 patients treated at RMH between 1962 and 1979 [32]. On the basis of these observations, radiotherapy is advocated for stages IIA and IIB, whereas chemotherapy should be employed for stage IIC patients.

Metastatic seminoma is extremely sensitive to chemotherapy, with excellent survival figures being achieved using the drug combinations employed to treat advanced testicular non-seminomas. In a series of patients treated with cisplatin-containing combination chemotherapy, 91% survived and were disease free at 12–73 (median 36) months [33]. Good results have also been reported with carboplatin (JM8) monotherapy [34].

Non-seminomatous germ-cell tumours (NSGCT): stage I
Clinical stage I NSGCT disease may be cured by orchiectomy alone [35]; relapse rates of 27% at 2–31 months have been reported, with most appearing within the first year. Surveillance allows about two-thirds of stage I NSGCT patients to escape further treatment after orchiectomy, and survival is nearly (but not quite) 100% [36]. A higher relapse rate has been found for embryonal carcinoma than for teratocarcinoma, and in the presence of vascular or lymphatic invasion. Careful histological assessment can thus identify a group of patients, around 20% of the total, with a much higher chance of relapse [37]. Two cycles of adjuvant chemotherapy will prevent relapse in almost all of these high-risk patients [38].

NSGCT: stage II
The management of stage IIA and IIB NSGCT disease is controversial. In the USA, radical lymph node dissection is the preferred initial treatment with a view to avoidance of chemotherapy in patients cured by surgery. In a recent experience, the overall survival rate was 98% [39], although approximately 50% of patients eventually did require chemotherapy. Patients with clinical stage II disease treated at RMH receive primary chemotherapy following orchiectomy; 17% of stage IIA and 39% of stage IIB patients have required lymphadenectomy for post-chemotherapy residual masses and 97% were disease free at a median follow-up of 5 years [40].

NSGCT: stages III and IV
Chemotherapy
Chemotherapy is the treatment of choice for men with metastatic disease, and the development of effective chemotherapy for testicular cancer has been one of the most dramatic advances in oncology. The introduction of the combination of vinblastine and bleomycin (VB) was an important milestone [41]. The combina-

tion of cis-platin with VB (PVB) has resulted in cure in approximately 75% of patients and for a number of years was the most widely used form of chemotherapy for patients with metastatic malignant teratoma. The combination of bleomycin, etoposide and cis-platin (BEP) has been evaluated as first-line treatment and was shown to be as effective as PVB but with less toxicity [42].

Para-aortic lymphadenectomy

One-quarter of patients who complete chemotherapy for advanced disease have residual masses in the para-aortic region (Fig. 4.2) or in the chest, or in both sites. When resected, this tissue has been found to contain residual undifferentiated malignancy (MTU) in one in five cases (Fig. 4.2) [43]. In a study of 231 consecutive patients undergoing para-aortic lymphadenectomy after chemotherapy, MTU was identified in 21%, differentiated teratoma in 57% and fibrosis/necrosis in 22% [44]; the overall 5-year survival rate was 80%. Histological findings have a profound effect on prognosis, as does completeness of surgical excision. The outlook was worse for those with residual MTU, only half of whom survived after complete excision. The significance of leaving differentiated teratoma behind is not clear, although there is evidence that this tissue is unstable [45,46]. The technical aspects of removal of these masses have been described elsewhere, and the potential hazards are well documented [47,48].

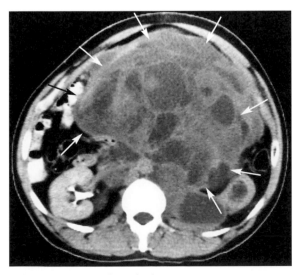

Figure 4.2. *Typical residual para-aortic mass present after chemotherapy and requiring lymphadenectomy, indicated by arrows.*

Side effects of therapy

Loss of ejaculation

Loss of ejaculation after para-aortic lymphadenectomy is caused by division of the sympathetic nerves, which lie beside the great vessels, or removal of the hypogastric plexus just below the bifurcation of the aorta [49]. A nerve-sparing operative technique can lead to a significant reduction in ejaculatory dysfunction. Loss of ejaculation has been found to occur significantly more often after bilateral dissection (46%) than after unilateral (14%) dissection, and has been related to the size of the excised mass (< 4 cm, 4%; 4–8 cm, 19%; > 8 cm, 60%) [50]. Return of ejaculation after the use of drugs such as ephedrine [51] or imipramine [52], as well as after electroejaculation [53], has been reported.

Infertility

Increasingly successful therapy, a more open society and legal precedent all now demand that reproductive function and future fertility are kept in mind, and fully discussed with both patient and relatives before, during and after treatment [54]. Many men presenting with testicular tumours are infertile, but it is not always clear whether this preceded the development of the tumour or was due to the tumour itself or its treatment [55]. At presentation, only one-quarter of these men have normal semen quality [56] and one-quarter have severe irreversible impairment of spermatogenesis demonstrable on testicular biopsy [57]. There is the potential for recovery of normal spermatogenesis among the remainder and it is therefore very important to limit toxicity of treatment in these men. The chemotherapy combinations used for treatment of metastatic testicular tumours, such as BEP, provide a good chance of recovery of spermatogenesis after a period of 1–2 years [42]. It is important that patients at high risk of loss of ejaculation should be recognized early in the course of their treatment so that seminal analysis and cryopreservation of semen can be arranged in suitable cases. Excellent results have been reported with artificial insemination using cryopreserved semen [58].

Conclusions

Effective chemotherapy has had a profound effect on the prognosis of patients with testicular cancer and on overall treatment philosophy. This, together with improved accuracy of non-invasive staging techniques, has facilitated the management of stage I testicular non-seminoma. Surgery has an important role in patients treated with chemotherapy for advanced NSGCT: residual masses require excision in approximately 25% of patients. Post-chemotherapy surgery has a therapeutic as well as a diagnostic role: patients in whom all disease has been excised have a significantly better prognosis than those in whom residual tissue has been left behind. It is most gratifying to see the vast majority of these men cured of a disease which not infrequently led to their death as recently as 20 years ago.

References

1. Mead GM, Stennings SP, Parkinson MC. The second Medical Research Council Study of prognostic factors in nonseminomatous germ cell tumors. *J Clin Oncol* 1992; 10: 85–94

2. Harding MJ, Paul J, Gillis CR, Kaye SB. Management of malignant teratoma: does referral to a specialist unit matter? *Lancet* 1993; 341: 999–1002

3. Daniels JL, Stutzman RE, McLeod DG. A comparison of testicular tumors in black and white patients. *J Urol* 1981; 125: 341–342

4. Davies JM. Testicular cancer in England and Wales: some epidemiological aspects. *Lancet* 1981; 1: 928–932

5. Pike MC, Chilvers C, Peckham MJ. Effect of age at orchidopexy on risk of testicular cancer. *Lancet* 1986; 1: 1246–1248

6. Martin DC. Malignancy and the undescended testis. In: Fonkalsrud EW, Mengel W (eds) The undescended testis. Chicago: Year Book Medical, 1981: 144–156

7. Gehring GG, Rodriguez FR, Woodhead DM. Malignant degeneration of cryptorchid testes following orchiopexy. *J Urol* 1974; 112: 354–356

8. Giwercman A, Grindsted J, Hansen B *et al.* Testicular cancer risk in boys with maldescended testis: a cohort study. *J Urol* 1987; 138: 1214–1216

9. Chilvers CED, Pike MC, Peckham MJ. Torsion of the testis: a new risk factor for testicular cancer. *Br J Cancer* 1987; 55: 105–106

10. Hausfeld KF, Schrandt D. Malignancy of testis following atrophy: report of three cases. *J Urol* 1965; 94: 69–72

11. Skakkebaek NE, Keiding N. Changes in semen and the testis. *Br Med J* 1994; 309: 1316–1319

12. Loughlin JE, Robboy SJ, Morrison AS. Risk factors for cancer of the testis. *N Engl J Med* 1980; 303: 112–113

13. Stephen RA. The clinical presentation of testicular tumours. *Br J Urol* 1962; 34: 448–450

14. Sandeman JF. Symptoms and early management of germinal tumours of the testis. *Med J Aust* 1979; 2: 281–284

15. Sokal M, Peckham MJ, Hendry WF. Bilateral germ cell tumours of the testis. *Br J Urol* 1980; 52: 158–162

16. Fordham MVP, Mason MD, Blackmore C, Hendry WF, Horwich A. Management of the contralateral testis in patients with testicular germ cell cancer. *Br J Urol* 1990; 65: 290–293

17. Vick CW, Brid KI, Rosenfield AT *et al.* Ultrasound of the scrotal contents. *Urol Radiol* 1982; 4: 147–153

18. Tiptaft PC, Nicholls BM, Hately W, Blandy JP. The diagnosis of testicular swellings using water-path ultrasound. *Br J Urol* 1982; 54: 759-764

19. Powell S, Hendry WF, Peckham MJ. Occult germ-cell testicular tumours. *Br J Urol* 1983; 55: 440–444

20. Azzopardi JG, Mostofi FK, Theiss EA. Lesions of testes observed in certain patients with widespread choriocarcinoma and related tumors. *Am J Pathol* 1961; 38: 207–225

21. Daugaard G, von der Maase H, Olsen J *et al.* Carcinoma in situ testis in patients with assumed extragonadal germ cell tumours. *Lancet* 1987; 2: 528–529

22. Mason MD. Tumour markers. In: Horwich A (ed) Testicular cancer: investigation and management, 2nd edn. London: Chapman and Hall, 1996: 35–51

23. Pugh RCB. In: Pugh RCB (ed) Pathology of the testis. Oxford: Blackwell, 1976: 144–146

24. Husband JE, Peckham MJ, Macdonald JS, Hendry WF. The role of computed tomography in the management of testicular teratoma. *Clin Radiol* 1979; 30: 243–252

25. Peckham MJ. Investigation and staging; general aspects and staging classification; non-seminomas: current treatment results and future prospects. In: Peckham MJ (ed) The management of testicular tumours. London: Arnold, 1981: 89–239

26. Medical Research Council Working Party on Testicular Tumours. Prognostic factors in advanced nonseminomatous germ cell testicular tumours: results of a multicentre study. *Lancet* 1985; 1: 8–11

27. Bosl GJ, Vogelzang NJ, Goldman A *et al.* Impact of delay in diagnosis on clinical stage of testicular cancer. *Lancet* 1981; 2: 970–973

28. Ekman P. Delay in the diagnosis of testicular cancer. *Lakartidningen* 1980; 77: 4275–4277

29. Horwich A, Brada M, Nicholls JEA. Intensive induction chemotherapy for poor risk non seminomatous germ cell tumours. *Eur J Cancer Clin Oncol* 1989; 25: 177–184

30. Hamilton C, Horwich A, Easton D, Peckham MJ. Radiotherapy for stage I seminoma testis: results of treatment and complications. *Radiother Oncol* 1986; 6: 115–120

31. Zagars GK. Management of stage I seminoma: radiotherapy. In: Horwich A (ed) Testicular cancer: investigation and management. 2nd edn. London: Chapman and Hall, 1996: 98–121

32. Ball D, Barrett A, Peckham MJ. The management of metastatic seminoma testis. *Cancer* 1982; 50: 2289–2294

33. Peckham MJ, Horwich A, Hendry WF. Advanced seminoma: treatment with cis-platinum-based combination chemotherapy or carboplatin (JM8). *Br J Cancer* 1985; 52: 7–13

34. Horwich A, Dearnaley DP, A'Hern R *et al.* The activity of single-agent carboplatin in advanced seminoma. *Eur J Cancer* 1992; 28: 1307–1310

35. Peckham MJ, Barrett A, Horwich A, Hendry WF. Orchiectomy alone for Stage I testicular non-seminoma. A progress report on the Royal Marsden Hospital study. *Br J Urol* 1983; 55: 754–759

36. Read G, Stenning SP, Cullen MH *et al.* Medical Research Council prospective study of surveillance for stage I testicular teratoma. *J Clin Oncol* 1992; 10: 1762–1768

37. Freedman LS, Parkinson MC, Jones WG *et al.* Histopathology in the prediction of relapse in patients with stage I testicular teratoma treated by orchiectomy alone. *Lancet* 1987; 2: 294–298

38. Cullen M. Adjuvant chemotherapy in high risk stage I non-seminomatous germ cell tumours of the testis. In: Horwich A (ed) Testicular cancer: investigation and management, 2nd edn. London: Chapman and Hall, 1996: 180–191

39. Donohue JP, Thornhill JA, Foster RS *et al.* The role of retroperitoneal lymphadenectomy in clinical stage B testis cancer: the Indiana University experience (1965 to 1989). *J Urol* 1995; 153: 85–89

40. Horwich A, Norman A, Fisher C *et al.* Primary chemotherapy for stage II nonseminomatous germ cell tumors of the testis. *J Urol* 1994; 151: 72–78

41. Samuels ML, Lanzotti VJ, Holoye PV *et al.* Combination chemotherapy in germinal cell tumors. *Cancer Treat Rev* 1976; 3: 185–204

42. Dearnaley DP, Horwich A, A'Hern R *et al.* Combination chemotherapy with bleomycin, etoposide and cisplatin (BEP) for metastatic testicular teratoma: long term follow-up. *Eur J Cancer* 1991; 27: 684–691

43. Bosl GJ. Management of metastatic germ cell tumours: toxicity reduction and the use of bleomycin. In: Horwich A (ed) Testicular cancer: investigation and management. 2nd edn. London: Chapman and Hall, 1996: 251–257

44. Hendry WF, A'Hern RP, Hetherington JW *et al.* Para-aortic lymphadenectomy after chemotherapy for metastatic non-seminomatous germ cell tumours: prognostic value and therapeutic benefit. *Br J Urol* 1993; 71: 208–213

45. Loehrer PJ, Williams SD, Clark SA. Teratoma following chemotherapy for non-seminomatous germ cell tumor: a clinicopathologic correlation. *Proc Am Soc Clin Oncol* 1983; 2: 139–142

46. Logothetis CJ, Samuels ML, Trindale A, Johnson DE. The growing teratoma syndrome. *Cancer* 1982; 50: 1629–1635

47. Baniel J, Foster RS, Rowland RG *et al.* Complications of post-chemotherapy retroperitoneal lymph node dissection. *J Urol* 1995; 153: 976–980

48. Skinner DG, Melamud A, Lieskovsky G. Complications of thoracoabdominal retroperitoneal lymph node dissection. *J Urol* 1982; 127: 1107–1110

49. Leiter E, Brendler H. Loss of ejaculation following bilateral retroperitoneal lymphadenectomy. *J Urol* 1967; 98: 375–378

50. Jones DR, Norman AR, Horwich A, Hendry WF. Ejaculatory dysfunction after retroperitoneal lymphadenectomy. *Eur Urol* 1993; 23: 169–171

51. Lynch JH, Maxted WC. Use of ephedrine in post-lymphadenectomy ejaculatory failure: a case report. *J Urol* 1983; 129: 379–383

52. Nijman JM, Jager S, Boer PW *et al.* The treatment of ejaculation disorders after retroperitoneal lymph node dissection. *Cancer* 1982; 50: 2967–2971

53. Ohl DA. Electroejaculation. *Urol Clin North Am* 1993; 20: 181–188

54. Hendry WF. Cancer therapy and fertility. In: Horwich A (ed) Oncology — a multidisciplinary textbook. London: Chapman and Hall, 1995: 213–223

55. Schilsky RL. Infertility in patients with testicular cancer: testis, tumour or treatment? *J Natl Cancer Inst* 1989; 81: 1204–1205

56. Hendry WF, Stedronska J, Jones CR *et al.* Semen analysis in testicular cancer and Hodgkin's disease: pre- and post-treatment findings and implications for cryopreservation. *Br J Urol* 1983; 55: 769–773

57. Berthelsen JG, Skakkebaek NE. Gonadal function in men with testis cancer. *Fertil Steril* 1983; 39: 68–75

58. Scammell GE, White N, Stedronska J *et al.* Cryopreservation of semen in men with testicular tumour or Hodgkin's disease: results of artificial insemination of their partners. *Lancet* 1985; 2: 31–32

CHAPTER 5

Duodenal and gastric ulcer disease

S. E. Patchett and M. J. G. Farthing

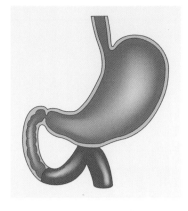

Introduction

The term peptic ulcer disease is often used to refer to both duodenal and gastric ulcers, although these disorders vary in many respects. Peptic ulcers can also occur in the oesophagus in association with gastroesophageal reflux, in the jejunum owing to the Zollinger–Ellison syndrome, or at the anastomotic site of a gastroenterostomy following gastric surgery.

Peptic ulcer disease is very common, affecting about 10% of the population at some point in their lives [1–3]; the disease is increasingly common in older age groups. There is also considerable geographic variation in incidence, with ulcer disease being more common in Scotland and the north of England than in southern England [4]. Epidemiological studies have suggested that duodenal ulcers occur three to four times more commonly than gastric ulcers and that both forms of ulcer disease occur more commonly in men than in women [5]. This pattern was particularly marked for duodenal ulcer disease, where the male:female ratio incidence was 4:1. There has been a steep decline in the incidence of peptic disease in recent years, particularly for duodenal ulcer disease, and particularly in men [6,7]. Certain characteristics of the disease have also changed, such that ulcer perforation in men appears to be decreasing, whereas there is an increasing incidence of ulceration in postmenopausal women.

Aetiology

A great many factors have been associated with the development of peptic ulceration including increased acid secretion, genetic factors, drugs, diet, and stress and lifestyle [4,7]. The multifactorial nature of the disease has resulted in no firm conclusion as to why only certain individuals develop ulcers.

Genetic factors

Genetic predisposition to ulcer disease probably remains an important factor in peptic ulceration, with approximately 20–50% of duodenal ulcer patients having a family history of duodenal ulcers [8]. Duodenal ulcers are also associated with the inheritance of blood group O [9], with certain HLA subtypes and in non-secretors of blood group substances [9]. Additionally, concordance for disease is greater in monozygotic twins than dizygotic twins [10], *Helicobacter pylori* infection can appear as clusters within families [11], and it has been suggested that much of the genetic predisposition to ulcer disease is related to this phenomenon.

Gastric acid and pepsin

Gastric acid and pepsin are both essential for the development of peptic ulceration, although the disturbances in acid secretion observed in peptic ulceration are complex. There is no apparent difference in gastric acid secretion or fasting gastric or duodenal pH between men and women [12]. In general, patients with *H. pylori*-positive duodenal ulceration have increased serum gastrin, an increased parietal cell mass and increased basal and maximal acid secretion compared with *H. pylori*-negative controls [13]. Many of these abnormalities disappear after eradication of *H. pylori*.

Non-steroidal anti-inflammatory drugs (NSAIDs)

Chronic NSAID ingestion has been reported to cause gastroduodenal ulceration, although the relative risk is uncertain and the evidence linking chronic duodenal ulceration with NSAIDs is not convincing. In various studies, the prevalence of gastric ulceration in NSAID users is 9–31% and the prevalence of duodenal ulcers is 0–19% [14,15]. NSAID ingestion is associated with a significantly increased risk of complicated peptic ulcer disease, particularly gastrointestinal haemorrhage [16]. The risk of complications is most notable at 1–3 months after the initiation of NSAID therapy [17].

Helicobacter pylori

The importance of H. pylori as a cause of peptic ulcer disease is now accepted worldwide. Indeed, the National Institutes of Health consensus conference in February 1994 came to the conclusion that peptic ulcer disease is largely an infective disease and that all patients with proven peptic ulceration should receive treatment directed at eradication of the organism [18]. The most persuasive evidence supporting this statement comes from the many long-term follow-up studies in peptic ulcer disease following successful eradication (Table 5.1). Healing of ulcer disease with acid-suppression therapy alone results in a 60–70% recurrence rate within 12 months. However, if the organism is successfully eradicated, ulcer recurrence is significantly reduced and often abolished.

It is now realized that this organism is one of the most common chronic infections of humans. As well as its role in duodenal and gastric ulcers, it probably also has a pivotal role in other gastrointestinal diseases, such as non-ulcer dyspepsia and gastric cancer. Eradication of the organism significantly alters the natural history of peptic ulcer disease, with a very real possibility of abolishing recurrence and curing the ulcer diathesis [19,20]. This has highly significant implications, both for the reduction of mortality and morbidity of peptic disease and in reducing the requirement for long-term maintenance therapy.

H. pylori is a Gram-negative spiral-shaped bacterium found only in association with gastric epithelium (Fig. 5.1). It tends to cluster below

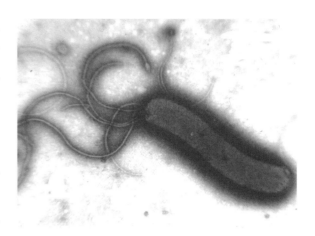

Figure 5.1. Helicobacter pylori.

the gastric mucus and around the junctions between cells, although rarely penetrating the cells themselves. Survival in the hostile, acidic environment of the stomach is facilitated through production of the enzyme urease, which hydrolyses urea to form ammonia and bicarbonate, thereby providing an alkaline micro-environment. Patients with H. pylori in the stomach may also harbour organisms in metaplastic gastric epithelium in the oesophagus or duodenum, although the organisms are not found in the blood or, with rare exceptions, in other parts of the body.

There is substantial variation in H. pylori prevalence, both between and within populations. In the Western World, the prevalence of infection in healthy persons younger than 30 years is 10%, whereas over the age of 60 years infection rates approach 60%. In all populations studied so far, there is also a close relationship between H. pylori prevalence and economic status, prevalence being significantly higher in the lower socio-economic groups. Almost all patients (> 95%) with proven duodenal ulcer disease will

Table 5.1. Helicobacter pylori *eradication and ulcer recurrence rates*

Study	Year	Follow-up (months)	Ulcer relapse (%)	
			H. pylori +ve	*H. pylori* –ve
Coughlan *et al.* [39]	1987	12	76	10
Marshall *et al.* [40]	1988	12	81	22
Rauws and Tyrgat [20]	1990	12	81	0
Patchett *et al.* [19]	1992	12	31	0

have evidence of *H. pylori* infection [22]. Similarly, *H. pylori* is present in more than 90% of patients with gastric ulceration, particularly when NSAID ingestion has been excluded [22]. There appears to be no difference, however, in *H. pylori* incidence between men and women [23].

It is now widely accepted that person-to-person transmission of *H. pylori* occurs, though the precise mode of transmission remains speculative. Reports of successful culture of the organism from stools support faecal–oral transmission [24], although the oral–oral and/or gastro–oral routes may yet prove to be at least as important [25].

Mechanism of ulcer formation

The mechanisms by which *H. pylori* induces peptic ulceration are varied and complex; some of these are listed in Table 5.2. Chronic antral infection is almost always associated with inflammation, although peptic ulcer disease and gastric carcinoma occur only in a subset of patients. Clearly, both bacterial and host factors are likely to contribute to this differential response. A number of histological and functional abnormalities have been described in chronic *H. pylori* infection. As mentioned earlier, both basal and meal-stimulated serum gastrin concentrations tend to be higher in infected patients than in non-infected controls. In addition, stimulated acid secretion is significantly higher in infected patients, and has been shown to return to normal

Table 5.2. *Pathogenetic mechanisms of* Helicobacter pylori *in peptic ulcer disease*

Toxin production	Urease
	Mucinase
	Lipase
	Phospholipase
	Cytotoxins (e.g. VacA)
Inflammation	Mucosal inflammation
	Neutrophil activation
	Macrocyte/monocyte activation
	Leukotrienes B_4 synthesis
Increased gastrin production	—

following eradication of the organism [26]. These changes are thought to result from interference with the physiological role of somatostatin in the control of gastrin release. In addition, *H. pylori* is capable of producing a range of potentially toxic enzymes including urease, mucinase, lipase and phospholipase, each of which may have direct toxic effects on gastric cells and on gastric mucus production. Furthermore, approximately 50–60% of *H. pylori* isolates produce a toxin that induces non-lethal vacuolation in a variety of cell lines [27]. This toxin, known as the vacuolating cyto-toxin or VacA, interestingly is more prevalent in isolates from individuals with peptic ulcer disease than in isolates from those with only gastritis, and thus the production of this protein may represent an important virulence factor [28]. Although many of these putative pathogenic factors have been identified in vitro, however, their significance in vivo is largely unknown and remains to be clarified.

Diagnosis of H. pylori

Several tests are available for diagnosis of *H. pylori* infection, although the choice of test largely depends on the question being asked and on local availability. Serological testing is probably the simplest non-invasive method available to detect primary *H. pylori* infection and several sensitive and specific tests are currently commercially available. Although these assays were originally designed for use in the laboratory, the advent of 'desk-top' whole-blood enzyme-linked immuno-sorbent assay (ELISA) kits for use by individual clinicians in primary care will undoubtedly increase the availability and value of serology as a diagnostic test. Positive serological tests strongly suggest current infection, as spontaneous clearance of infection is unusual. However, after successful treatment, antibody levels remain positive in most cases for several years, thereby limiting the usefulness of blood testing for the follow-up of treatment response.

For confirmation of eradication of infection, the [^{13}C]- or [^{14}C]urea breath test is preferable (Fig. 5.2). Following ingestion of a test meal containing labelled urea, *H. pylori* metabolizes the urea, liberating ^{13}C or ^{14}C-labelled carbon dioxide. This is exhaled, collected in a test-tube and quantified. Sensitivity and specificity of this test is high and although false negatives do occur (e.g. following recent antibiotic or omeprazole therapy), this test is now currently considered the gold standard for the follow-up of patients after treatment.

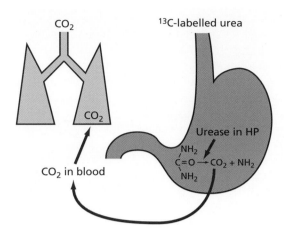

CO_2 ¹³C-labelled urea

CO_2

CO_2 in blood

Urease in HP

NH₂
C=O → CO_2 + NH₂
NH₂

Figure 5.2. *Diagrammatic representation of ¹³C breath test. HP, Helicobacter pylori.*

If the patient is undergoing endoscopy, antral biopsy specimens can be obtained enabling direct bacterial culture and histological detection of *H. pylori* in gastric mucosa. An alternative, less expensive endoscopic method is to test for bacterial urease in the biopsy sample. In this test, the gastric antral biopsy specimen is placed in a solution of urea containing a pH indicator. Metabolism of the urea by bacterial urease changes the pH of the solution, thereby producing a colour change within minutes [29,30].

Treatment decisions

Although it is now possible to diagnose and treat *H. pylori* infection rapidly and effectively, there remains considerable controversy as to who should be treated. The scene is constantly changing, as treatment strategies encompass both the potential implications of long-term infection and the considerable financial implications. In patients in whom a diagnosis has been established, there is at least some consensus with regard to indications for treatment. It is clear that patients with proven duodenal ulceration or *H. pylori*-positive gastric ulceration should have eradication therapy, as this permanently cures the condition in the majority of patients and probably also prevents life-threatening complications, such as peptic ulcer haemorrhage [31]. On the other hand, there is no evidence that patients with a firm diagnosis of gastro-oesophageal reflux disease benefit from *H. pylori* eradication; thus, testing for the presence of the organism in this group of patients is probably not indicated. Patients with non-ulcer dyspepsia in whom other causes of dyspepsia have been

excluded form a heterogeneous group. Therefore, perhaps unsurprisingly, firm recommendations with regard to *H. pylori* eradication in this group are lacking. The literature supporting eradication therapy in patients with non-ulcer dyspepsia is not convincing [32,33]. However, it is possible — or even probable — that a subgroup of these patients will benefit from eradication. Many clinicians will therefore advocate treatment of *H. pylori* if other investigations have excluded alternative causes for their patients' symptoms.

Clinical features of peptic ulcer disease

The clinical hallmark of peptic ulcer disease is pain. This is typically described as a burning pain localized to the epigastrium and relieved by antacids. The pain of duodenal ulceration is often worse at night and when the patient is fasting. The relationship to food is variable, however, and not helpful in diagnosis. Nausea and vomiting are uncommon features unless the pain is severe, or gastric outlet obstruction is present. Persistent severe pain or back pain may suggest perforation or penetration of other organs, such as the pancreas. Haemorrhage may present with haematemesis and/or melaena, and pain in this situation may often be absent. Patients with severe ulceration, however, may be completely asymptomatic: 50% of patients who die from peptic ulceration are unaware of their diagnosis prior to the final event. It is also difficult to distinguish between gastric ulceration and duodenal ulceration on clinical features alone.

Typically, the clinical course of untreated peptic disease is one of remission and relapse. Spontaneous healing is not uncommon, but may be delayed by smoking or by taking NSAIDs. Data from the 'pre-*H. pylori*' era suggest that the natural history is for the disease to remit over many years owing to the development of gastric atrophy and the consequent reduction in acid output [4].

Investigations

A confident diagnosis of peptic ulcer disease cannot be made from a history and physical examination alone, as the clinical picture overlaps closely with other causes of dyspepsia, such as gastro-oesophageal reflux, non-ulcer dyspepsia and, occasionally, gastric cancer. Gastroscopy is now the preferred method of diagnosis, as this method not only allows direct visualization of the ulcer but also enables the clinician to obtain mucosal biopsy samples where appropriate. Duodenal ulcers appear as discrete, often single areas of ulceration resembling an aphthous ulcer (Fig. 5.3). They are often associated with surrounding inflammation (duodenitis) or with duodenal deformity suggesting chronic disease. Gastric ulcers most commonly occur on the lesser curve or antrum of the stomach; ulceration in other areas suggests an alternative disease process, such as malignancy. Because benign gastric ulceration and gastric malignancy can appear identical endoscopically, it is mandatory to obtain multiple targeted biopsy samples from the ulcer margin to exclude malignancy. Follow-up endoscopy subsequent to a course of medical treatment is also strongly recommended.

Duodenal and gastric ulceration can also be successfully diagnosed using a double-contrast barium meal, although in the duodenum it is sometimes difficult to differentiate between inactive ulcer scarring and active ulceration. Although histology is usually required to confirm the presence of gastric malignancy, expert radiologists can almost always differentiate between benign and malignant gastric disease.

Most patients who present to their doctors with symptoms suggestive of an ulcer can be managed in the primary care setting and do not

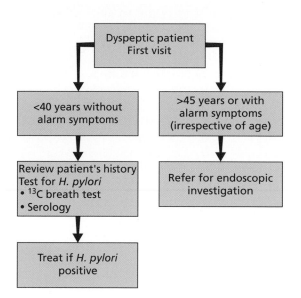

Figure 5.4. *Recommended approach to dyspepsia in the community.*

require referral to hospital for investigation. The decision to refer a patient for further investigation depends principally on the clinical presentation and on the age of the patient. A recent European consensus meeting suggested that patients with dyspeptic symptoms, who are under 40 years of age and are without 'alarm' symptoms (e.g. anaemia, weight loss, dysphagia, palpable mass), should be tested for the presence of *H. pylori* using a non-invasive method, such as a serological test or breath test, and, if positive, treated without further investigations [34] (Fig. 5.4).

It is strongly recommended, however, that patients over 45 years with severe dyspeptic symptoms, or those with 'alarm' symptoms, are referred for endoscopic investigation. Patients with proven peptic ulceration who are not taking NSAIDs and who are *H. pylori* negative, or those who have severe, unresponsive or atypical ulceration, should have a fasting plasma gastrin measured to exclude the Zollinger–Ellison syndrome.

Management of duodenal and gastric ulcer disease

The vast majority of peptic ulcers are now successfully treated medically, with surgery being reserved largely for the management of the complications of peptic disease. The aims of treatment are to relieve symptoms, heal the ulcer,

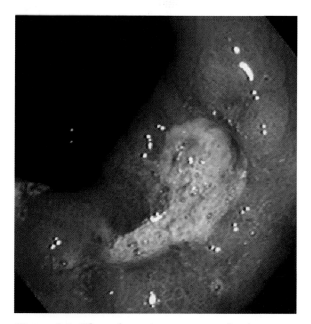

Figure 5.3. *The endoscopic appearance of a chronic duodenal ulcer.*

prevent recurrence and prevent complications. The first three of these aims can usually be achieved with *H. pylori* eradication in patients with *H. pylori* infection or with acid suppression in those who are *H. pylori* negative.

With the introduction of modern drugs for the treatment of peptic disease, there is no longer any indication to impose dietary restrictions, as this approach does not alter the natural history of the disease. It is sensible to advise the patient to give up smoking, not only because of the beneficial effects that this will have on general health but also because there is some evidence that continued smoking slows healing [35]. There is little evidence that alcohol ingestion impacts in any way on the natural history of peptic disease, and abstinence is unnecessary.

Peptic ulcers associated with *H. pylori*

The aim of treatment of *H. pylori* is to eradicate the organism from the foregut. This is currently defined as absence of the organism for at least 28 days after the end of antimicrobial therapy. Successful eradication of the organism will result in healing of the ulcer in over 90% of cases and prevention of recurrence of the ulcer. Treatment of *H. pylori* can be difficult and requires the use of combination therapy. This is because the organism lives under a mucous layer in the stomach, which restricts access of antimicrobials. In addition, the organism may acquire resistance to antimicrobials, particularly the imidazole derivatives. The ideal treatment should be simple, safe, free from side effects and 100% effective, but modern therapy still falls short of these ideals. Regimens for treatment are constantly changing, but currently recommended treatment schedules are given in Table 5.3.

Peptic ulcers not associated with *H. pylori*

Most *H. pylori*-negative ulcers are caused by NSAID ingestion. In this group of patients, the NSAID should be discontinued, if at all possible, and treatment with an acid-suppressing drug should be commenced. Options for treatment include proton pump inhibitors, H2-receptor antagonists and prostaglandin E_1 (PGE_1) analogues.

Proton pump inhibitors

Drugs in this category include omeprazole 20 mg daily, lansoprazole 30 mg daily and pantoprazole 40 mg daily. These drugs stop acid secretion by irreversible inhibition of the proton pump in the gastric parietal cell. Proton pump inhibitors are probably the treatment of choice as they provide more rapid healing and faster relief of pain than H2-receptor antagonists. They are safe and extremely well tolerated, with a very low incidence of side effects. Proton pump inhibitors do, however, result in profound acid inhibition, which is associated with an increased susceptibility to enteric infection. Early studies in the rat suggested that the rise in serum gastrin induced by omeprazole was associated with an increased incidence of gastric carcinoids. However, gastric carcinoids have not been shown to develop in man after prolonged treatment with omeprazole.

H2-receptor antagonists

Drugs in this category include cimetidine 800 mg daily and ranitidine 300 mg daily. These agents result in healing of 80–90% of peptic ulcers although, with the introduction of more potent acid-inhibitory drugs, their use is less frequent at present.

Table 5.3. *Recommended treatment schedules for* Helicobacter pylori; *drugs are taken concurrently over the course of 7 days*

Drug	Dosing	Duration	Efficacy
Omeprazole (20 mg)/lanzoprazole (30 mg)	Twice daily	7 days	90%
Clarithromycin (250 mg)	Twice daily	7 days	–
Metronidazole (400 mg)	Twice daily	7 days	–
Omeprazole (20 mg)/lanzoprazole (30 mg)	Twice daily	7 days	90%
Clarithromycin (500 mg)	Twice daily	7 days	–
Amoxycillin (1 g)	Twice daily	7 days	–

PGE₁ analogues

Misoprostol is a synthetic analogue of PGE_1 that reduces gastric secretory activity and enhances gastric mucosal defence. This agent has no place in the routine treatment of peptic disease, principally because of its unimpressive healing rates and its relatively frequent side effects (diarrhoea and abdominal pain). Its principal use is as a cytoprotective agent against NSAID-associated peptic ulcers, particularly in the elderly.

Surgical treatment

Surgery is now rarely required for the management of peptic ulceration, largely owing to the efficacy of modern therapies. It is reserved principally to treat the complications of ulcer disease — namely, recurrent and uncontrolled haemorrhage, particularly following failed endoscopic haemostasis — or for ulcer perforation. Ligation of the bleeding vessel or oversewing the perforation is all that is required. Procedures commonly used in the past, such as partial gastrectomy or vagotomy, are now almost obsolete.

Follow-up

In general, the effectiveness of treatment should be assessed symptomatically. Follow-up endoscopy is not indicated in duodenal ulcer disease, but is strongly recommended in gastric ulceration to ensure healing of the ulcer. The importance of routinely confirming the success or otherwise of *H. pylori* eradication following treatment is contentious. Confirmation of eradication is appropriate in patients who present with complications, or in those whose symptoms return or fail to resolve following a course of treatment. Recent data suggest that disappearance of dyspepsia following a course of therapy is a powerful predictor of successful *H. pylori* eradication [36].

Complications of peptic ulcer disease

The principal complications of peptic disease are perforation, haemorrhage and gastric outflow obstruction.

Perforation

Ulcer perforation is thought to occur in about 5–10% of patients with peptic ulcer disease; it is more common in men than in women and in duodenal than in gastric ulcers. Approximately 50% of patients will have no previous history of dyspepsia at the time of perforation. Typically, the patient presents with sudden onset of abdominal pain and examination reveals abdominal rigidity, rebound tenderness and absent bowel sounds. Plain abdominal radiographs may show free intraperitoneal air, and the white cell count is usually elevated. Treatment involves oversewing the ulcer surgically and eradication of *H. pylori* if present.

Haemorrhage

Approximately 10–15% of peptic ulcers manifest as a clinically apparent haemorrhage. Despite the reduced prevalence of peptic ulcer disease, the number of hospitalizations for peptic ulcer bleeding has changed relatively little in recent years, largely because of the increasing age of patients with ulcer bleeding [2]. For similar reasons, the overall mortality has changed little over the last 30 years and remains at 6–7%.

There appears to be no difference in ulcer bleeding rates between men and women; likewise, there is no difference in acid secretion between bleeding and non-bleeding ulcers [37]. The prevalence of *H. pylori* may be 15–20% lower in ulcers that bleed. Conversely, several studies have indicated that NSAIDs are an important risk factor for ulcer bleeding. Thus, these drugs not only induce ulcers but also increase the chance of complications such as bleeding [15,16].

Clinically, most patients with a bleeding peptic ulcer present with haematemesis, melaena, or both. Management involves resuscitation of the patient, confirmation of the exact diagnosis and specific treatment of the bleeding ulcer. Endoscopy is an essential step as it identifies the point of bleeding, permits therapy with injection of adrenaline or heat coagulation, and provides important prognostic information. Ulcer size or the presence of stigmata of bleeding can predict the risk of rebleeding; thus, subsequent management should be tailored to the endoscopic findings. Most studies have shown that patients with no evidence of clot or visible vessel in the ulcer base have a low risk of further bleeding and are thus candidates for early discharge [38]. There is little evidence that drug therapy is beneficial in arresting bleeding or preventing rebleeding. Treatment to induce ulcer healing should be commenced as soon as practical after diagnosis, and *H. pylori* should be eradicated if present.

Gastric outflow obstruction

Gastric outflow obstruction due to stenosis of a chronically scarred pylorus is occasionally seen in recurrent peptic disease. A history of long-standing dyspeptic pain with recent onset of projectile vomiting is typical. Diagnosis is confirmed with endoscopy or barium meal, which will usually show a dilated stomach with copious gastric residue. It is important to differentiate outlet obstruction due to peptic disease from malignant obstruction due to cancer of the gastric antrum or (occasionally) the pancreas. Although endoscopic balloon dilatation of the pylorus is feasible, stenosis usually recurs and treatment is most commonly surgical following correction of fluid and electrolyte abnormalities.

Conclusions

The last 25 years have seen dramatic changes in the ability of clinicians to diagnose and treat duodenal and gastric ulcer disease. Surgery, once the mainstay of treatment, is now reserved largely for the management of complications. Medical treatment is effective and safe, but much needs to be done to resolve the debate about who should be treated and how.

References

1. Kurata JH, Nogawa AN, Abbey DE, Petersen F. A prospective study of risk for peptic ulcer disease in Seventh-Day Adventists. *Gastroenterology* 1992; 102: 902–909

2. Kurata JH, Corboy ED. Current peptic ulcer time trends. An epidemiological profile. *J Clin Gastroenterol* 1988; 10: 259–268

3. Kurata JH, Haile BM. Epidemiology of peptic ulcer disease. *Clin Gastroenterol* 1984; 13: 289–307

4. Misiewciz JJ, Pounder RE. Peptic ulceration. In: Weatherall DJ, Ledingham JGC, Warrell DA (eds) Oxford textbook of medicine. Oxford: Oxford University Press, 1996: 1877–1891

5. Kurata JH, Haile BM, Elashoff JD. Sex differences in peptic ulcer disease. *Gastroenterology* 1985; 88: 96–100

6. Sonnenberg A, Everhart JE. The prevalence of self-reported peptic ulcer in the United States. *Am J Public Health* 1996; 86: 200–205

7. Rosenstock SJ, Jorgensen T. Prevalence and incidence of peptic ulcer disease in a Danish County: a prospective cohort study. *Gut* 1995; 36: 819–824

8. Tarpila S, Samloff IM, Pikkarainen P *et al.* Endoscopic and clinical findings in first-degree relative of duodenal ulcer patients and control subjects. *Scand J Gastroenterol* 1982; 17: 503–506

9. Odeigah PG. Influence of blood group and secretor genes on susceptibility to duodenal ulcer. *East Afr Med J* 1990; 67: 487–500

10. Raiha I, Kemppainen H, Kaprio J *et al.* Lifestyle, stress, and genes in peptic ulcer disease. *Arch Intern Med* 1998; 158: 698–704

11. Drumm B, Perez-Perez GI, Blaser MJ, Sherman PM. Intrafamilial clustering of Helicobacter pylori infection. *N Engl J Med* 1990; 322: 359–363

12. Russell TL, Berardi RR, Barnett JL *et al.* Upper gastro-intestinal pH in seventy-nine healthy, elderly, North American men and women. *Pharmacol Res* 1993; 10: 187–196

13. El-Omar E, Penman ID, Ardill JE *et al.* Helicobacter pylori infection and abnormalities of acid secretion in patients with duodenal ulcer disease. *Gastroenterology* 1995; 109: 681–691

14. McCarthy DM. Nonsteroidal antiinflammatory drug-induced ulcers: management by traditional therapies. *Gastroenterology* 1989; 96: 662–674

15. Graham DY. The relationship between nonsteroidal anti-inflammatory drug use and peptic ulcer disease. *Gastroenterol Clin North Am* 1990; 19: 171–182

16. Hawkey CJ. Gastroduodenal problems associated with non-steroidal, anti-inflammatory drugs (NSAIDs). *Scand J Gastroenterol Suppl* 1993; 200: 94–95

17. Gabriel SE, Jaakkimainen L, Bombardier C. Risk for serious gastrointestinal complications related to use of nonsteroidal anti-inflammatory drugs. A meta-analysis. *Ann Intern Med* 1991; 115: 787–796

18. NIH Consensus Conference. Helicobacter pylori in peptic ulcer disease. NIH Consensus Development Panel on Helicobacter pylori in peptic ulcer disease. *JAMA* 1994; 272: 65–69

19. Patchett S, Beattie S, Leen E *et al.* Helicobacter pylori and duodenal ulcer recurrence. *Am J Gastroenterol* 1992; 87: 24–27

20. Rauws EA, Tytgat GN. Cure of duodenal ulcer associated with eradication of Helicobacter pylori. *Lancet* 1990; 335: 1233–1235

21. Sitas F, Forman D, Yarnell JW *et al.* Helicobacter pylori infection rates in relation to age and social class in a population of Welsh men. *Gut* 1991; 32: 25–28

22. Rauws EAJ, Langenberg W, Houthoff HJ *et al.* Campylobacter pyloridis associated chronic active antral gastritis. *Gastroenterology* 1988; 94: 33–40

23. Graham DY, Malaty HM, Evans DG *et al.* Epidemiology of Helicobacter pylori in an asymptomatic population in the United States. Effect of age, race, and socioeconomic status. *Gastroenterology* 1991; 100: 1495–1501

24. Thomas JE, Gibson GR, Darboe MK *et al.* Isolation of Helicobacter pylori from human faeces. *Lancet* 1992; 340: 1194–1195

25. Axon AT. Review article: is Helicobacter pylori transmitted by the gastro-oral route? *Aliment Pharmacol Therapeut* 1995; 9: 585–588

26. El-Omar E, Penman I, Dorrian CA *et al.* Eradicating Helicobacter pylori infection lowers gastrin mediated

acid secretion by two-thirds in patients with duodenal ulcer. *Gut* 1993; 34: 1060–1065

27. Cover TL, Dooley CP, Blaser MJ. Characterization of and human serologic response to proteins in Helicobacter pylori broth culture supernatants with vacuolizing cytotoxin activity. *Infect Immun* 1990; 58: 603–610

28. Crabtree JE, Taylor JD, Wyatt JI *et al.* Mucosal IgA recognition of Helicobacter pylori 120 kDa protein, peptic ulceration, and gastric pathology. *Lancet* 1991; 338: 332–335

29. Thillainayagam AV, Arvind AS, Cook RS *et al.* Diagnostic efficiency of an ultrarapid endoscopy room test for Helicobacter pylori. *Gut* 1991; 32: 467–469

30. Katelaris PH, Lowe DG, Norbu P, Farthing MJ. Field evaluation of a rapid, simple and inexpensive urease test for the detection of Helicobacter pylori. *J Gastroenterol Hepatol* 1992; 7: 569–571

31. Graham DY, Hepps KS, Ramirez FC *et al.* Treatment of Helicobacter pylori reduces the rate of rebleeding in peptic ulcer disease. *Scand J Gastroenterol* 1993; 28: 939–942

32. Talley NJ, Hunt RH. What role does Helicobacter pylori play in dyspepsia and non-ulcer dyspepsia? Arguments for and against H. pylori being associated with dyspeptic symptoms. *Gastroenterology* 1997; 113: S67–77

33. Talley NJ. A critique of therapeutic trials in Helicobacter pylori-positive functional dyspepsia. *Gastroenterology* 1994; 106: 1174–1183

34. Malfertheiner P, Megraud F, O'Morain C *et al.* Current European concepts in the management of Helicobacter pylori infection: the Maastricht Consensus Report. The European Helicobacter Pylori Study Group (EHPSG). *Eur J Gastroenterol Hepatol* 1997; 9: 1–2

35. Eastwood GL. The role of smoking in peptic ulcer disease. *J Clin Gastroenterol* 1988; 10: S19–23

36. McColl KE, El-Nujumi A, Murray LS *et al.* Assessment of symptomatic response as predictor of Helicobacter pylori status following eradication therapy in patients with ulcer. *Gut* 1998; 42: 618–623

37. Laine L, Peterson WL. Bleeding peptic ulcer. *N Engl J Med* 1994; 331: 717–727

38. Rockall TA, Logan RF, Devlin HB, Northfield TC. Risk assessment after acute upper gastrointestinal haemorrhage. *Gut* 1996; 38: 316–321

39. Coughlan JG, Gilligan D, Humphries H *et al.* Campylobacter pylori and recurrence of duodenal ulcers — a 12-month follow-up study. *Lancet* 1987; 2: 1109–1111

40. Marshall BJ, Goodwin CS, Warren JR *et al.* Prospective double-blind trial of duodenal ulcer relapse after eradication of Campylobacter pylori. *Lancet* 1988; 2: 1437–1442

CHAPTER 6

Groin hernias

H. B. Devlin

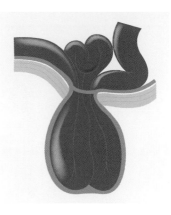

Introduction

Surgery for groin hernias in men is one of the commonest general surgical procedures. In the UK, one in eight males is likely to have an operation for an inguinal hernia; in Europe, 8–10% of males will have had a groin hernia operation during their lifetime [1].

Epidemiology

Inguinal hernias

In the adult UK population 3% will require an operation for inguinal hernia, with the peak incidence occurring in the sixth decade. The ratio of elective to emergency operations is 12:1 and the male to female ratio is 12:1. Indirect inguinal hernias make up 65% of all hernia cases.

In Africans, the incidence of indirect inguinal hernia is three times greater than in Europeans and the patients are, on average, 40 years younger at presentation than in Europe. There are also differences in the incidence of groin hernias between different African tribes: 30% of adult males in the African community on the Isle of Pemba off the coast of Madagascar develop a hernia, whereas in Tanzanians the figure is 16%, in Rhodesian miners it is 9% and in Southern Ghanaians it is 7.7% [1]. Similarly, groin hernias are extremely common in Afro-Caribbean males, probably because of the different anatomy of the pelvis and the internal oblique muscle in Negroid persons [1].

Femoral hernias

The ratio of the incidence of femoral hernias in females and males is 4:1. Femoral hernias are most common in middle-aged and elderly women, especially after weight loss, and in multiparous women. In women, femoral hernias are less common than inguinal hernias (femoral/inguinal hernia ratio 1:18); however, in older women the situation is reversed, with femoral hernias becoming more common.

Anatomy and aetiology

In anatomical terms, the formation of the groin in males differs completely from that in females: in females, the generative organs are internal; in males, they are essentially external. It is this externality that leads to the weakness in the groin that, in turn, predicts the development of groin hernias in males. Modern concepts of groin herniation stress the laminar musculo-aponeurotic structure of the groin region. Disruption or stretching of one or more of these laminae gives rise to a groin hernia (Fig. 6.1). The essential goal of hernia repair is, therefore, to restore the structural integrity of these layers.

In the groin, inguinofemoral hernias result from the breakdown of the fascia transversalis, the investing fascia of the deep surface of the transversalis muscle. The fascia covers the transversalis muscle and its aponeurotic tendon of insertion, and forms the posterior wall of the inguinal canal. Fruchaud has created an entirely new concept, 'the myopectineal orifice', which combines the traditionally separate inguinal and femoral canals to form a unified highway from the abdomen to the thigh and the scrotum [2]. The abdominocrural tunnel of fascia transversalis extends through the myopectineal orifice. All inguinal and femoral hernias pass through this orifice, as do the iliofemoral vessels and vessels to the lower limb and the spermatic vessels to the scrotum. On the basis of this anatomical concept, Fruchaud recommended complete reconstruction of the endofascial wall (fascia transversalis) of the myopectineal orifice. This unifying concept forms the basis for all extraperi-

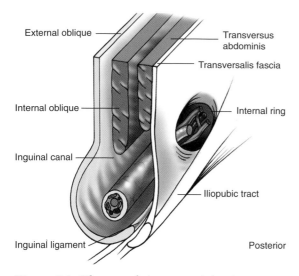

Figure 6.1. *The musculo-aponeurotic laminar structure of the groin region and its distortion by a hernia sac.*

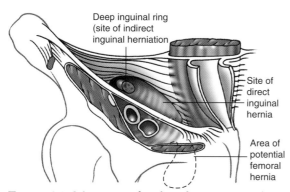

Figure 6.2. *Myopectineal orifice, demonstrating the congenital indirect inguinal hernia, which protrudes through to the deep inguinal ring; the acquired direct inguinal hernia, which bulges through the posterior wall of the inguinal canal; and the femoral hernia, which plunges through the potential weakness alongside the femoral vein.*

toneal mesh repairs, open or laparoscopic, of groin hernias (Fig. 6.2).

Although many groin hernias are first noticed after a strain, injury is an uncommon cause of such hernias. Early operation after injury fails to show any bruising or signs of tissue trauma. Fractures of the bony pelvis are seldom followed by groin herniation [3]. Raised intra-abdominal pressure from ascites, malignancy, liver or heart failure, or continuous ambulatory perfusion for renal failure, often causes a persistent, and previously closed, processus vaginalis to reopen and present as an indirect hernia. Abdominal disease can present as a groin hernia:

for example, in appendicitis or inflammatory disease, pus can distend a hernia sac; malignant deposits from stomach and colon cancer can each first present as deposits in a hernia sac.

Indirect inguinal hernia

An indirect inguinal hernia is due to dilatation of the fascia transversalis at the deep ring and is classified as a congenital defect. Failure of closure of the processus vaginalis allows abdominal contents, omentum and small gut to move into and out of the deep ring, which is then repeatedly stretched. The Australian surgeon Russell was responsible for clearly defining the process [4]. Failure of the closure of the deep ring at the peritoneal level causes this congenital type of hernia seen in premature babies, in young boys and young men. Indirect inguinal hernias are a polygenic defect in the development of the groin and, as mentioned earlier, the increased incidence in certain African tribes is due to their carrying this defect.

Direct inguinal hernia

A direct inguinal hernia is a weakening of the fascia transversalis in the posterior wall of the inguinal canal medial to the deep epigastric vessels (Hesselbach triangle); this type of hernia is acquired. Chronic smokers exhibit circulating proteases of pulmonary origin, giving rise to increased serum elastolytic activity. This is associated with a qualitative defect in the inhibitory capacity of α_1-antitrypsin. Changes in the fascia transversalis lamina ('metastatic emphysema') occur in these patients, leading to direct inguinal herniation. This qualitative abnormality of the endofascia of the abdomen was discovered by Read [5] and Peacock [6]. It also occurs in some congenital defects of the mesenchyme, mainly Marfan's syndrome and prune-belly syndrome, which are very rare. In these patients, the fascia transversalis gives way and the hernia bulges out through it. Persistent poor nutrition and constant straining may be cofactors. In case–control studies, such hernias were shown to be more common in labouring men who strained a great deal [1].

Femoral hernia

A femoral hernia is caused by atrophy or dilatation of the femoral ring. This allows the fascia transversalis, which impinges on the ring from above, to be forced into it. As the fascia transversalis stretches and traverses the femoral canal, extraperitoneal fat and peritoneum follow to give the classic thick-walled, fatty, femoral hernia sac.

Embryology

Embryologically, the gonads develop at the caudal pole of the primitive kidneys at 7–14 days. Primitive gonads in the female migrate down into the pelvis where they remain. In contrast, in the male, the gonads (testicles) undergo a complex migration: first, they descend towards the pelvis; then they move towards the anterior abdominal wall, then out through the anterior abdominal wall at the site of the inguinal canal and down into the scrotum (Fig. 6.3). This migration leads to the different development of the groin muscles in the male.

The groin muscles arch over the developing testicles and associated vessels. As the testicles migrate caudally from the posterior abdominal wall, they are surrounded initially by a pouch or out-pocket of peritoneum. This out-pocket of peritoneum continues down into the scrotum, where it forms a covering of the testicles. The out-pocket normally becomes closed completely in the foetus some weeks before birth. It is interesting that, in premature babies, often this out-pocketing or diverticulum of peritoneum remains open until after the birth of the baby.

The baby is born with a hernia in the initial premature state and this can result in perinatal complications.

Diagnosis

Diagnosis is made by visualization of the hernia. The patient may notice a lump in the groin, which is often visible long before it is palpable. Once a hernia has been diagnosed, the traditional treatment is to operate and repair it. However, a number of considerations are first necessary.

A hernia is a reducible expansile lump that varies in size. Other lumps in the groin, such as aneurysms of the iliac/femoral vessels, saphenovarix of the saphenous vein, enlarged groin lymph nodes due to inflammation or tumour metastasis and the ubiquitous lipoma, must be considered in the differential diagnosis. Additional information on the anatomy of the groin may be found by ultrasound scanning, by computed tomography or by nuclear magnetic resonance imaging. However, this information often does not assist the therapeutic decisions regarding the hernia. The only certain diagnostic

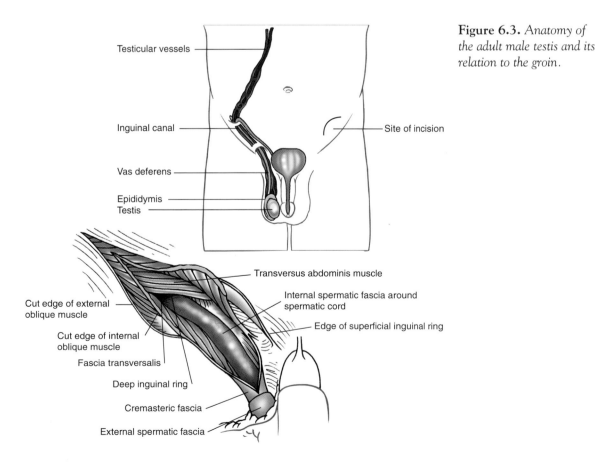

Figure 6.3. *Anatomy of the adult male testis and its relation to the groin.*

Testicular vessels

Inguinal canal

Site of incision

Vas deferens

Epididymis
Testis

Transversus abdominis muscle

Internal spermatic fascia around spermatic cord

Cut edge of external oblique muscle

Edge of superficial inguinal ring

Cut edge of internal oblique muscle

Fascia transversalis

Deep inguinal ring

Cremasteric fascia

External spermatic fascia

modality is herniography; this is performed by injecting a non-irritant contrast medium into the peritoneal cavity and taking prone radiographs of the groin while the patient strains [7].

Treatment

An absolute indication for operation is obstruction or strangulation of the hernia. Congenital and indirect hernias tend to strangulate more easily than other hernias and should be operated on at all ages (Fig. 6.4). In particular, indirect hernias in preterm babies of low birth weight require urgent operation to prevent strangulation.

Direct hernias do not have such clear-cut requirements for operation. Indirect hernias, which have episodes of becoming irreducible, certainly need surgery fairly soon. If there is an episode of obstruction and strangulation, imme-

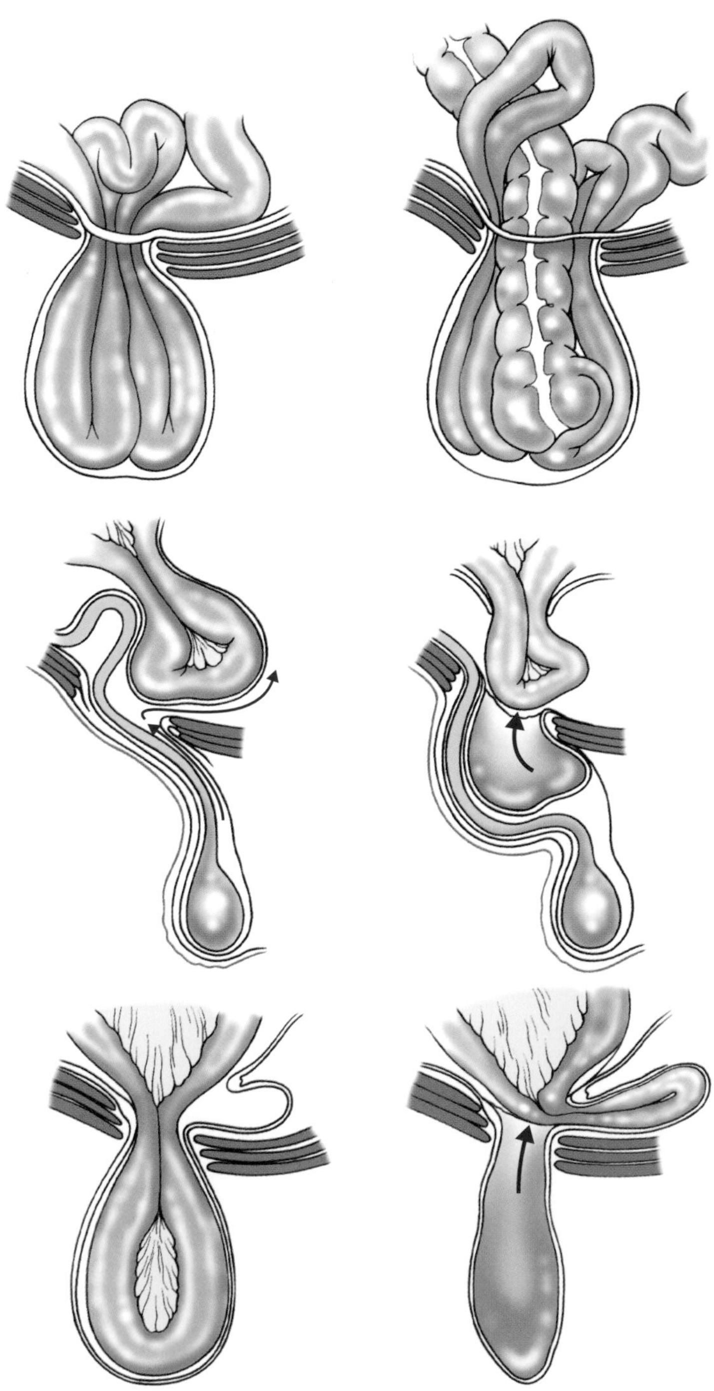

Figure 6.4. *Small and large bowel may prolapse and either are susceptible to strangulation or obstruction.*

diate surgery is always indicated. The direct hernia in the elderly man, which reduces spontaneously when the man relaxes and lies down, has a relatively low incidence of strangulation and does not inevitably need surgery. Surgery may also be indicated if the hernia is painful or uncomfortable for the patient. Repairing a direct hernia in an elderly, unfit man will not necessarily increase his longevity.

All patients need assessment prior to surgery. First, the patient must be fit for operation. In urgent cases where strangulation or obstruction have occurred, resuscitation is always needed. All patients, especially older patients, need management, during surgery, of any co-morbidities, such as heart disease and renal disease.

Surgical procedures

There is no universal surgical procedure for groin hernia repair: treatment should be carefully tailored to the anatomical findings in the groin. There are various classifications for surgeons to adopt when looking at inguinal hernias and deciding what operation to perform, but essentially the anatomy of the fascia transversalis defines what to do. Reduction of the peritoneum sac and replacement or reinforcement of the fascia transversalis by non-absorbable sutures or by prosthetic non-absorbable mesh is the current treatment of choice.

Adopting the policy of individualized hernia repair, four operative treatments of hernias can be defined:

1. If the deep ring is of normal diameter and the fascia transversalis of normal strength, disruption by surgery is not necessary. Instead, a simple excision of the peritoneal indirect sac, herniotomy, will suffice to cure the condition.
2. If the deep ring is stretched, but the remainder of the posterior wall is normal, a simple operation to tighten the deep ring and resect the indirect hernia sac will suffice: a Marcy or Lytle operation is appropriate.
3. In cases where the posterior wall is deficient, there is a direct hernia, or the deep ring is dilated by a substantial indirect hernia in a young man or in an elderly man, a repair of the defect with reinforcement, by either the Bassini–Shouldice procedure or the Lichtenstein operation, is needed.
4. With recurrent hernias, especially with complex ones, an extraperitoneal mesh replacement, the Stoppa or Wantz operation, will be necessary.

Surgical techniques

There are three repair operations that are recommended for inguinal hernias. All of them involve surgical closure or occlusion of the defect through which the hernia has appeared.

Bassini–Shouldice operation

The Bassini–Shouldice operation (Fig. 6.5) involves carefully dividing and separating out the fascia transversalis and then closing it with an overlap using non-absorbable sutures. This technique has stood the test of time and has the lowest incidence of complications in a large series of patients [8].

Lichtenstein technique

A second and very acceptable method of treating hernias is to place the new mesh plastic reinforcement for the fascia transversalis anterior to the fascia transversalis — the Lichtenstein technique (Fig. 6.6) [9]. This is the 'tensionless' plastic repair and is currently the most popular operation, particularly in US and UK 'hernia centres' [10]. It can be readily carried out under local anaesthesia [11]. Excellent results of using this operation have been described by both specialist and generalist hernia surgeons.

Stoppa (French) operation

A third technique, the Stoppa (French) operation, is particularly suited to recurrent complicated groin hernias [11]. The extraperitoneal plane is opened up through either a midline or a Pfannenstiel incision, allowing bilateral hernias to be repaired simultaneously. In a modification to the procedure — the Wantz operation — a horizontal incision is made on one side of the abdomen just above the iliac spine (Fig. 6.7) [12]. The rectus muscle is retracted and the extraperitoneal plane exposed and developed. The peritoneal sacs of any hernia are milked back from the parietal openings and are then divided off and sutured flush with the peritoneum. Indirect and direct inguinal and femoral hernias can each be dealt with simultaneously.

A patch of polypropylene or Marlex mesh is the best prosthesis to use. For bilateral hernias, a double-chevron piece of mesh is used; for unilateral hernias, a single piece is cut appropriately. The important points are that the mesh must overlap the defect (i.e. the deep ring), the direct area (Hesselbach triangle) and the femoral ring by at least 2 cm in each direction. Furthermore, the mesh must extend down into the pelvis behind the superior ramus of the pubis and must

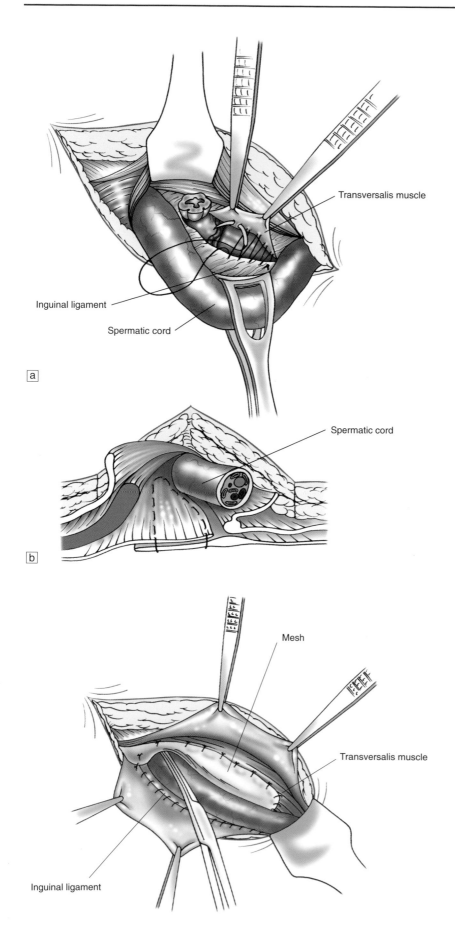

Transversalis muscle

Inguinal ligament

Spermatic cord

a

Figure 6.5. *The Bassini–Shouldice operation to repair the fascia transversalis. (a) Transversalis muscle is approximated to the inguinal ligament. (b) Care is taken not to constrict the spermatic cord.*

Spermatic cord

b

Mesh

Transversalis muscle

Inguinal ligament

Figure 6.6. *The Lichtenstein operation to patch the fascia transversalis by placing a prosthetic mesh anterior to the defect.*

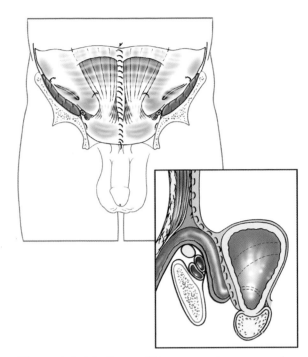

Figure 6.7. *The Stoppa–Wantz operation to strengthen the fascia transversalis from behind with a patch of prosthetic mesh.*

overlap and lie on the femoral vessels; thus, the mesh covers and overlaps all the myopectineal orifice of Fruchaud. It is advisable to mark out the optimum dimensions of the mesh with a skin pencil on the patient pre-operation as the incision distorts the anatomy. The mesh is cut to the previously defined dimensions and held in place by the pressure of the intact peritoneum from behind and by the sutured parietes in front.

Some fixation is, however, necessary, particularly to prevent mesh displacement when the retractors are removed during wound closure. It is usual, therefore, to suture (with a single suture at each site) the mesh to the pectineal ligament, the conjoint tendon at its medial attachment to the pubis, and the deep surface of the transversus muscle lateral to the deep ring. In reality, the mesh is held in place by anatomical forces, re-inforcing the fascia transversalis, like 'ham in the sandwich'. The extraperitoneal operation, which does not involve dissection of the inguinal canal and cord, has enormous advantages for repairing a recurrent groin hernia.

This procedure can now be conducted laparoscopically, which is relatively painless in the short term. However, this is still a new operation and the long-term results of it are unknown. Full-scale mesh replacement can be done on both sides simultaneously. If the operation is entirely extraperitoneal, any danger to abdominal organs is avoided and any risk of adhesion formation minimized. However, laparoscopic surgery takes time and does require a general anaesthetic; it also requires a skilled laparoscopic surgeon [13]!

Hospitalization or ambulatory care

Where and how the operation should be done is another key question to which patients want an answer. Should it be done on an ambulatory day-care basis or should the patient be admitted to hospital? For all three surgical techniques detailed above, ambulatory surgery is recommended. Provided that adequate reassurance is given to the patient that catastrophic complications such as bleeding will not occur, home care is the ideal. Adequate arrangements should be made to control pain in the postoperative period, and the patient should be sent home with optimum pain control. Ambulatory surgery under local or spinal anaesthesia is a way forward and a treatment of choice. However, many surgeons and many patients prefer general anaesthesia and, for this reason, admission to hospital for some hernia repairs still persists.

Complications

Complications of hernia operations are local bruising and haematoma formation, which is almost inevitable in some form in every hernia operation. Frank bruising (i.e. swelling in haematoma formation beneath the skin) should be rare with careful surgery. Infection at the wound site should be very rare with modern surgery. Avoidance of haematoma formation means avoidance of sepsis, as one usually leads to the other. Infection rates of under 1% are now recorded at good clinics.

The very rare complications of damage to the blood supply to the testicle should not occur with primary hernias and, certainly, in large series, rates of testicular blood supply compromise are well under 1%. Recurrence of hernias in primary hernia repairs should be under 1% with modern techniques. A more common complication of hernia operations is to miss a concomitant hernia elsewhere in the groin: a femoral hernia may be overlooked when repairing an indirect hernia. This is a common mistake for surgeons to make and all the hernia sites should be checked before operating. Very rare complications of open surgery are persistent pain due to local nerve trauma at operation.

Mortality with elective hernia operations is currently extremely rare. In elderly patients with strangulated hernias, co-morbidities, rather than the hernia itself, often lead to death. A co-morbidity of chronic obstructive airways disease, heart failure or pulmonary embolus may occur in the older patient and, unless the patient is managed appropriately, can cause death.

Conclusions

Overall, the objective in hernia management is to achieve a good outcome for the patient, who should be mobilized quickly, with little pain, and enabled to return to normal employment or work within a week. From the medical point of view, there should be no complications and no recurrence.

Finally, the outcome from the population point of view should be rapid return to gainful employment and a vast reduction on a national scale of the numbers of cases of hernia coming to strangulation — necessitating an urgent operation with a significant mortality. With good surgery, recurrent inguinal hernias should be banished to history.

References

1. Devlin HB, Kingsnorth AN. Management of abdominal hernias, 2nd edn. London: Chapman and Hall, 1997

2. Fruchaud H. L'Anatomie chirurgicale de la région de l'aine. Paris: C Dion & Co., 1956

3. Ryan EA. Hernias related to pelvic fractures. *Surg Gynecol Obstet* 1971; 133: 440–446

4. Russell RH. The saccular theory of hernia and the radical operation. *Lancet* 1906; 3: 1197–1203

5. Cannon DJ, Read RC. Metastatic emphysema. A mechanism for acquiring inguinal herniation. *Ann Surg* 1981; 194: 270–276

6. Peacock EE, Madden JW. Studies on the biology and treatment of recurrent inguinal hernia: II. Morphological changes. *Ann Surg* 1974; 179: 567–571

7. Gullmo A. Herniography. *World J Surg* 1989; 13: 560–568

8. Schumpelick V, Treutner KH, Arit G. Inguinal hernia repair in adults. *Lancet* 1994; 344: 375–379

9. Amid PK, Shulman AG, Lichtenstein IL. Critical suturing of the tension-free hernioplast. *Am J Surg* 1993; 165: 369–372

10. Kark AE, Kurzer M, Waters KJ. Tension-free mesh hernia repair: review of 1098 cases under local anaesthesia in a day unit. *Ann R Coll Surg Engl* 1995; 77: 299–304

11. Stoppa R, Warlaumont CR, Verhaeghe PJ *et al.* Comment, pourquoi, quand utiliser les prosthèses de tulle de Dacron pour trainer les hernies et les éventrations. *Chirurgie* 1982; 108: 570–575

12. Wantz GE. Atlas of hernia surgery. New York: Raven Press, 1991

13. O'Dwyer PJ. In: Devlin HB, Kingsnorth AN (eds) Management of abdominal hernias, 2nd edn. London: Chapman and Hall, 1997: 177–184

CHAPTER 7

Colorectal cancer

J. Northover

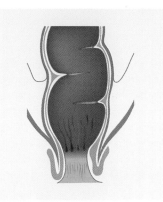

Introduction

Colorectal cancer is very common in Western countries, being the second most prevalent malignancy in men after lung cancer. In non-smoking males it is the major cause of cancer mortality. Globally, colorectal cancer is fourth in the league of cancers causing death [1]; in 1996, there were 510 000 colorectal cancer deaths worldwide, which represented 7.2% of all cancer deaths. In the UK, there are around 30 000 new cases annually, of whom nearly 20 000 are destined to die of the disease. In many Western countries, colorectal cancer is even more common; in many developing countries, the incidence and, hence, the importance as a public health issue, is increasing.

Pathogenesis

Understanding of the pathogenesis of colorectal cancer at the molecular level has increased over the past 10 years. Unlike the other common cancers, colorectal cancer usually passes through an orderly sequence — the adenoma–carcinoma sequence (ACS). Normal mucosa first becomes dysplastic, then small benign adenomas develop. These usually become raised, making them visible macroscopically [2]. A proportion of adenomas go on to become larger adenomas, while others may undergo malignant change, ultimately metastasizing to lymph nodes and distant sites [3]. Probably less than 1% of adenomas progress to malignancy [4].

More recently, a series of genetic alterations have been identified which are causally related to the macroscopic elements of the ACS [5]. These mostly occur at a somatic level as a result of damage due to environmental factors, but some relate to inherited mutations. In a small proportion of individuals, perhaps around 5%, dominantly inherited mutations induce a very high risk of colorectal cancer at an early age (Fig. 7.1) [6–8].

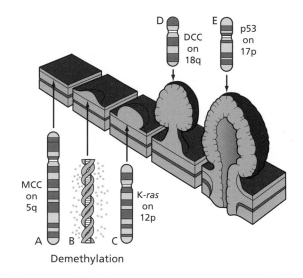

Figure 7.1. *The adenoma–carcinoma sequence and its associated genomic mutations — the 'Vogelgram'.*

Both the carcinoma and its precursor lesion, the adenoma, have a predilection for the distal third of the large bowel; 75% of colorectal neoplasms occur in this segment, with the caecum as the next most prevalent site, harbouring around 10% of tumours. In the latter part of the 20th century there has been a rightward shift in subsite distribution of this disease, which is more apparent in women than in men [9].

Predispositions: gender and race

The most comprehensive data on gender differences in colorectal cancer incidence and mortality are available from the USA. Data derived from the Surveillance, Epidemiology and End Results (SEER) Program indicate that there are significant differences in age-adjusted colorectal cancer mortality between men and women, and that Blacks are more frequently affected than

Whites (Table 7.1) [10]. The SEER data indicate that the incidence of colorectal cancer increased in male patients in the period 1950–1984, while falling slightly in female patients. From the mid-1980s there has been a steady decline in incidence in both sexes [11].

There are enormous variations in colorectal cancer incidence between countries: a 200-fold variation in rectal cancer incidence and sixfold variation in that of colon cancer exists in men (Figs. 7.2 and 7.3) [12]. Japanese men in Hawaii, the descendants of migrants, are twice as likely to develop rectal or colon cancer as their cousins in Japan. These classic observations were part of the evidence that environmental factors and, in particular, diet play a major part in the aetiology of colorectal cancer. Although worldwide, colon cancer affects the genders equally, in countries with the highest incidence (North America and Australia), and those with a rapidly increasing incidence (Japan and Italy), there is an age-adjusted 20% excess in males; this difference is less marked in the UK. The greatest male–female difference is seen in Hawaiian Polynesians (28 and 14 cases per 100 000, respectively) [13]. In general, there is a tendency for colon cancer to be more common in women than in men below the age of 50, but more common in men after that age [14].

Aetiology

Diet

The most consistent dietary observation is that vegetable consumption is inversely proportional to colorectal cancer risk [15]. High fibre intake appears to be similarly protective, although

Table 7.1. *Age-adjusted mortality and incidence rates per 100 000 population for colorectal cancer: Whites and Blacks, men (M) and women (F), USA, 1985–1989 [10]*

	Whites		Blacks	
	M	**F**	**M**	**F**
Mortality	24.2	16.4	27.6	20.8
Incidence	61.0	42.1	60.5	46.4

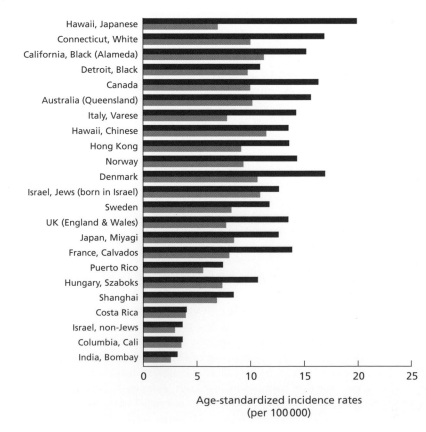

Figure 7.2. *Incidence of rectal cancer by gender (■ male; ■ female) and geographical location, 1992 [12].*

Age-standardized incidence rates (per 100 000)

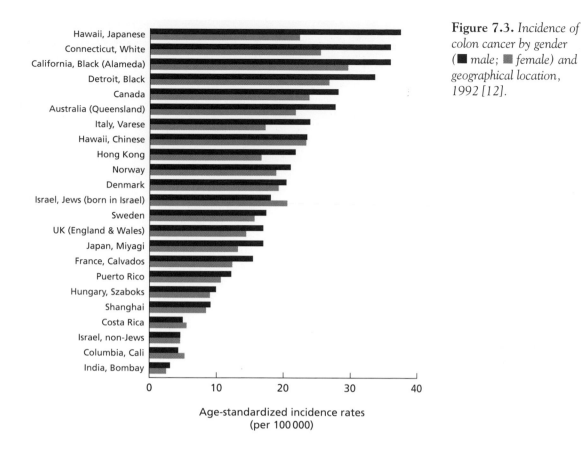

Figure 7.3. *Incidence of colon cancer by gender (■ male; ■ female) and geographical location, 1992 [12].*

Age-standardized incidence rates
(per 100 000)

cereal intake appears proportionately related to cancer risk in Italy and Japan [14]. Data on the protective effects of fruit are more limited and inconsistent [1]. Animal protein consumption is generally associated with colorectal cancer risk, although fish and seafood consumption may be inversely related [15]. The specific mechanisms whereby animal fat predisposes to colorectal cancer are unclear; however, the presence of fat, as well as processing and cooking methods, may be factors [1]. Heavily browned meat, with a consequent excess of mutagenic heterocyclic amines, may be an important meat-related factor [16].

Evidence on calcium and vitamin D intake has been conflicting. The intake of various micronutrients, such as selenium and the carotenoids, has been said to be protective, but the current evidence is not conclusive [14].

Physical activity

It has become apparent in both sexes that physical inactivity is associated with increased colon cancer risk [17]. Lifetime patterns are probably more important than the effect of a relatively recent change in lifestyle. The association with rectal cancer, although not as well studied, is less apparent.

Occupation

Certain occupations may expose workers to specific substances that produce an increased risk for colorectal cancer. Asbestos, with a twofold colon cancer risk excess, is the best documented; pesticide and herbicide exposure may also carry some risk [14]. Painters; printers; railwaymen; and wood, metal and car workers, have all been shown to be at increased risk for colorectal cancer [14].

Smoking

Cigarette smoking has not been implicated in colon cancer, whereas cigar and pipe smoking have been shown to be more common in case–control studies [14].

Alcohol

Of 19 population studies, the slight majority have shown a positive correlation between colon cancer risk and alcohol intake [14]. Beer consumption appears to be more positively correlated with rectal cancer in men than in women. It is likely that the association is related to total ethanol intake rather than to the type of drink [1].

Caffeine

The few studies in this area have produced conflicting data [14]. Taken together, evidence suggests that coffee may decrease colorectal cancer risk [1].

Clinical presentation

Symptoms

Colorectal cancer often presents with symptoms at a late stage in the evolution of the disease: in some series, as many as 50% of cases were manifestly beyond cure by the time that symptoms compelled sufferers to seek help. In part, this is due to the lack of symptoms until an advanced disease stage; however, it is also due to a delay in presentation after symptom onset. The symptoms of colorectal cancer may be mistaken for those of more minor conditions, such as haemorrhoids or irritable bowel syndrome, leading to further delay [18,19]. The commonest symptoms are listed below. Any of these symptoms should lead the patient, particularly the middle-aged and elderly, to seek medical advice.

Change of bowel habit

Change of bowel habit may be a minor change in frequency or timing of defaecation, or an unexplained change in the consistency of the stool. Moreover, there is often variation and irregularity in both the frequency and consistency of the stool. This symptom has been shown to be the best diagnostic discriminator in a recent case–control study [20].

Bleeding

Blood may be seen to be mixed with the motion. Various shades of colour of the blood may be seen: it is often plum-coloured if the tumour is proximal or bright red if in the rectum, but no shade is site specific. In people at and beyond middle age, rectal bleeding has a positive predictive value for cancer of at least 10% [21,22].

Mucous discharge

Mucous discharge may be a prominent feature, particularly in distal tumours, often stained by stool or blood.

Tenesmus

A rectal tumour can give a sensation of incomplete evacuation, as the 'malignant stool' remains firmly attached to the rectal wall.

Anaemia

Classically, anaemia may be the only feature of right-sided colonic tumours. Colorectal cancer is an important differential diagnosis of anaemia of unknown origin, especially after the age of 55.

Acute complications

Around 30% of all bowel tumours present as emergencies with obstruction or peritonitis [23–25].

Signs

General signs of anaemia and/or weight loss should be sought. Abdominal examination may reveal a mass, particularly in the presence of a large sigmoid or caecal tumour. The liver may be enlarged, owing to metastasis. As the predominant anatomical site of colorectal cancer is the distal segment, digital examination should always be a part of the examination of a patient presenting with any of the above symptoms. Rectal tumours up to 10 cm from the anus may be palpable as a firm, sometimes ulcerated, mass arising from the rectal wall. Even if the tumour is not palpable, blood or mucus on the glove may provide a clue. Rigid sigmoidoscopy is a routine part of the outpatient examination, permitting the distal 25 cm to be examined.

Investigations

The decision whether symptoms and signs require investigation may be difficult for the general practitioner. In general terms, if the clinical picture requires investigation, the whole length of the rectum and colon needs examination, although the surgeon to whom the patient is referred may feel that this can be avoided in some cases after sigmoidoscopic examination. The two major methods of investigation in cases of suspected colorectal cancer are endoscopy and radiology.

Endoscopy

Colonoscopy has become more widely used: it allows biopsy of any lesion identified and is more sensitive than contrast radiology in the detection of small cancers and adenomas, particularly in the sigmoid colon, where convolution and the presence of diverticular disease can make radiological interpretation difficult [26]. A small proportion of cancers are identified as malignant polyps on endoscopy and may be treated definitively by endoscopic polypectomy (Fig. 7.4). Colonoscopy carries a small but definite morbidity and mortality risk [26].

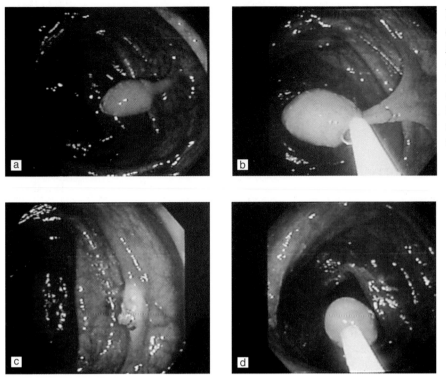

Figure 7.4. *Colon polyp at endoscopy: (a) stalked polyp; (b) snare placed around stalk; (c) diathermied stalk base after polyp excision; (d) excised polyp held in snare for transanal retrieval.*

Radiology

Double-contrast barium enema is still the commonest method of diagnosis of colon cancer in the UK (Fig. 7.5). Despite the shortcomings compared with endoscopy mentioned above, it has the advantage of sometimes being more precise in identifying the exact anatomical site of a tumour.

Preoperative staging

As planning of treatment becomes more complex, preoperative staging investigations to define the anatomy of the primary tumour and any locoregional or distant spread become more important. This process facilitates decisions, not only on the type of surgery to perform but also on the various preoperative adjuvant therapies.

The tumour can be scanned using whole body methods, such as computed tomography (CT) and magnetic resonance imaging (MRI), or more localized procedures, such as liver ultrasound (US) and intrarectal US or MRI [27]. Using intrarectal US, rectal tumours can be examined to provide reliable evidence regarding degree of spread through the rectal wall and possible involvement of contiguous organs (Fig. 7.6) [28].

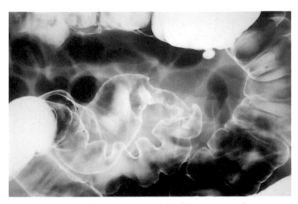

Figure 7.5. *Colon cancer on double-contrast barium enema. Irregular 'apple core' stricture due to carcinoma of sigmoid colon.*

Surgical treatment

Rectal cancer

There are three main categories of potentially curative surgery for rectal cancer:
1. Anterior resection: radical removal of the involved segment of bowel with subsequent anastomosis;
2. Abdominoperineal excision: the Miles' operation;
3. Transanal local excision: 'simple' removal via the anus of the disc of rectal wall harbouring the tumour.

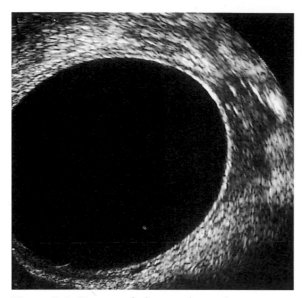

Figure 7.6. *Transrectal ultrasound scan showing locally advanced rectal cancer. The normal rectal wall comprises five layers, three white and two black, clearly seen for most of the circumference; on the right an irregular dark tumour mass can be seen penetrating all layers of the bowel wall.*

The choice of operation depends to a variable degree on a series of factors, including:

1. The size, site and apparent degree of advancement of the tumour;
2. The patient's general condition, age and physical stature;
3. The patient's and surgeon's preferences.

In some cases, the choice is obvious. With a high-sited, small tumour in a fit man, treatment is usually by anterior resection, whereas the very low, bulky, aggressive tumour, particularly in the unfit or obese man, is suited to the Miles' procedure. A small proportion (around 5%) of small, early tumours close to the anus may be suitable for transanal local excision. In many cases, however, the choice of procedure is less clear-cut, and is more likely to depend on the surgeon's experience and inclinations.

Complications of rectal surgery

Perhaps more than any other type of non-genital cancer surgery, that for rectal cancer harbours significant risk for sexual function in men. The nerve supply to the organs of sexual function and of the bladder lies in close proximity to the planes of surgical dissection. These comprise the sympathetic nerves in the hypogastric plexus and the sacral parasympathetic supply in the nervi erigentes (Fig. 7.7) [29]. Damage to the former may result in disorders of bladder emptying, while the latter are responsible for penile erection and ejaculation. Until relatively recently, many surgeons were fatalistic about nerve damage during such surgical procedures. Rectal cancer surgery was seen as carrying an almost inevitable risk of urinary problems and erectile dysfunction; rates of up to 50% have been reported. In recent times, as the anatomy of the nerves has become better understood and as the pattern of dissection and the methods of achieving it have been refined, the risk has fallen dramatically. Unless the nerves are actually invaded by the tumour, or the anatomy of the patient is such as to make visualization of the area at risk very difficult, it is usually possible to avoid these complications.

Nerve damage may be partial or complete, in terms of both the anatomy of the injury and the extent of functional deficit. If injury does occur, it is unlikely to recover completely. Methods of dealing with partial or complete erectile dysfunction are beyond the scope of this chapter, and are dealt with elsewhere in this book (see Ch. 12).

Colon cancer

In principle, the operations for tumours in different parts of the colon are similar: the affected segment and its lymphatic drainage are isolated by an appropriate dissection and then removed; subsequently, the two bowel ends are joined, usually using a hand-sutured technique.

Postoperative follow-up

It has become a convention that colorectal cancer patients are followed for 5 years after surgery. A majority of surgeons aim to see their patients 3-monthly for the first 2 years, 6-monthly thereafter until 5 years after surgery, then discharging the patient from further surveillance. This is based on two tenets: that the majority of the risk of recurrence has dissipated by the end of 2 years, and that the survival becomes parallel with the general population curve (and hence the risk of recurrence has gone) at 5 years.

The process of follow-up after cancer surgery has several aims [30], including the identification of postoperative complications, the provision of patient reassurance, audit of the surgeon's performance, detection of metachronous tumours and detection of recurrent cancer. Criticism of

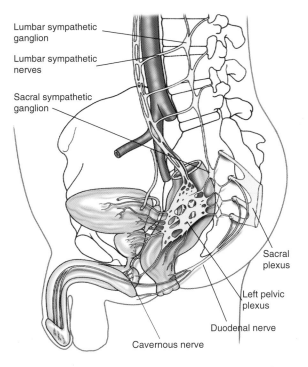

Lumbar sympathetic ganglion

Lumbar sympathetic nerves

Sacral sympathetic ganglion

Sacral plexus

Left pelvic plexus

Duodenal nerve

Cavernous nerve

Figure 7.7. *Anatomy of the pelvic autonomic supply.*

these objectives is based on the following observations: most postoperative complications, except perhaps incisional hernia, become manifest within the first year; many patients are alarmed rather than reassured by an impending outpatient follow-up visit; few surgeons make proper use of follow-up data to review, criticize and alter their cancer management strategies; in addition, only around 5% of colorectal cancer patients develop metachronous cancer. Consequently, detection of recurrent cancer should be the main reason for follow-up in most cases.

Reflecting the high cost and low evidence base for effectiveness of colorectal cancer follow-up, the UK Government's National Health Service Executive recently published recommendations that reflect appropriately the difficult and evolving balance between the advantages of postoperative vigilance and the costs (financial, emotional and physical) of surveillance and consequent interventions [31]. The follow-up procedures that are conducted are described below.

Clinical assessment

Clinical assessment is likely to be offered according to the schedule stated earlier. It includes questioning regarding symptoms, general physical examination and, particularly after rectal cancer surgery, rigid sigmoidoscopic examination.

Colonoscopy

Colonoscopy should have been performed perioperatively to exclude a synchronous second primary cancer and/or associated adenomata. Depending on the presence of associated neoplasia, the age of the patient and the enthusiasm of the clinician, repeated colonoscopy may be offered every 1–5 years in perpetuity after primary treatment.

Scanning procedures

As the liver is the most frequently affected distant site for metastasis, examination may be performed using US, CT or MRI, particularly in the first 2–3 years after surgery. The possibility of cure by resection of localized liver recurrence is quite high (in the region of 30%) [32–35], but whether presymptomatic diagnosis by regular scanning increases the proportion thus cured remains another area for debate in the controversy surrounding follow-up practice.

Serum marker assay

Although frequent blood sampling for carcinoembryonic antigen is widely practised, particularly in the USA, yet again there is no evidence of its value; indeed, preliminary data from the only randomized trial in this area strongly indicate no survival benefit [36].

Adjuvant therapy

Overall, surgery alone is curative in around 60% of those colorectal cancer cases in which a radical operation is performed. Although improvements in outcome may be possible through improvements in surgical technique, most effort to increase the cure rate has gone into adjuvant therapy — the addition of radiotherapy, chemotherapy or immunotherapy to surgery, either before, during or after the operation. Today there can be no doubt that at least some forms of adjuvant therapy can improve the outlook in this disease, although which patients are most likely to benefit and which modes or regimens of treatment should be used remain the focus of debate and widespread clinical research. Radiotherapy is essentially a locoregional modality, aimed mainly at reducing the risk of local cancer recurrence in rectal cancer cases, whereas chemotherapy is seen as a means of improving the chance of survival through its systemic effect.

Radiotherapy

Radiotherapy is used mainly in the management of rectal cancer. It may be delivered pre- or post-operatively; in a few centres, it can be delivered to the precise site at risk of recurrence with the abdomen open at operation. Given preoperatively, radiotherapy has been shown in randomized trials to downstage the disease [37,38]. Regimens range from high-dose therapy (4000–5000 cGy total dose, delivered over a 4–5-week period, followed by a 6-week rest prior to surgery) to low-dose, rapid courses (1000–2500 cGy in the week immediately prior to surgery) [39]. The major disadvantages of preoperative therapy include the delay in performing surgery and the blanket delivery of therapy to all cases in the absence of pathological staging information; its advantages include a lesser likelihood of radiation morbidity — in particular, of damage to the small intestine.

Postoperative radiotherapy can be used more selectively, owing to the availability of pathological staging information; surgical delays are also avoided. The major disadvantage of postoperative therapy is small bowel radiation damage, made more likely by operation-induced adhesions that cause the small bowel to be held inevitably in the field of treatment. This leads to significant morbidity, and occasional mortality, in around 5% of cases.

There are no widely accepted guidelines for the use of adjuvant radiotherapy in rectal cancer. Most surgeons would accept that, in cases of locally advanced rectal cancer in which the feasibility of surgical clearance appears marginal, preoperative radiotherapy is advisable. Many surgeons, particularly those whose local recurrence rate is favourably low, prefer to reserve adjuvant radiotherapy for those patients in whom pathological examination of the surgical specimen suggests a particular risk of recurrence; this group therefore favour a selective policy of postoperative therapy. Recent trials in Sweden have yielded persuasive evidence for the uniform use of short-course preoperative therapy, having demonstrated a decrease in local recurrence at all pathological stages, even the earliest [39].

Chemotherapy

Adjuvant chemotherapy for colon and rectal cancer has been investigated for more than 40 years, and has involved mainly the use of 5-fluorouracil (5-FU), either alone or in combination with other drugs. Until 10 years ago, the results were uniformly quite disappointing; however, since the late 1980s, a series of trials has shown promise, leading to much wider use of adjuvant chemotherapy. Opinions differ on its role in various clinical situations, but the evidence for its efficacy is sufficient for it to be seen as uniformly relevant therapy in the majority of cases, particularly by oncologists in the USA.

Much was made in the late 1980s and early 1990s of a regimen comprising 5-FU combined with the immunostimulatory agent levamisole. Data published almost 10 years ago were sufficiently persuasive that it was considered standard therapy in the USA for Dukes' C cases of colon cancer [40]. Evidence now suggests that levamisole plays no part in chemotherapy for this disease [41]. Other drug combinations, particularly 5-FU with folinic acid, may be more efficacious than 5-FU/levamisole, and trials of this combination continue in many countries [42].

In rectal cancer, chemotherapy may be used alone or in combination with radiotherapy. Again, trials in the early 1990s led to advice in the USA for the uniform use of combination therapy, at least in Dukes' C tumours [43]; again, many European commentators have not found the evidence sufficiently persuasive. Data from the Mayo Clinic indicate that side effects of adjuvant chemotherapy/radiotherapy in rectal cancer outweigh the benefits.

Prognosis

The main staging system for colorectal cancer is Dukes' classification. This is based on the depth of invasion by the primary tumour, lymph node involvement and tumour differentiation. Dukes' classification and its prognostic significance are shown in Table 7.2. As prognostic indicators, the classical Dukes' system and its various modifications leave much to be desired.

Prevention

Diet

A large proportion of colorectal cancer risk appears to be associated with dietary and other environmental/lifestyle factors. Consequently, a corresponding proportion of cases ought to be preventable by suitable alterations in diet and lifestyle. In order to provide evidence upon which to base dietary advice, various randomized controlled trials (RCTs) have been, or are being, performed. Because of the relative rarity of colorectal cancer in the general population (preva-

Table 7.2. *Dukes' classification system*

Dukes' classification	Criteria	Cases (%)	5-year survival (%)
A	▪ Confined to bowel wall	10	90
	▪ Lymph nodes clear		
B	▪ Penetrates bowel wall	45	60
	▪ Lymph nodes clear		
C	▪ Lymph nodes involved	45	30

lence around 1:500 at any one time), and despite its prominence in the league table of killing cancers, RCTs using cancer incidence or mortality as the endpoint are practically non-viable. Instead, adenoma incidence or recurrence have been generally used as measures of effect. The Women's Health Initiative in the USA, involving 63 000 randomized persons, is the largest study on lifestyle indicators using cancer itself as the measured endpoint [44]. Evidence should become available within the next decade upon which to develop dietary preventative advice, applicable to men as well as to women!

Screening

For screening to be considered worthwhile as a public health measure used as part of the overall strategy for coping with a particular condition, several criteria must be met. First, the condition must be sufficiently common, with the potential for earlier intervention to alter the outcome favourably. Second, the test must be safe, cheap and acceptable to the target population, easy to apply and sufficiently sensitive and specific. Third, there must be an infrastructure capable of coping with the management of all those found to have positive screen test results. The first two of these criteria have been broadly fulfilled in colorectal cancer, although a clear view of the effect on the incidence and mortality has required the performance of large RCTs. In a number of countries, including the UK, endoscopy and radiological services currently available would not be able to cope with the load generated by nationwide screening. Only in Germany has there been a national policy of bowel cancer screening (despite a deficient evidence base and poor population compliance, particularly among men). As data from RCTs have become available in the past few years, other countries are contemplating the issue seriously.

Two main approaches to screening have been investigated:

1. Tests looking for tumour products in the stool, principally occult blood [45] and, more recently, mutated genes in shed cancer cells [46];
2. Direct examination of the bowel mucosa using endoscopes, particularly the flexible sigmoidoscope but also the colonoscope.

High-risk groups
Certain groups are at increased risk for colorectal cancer, primarily those with an inheritable predisposition and those with long-standing inflammatory bowel disease.

Inherited predisposition
There are two principal dominantly inheritable conditions predisposing to colorectal cancer: these are familial adenomatous polyposis (FAP) and hereditary non-polyposis colorectal cancer (HNPCC) syndrome. Both are rare, accounting for no more than 5% of all colorectal cancers between them, and neither condition is gender linked, nor is there evidence of significant geographical variation.

FAP is characterized by the development in the teenage years of large numbers of adenomas on the colorectal mucosa, some of which progress to malignancy by 40 years of age if left untreated [47]. Associated lesions in affected individuals include duodenal adenomas, desmoid tumours (mainly affecting the abdomen) and various incidental abnormalities, such as benign osteomas, skin cysts and retinal pigmentation. FAP is caused by mutations in a gene located on the long arm of chromosome 5 [48]. Cancer preventative measures involve the removal of the bulk of the large intestine in affected individuals in their mid to late teens [47].

HNPCC produces a less obvious clinical picture in affected individuals: there is no carpet of adenomas to betray the diagnosis. There is, however, a predilection for right-sided tumours, occurring at a younger average age, and more frequently with multiple primary tumours [49]. The condition is caused by mutations in the mismatch repair genes which 'police' the process of cell division, usually identifying and rectifying chance mutations in the genome [8,50]. The resulting inefficiency in the process leads to the accumulation of the somatic mutations that underlie the ACS. In families harbouring this condition, regular colonoscopic surveillance is offered in order to identify and remove any adenomas before they progress to frank malignancy.

Certain families harbour an inheritable risk, but do not possess the currently understood predisposing mutations. If a family pedigree gives rise to sufficient suspicion of a predisposition, even in the absence of an identified genetic explanation, colonoscopic surveillance should be offered.

Inflammatory bowel disease

Colorectal cancer occurs more frequently in patients with ulcerative colitis (UC) or Crohn's disease than in the general population. The cancer risk is small in Crohn's patients, and in those with anatomically limited or recent-onset UC. In those with UC of 10 years' duration or more, and in whom the disease affects the majority of the large bowel, cancer risk rises sharply. In those with extensive colitis of more than 20 years' duration, the cancer risk exceeds 20%. Cancer is usually preceded by the development of dysplastic mucosal lesions; regular (1–2-yearly) colonoscopy to try to identify these premalignant lesions may lead to effective preventive surgical treatment, but debate continues over the efficacy of such surveillance programmes [51,52].

References

1. Potter J. Colon, rectum. In: Potter J (ed) Food, nutrition and the prevention of cancer: a global perspective. Washington: American Institute for Cancer Research, 1997
2. Muto T, Bussey H, Morson B. The evolution of cancer of the colon and rectum. *Cancer* 1975; 36: 2251–2270
3. Gutman M, Fidler I. Biology of human colon cancer metastasis. *World J Surg* 1995; 19: 226–234
4. Hamilton S. Pathology and biology of colorectal neoplasia. In: Young GP, Rozen P, Levin B (eds) Prevention and early diagnosis of colorectal cancer. London: Saunders, 1996: 3–21
5. Fearon E, Vogelstein B. A genetic model for colorectal tumorigenesis. *Cell* 1990; 61: 759–767
6. Bodmer W, Bailey C, Bodmer J et al. Localization of the gene for familial adenomatous polyposis on chromosome 5. *Nature* 1987; 328: 614–616
7. Fishel R, Lescoe M, Rao M. The human mutator gene homologue MSH2 and its association with hereditary nonpolyposis colon cancer. *Cell* 1993; 75: 1027–1038
8. Bronner C, Baker S, Morrison P. Mutation in the DNA mismatch repair gene homologue hMLH1 is associated with hereditary non-polyposis colon cancer. *Nature* 1994; 368: 258–261
9. Butcher D, Hassanein K, Dudgeon M et al. Female gender is a major determinant of changing subsite distribution of colorectal cancer with age. *Cancer* 1985; 56: 714–716
10. Schottenfeld D. Epidemiology. In: Cohen A, Winawer S (eds). Cancer of the colon, rectum and anus. New York: McGraw-Hill, 1995: 11–24
11. Chu K, Tarone R, Chow W et al. Temporal patterns in colorectal cancer incidence, survival and mortality from 1950 through 1990. *J Natl Cancer Inst* 1994; 86: 997–1006
12. Parkin D, Muir C, Whelan S et al. Cancer in five continents. Vol. VI. Lyon: International Agency for Research on Cancer, 1992
13. Parkin D, Muir C, Whelan S. Cancer incidence in five continents. Vol V. Lyon: International Agency for Research on Cancer, 1987
14. Potter J. Epidemiologic, environmental and lifestyle issues in colorectal cancer. In: Young, Rozen, Levin (eds) Prevention and early detection of colorectal cancer. London: WB Saunders, 1996: 23–43
15. Potter J, Slattery M, Bostick R, Gapstur S. Colon cancer: a review of the epidemiology. *Epidemiol Rev* 1993; 15: 499–545
16. Gerhardsson-de-Verdier M, Hagman U, Peters R. Meat, cooking methods and colorectal cancer: a case-referent study in Stockholm. *Int J Cancer* 1991; 49: 520–525
17. Slattery M, Abd-Elghany N, Kerber R, Schumacher M. Physical activity and colon cancer: a comparison of various indicators of physical activity to evaluate the association. *Epidemiology* 1990; 1: 481–485
18. Holliday H, Hardcastle J. Delay in diagnosis and treatment of symptomatic colorectal cancer. *Lancet* 1979; 1: 309–311
19. Crosland A, Jones R. Rectal bleeding: prevalence and consultation behaviour. *Br Med J* 1995; 311: 486–488
20. Curless R, French J, Williams G, James O. Comparison of gastrointestinal symptoms in colorectal carcinoma patients and community controls with respect to age. *Gut* 1994; 35: 1267–1270
21. Goulston K, Dent O. How important is rectal bleeding in the diagnosis of bowel cancer or polyps? *Lancet* 1986; 2: 261–265

22. Fitjen G, Starmans R, Muris J *et al*. Predictive value of signs and symptoms for colorectal cancer in patients with rectal bleeding in general practice. *Fam Pract* 1995; 12: 279–286

23. Goulston K. Role of diet in screening with fecal occult blood tests. In: Winawer SJ, Schottenfeld D, Sherlock P (eds) Colorectal cancer: prevention, epidemiology, and screening. New York: Raven Press, 1980: 271–274

24. Chester J, Britton D. Elective and emergency surgery for colorectal cancer in a district general hospital: impact of surgical training on patient survival. *Ann R Coll Surg Engl* 1989; 71: 370–374

25. Waldron R, Donovan I, Drumm J *et al*. Emergency presentation and mortality from colorectal cancer in the elderly. *Br J Surg* 1986; 73: 216

26. Winawer S, Fletcher R, Miller L *et al*. Colorectal cancer screening: clinical guidelines and rationale. *Gastroenterology* 1997; 112: 594–642

27. Malone D, McGrath F. Optimising the detection of colorectal liver metastases within the Canadian health care system. *Can Assoc Radiol J* 1993; 44: 5–13

28. Hildebrandt U, Feifel G. Preoperative staging of rectal cancer by intrarectal ultrasound. *Dis Colon Rectum* 1995; 28: 42–46

29. Scholefield J, Northover J. Surgical management of rectal cancer. *Br J Surg* 1995; 82: 745–748

30. Cochrane J, Williams JT, Faber R. Value of outpatient follow-up after curative surgery for carcinoma of the large bowel. *Br Med J* 1980; 280: 593–595

31. NHS Executive. Clinical guidelines: using clinical guidelines to improve patient care in the NHS. London: NHS Executive, 1997

32. Bradpiece H, Benjamin I, Halevy A, Blumgart L. Major hepatic resection for colorectal liver metastases. *Br J Surg* 1987;74:324–326

33. Fegiz G, Bezzi M, De Angelis R *et al*. Surgical treatment of liver metastases from colorectal cancer. *Ital J Surg Sci* 1985; 15: 259–265

34. Hughes KS, Rosenstein RB, Songhorabodi S *et al*. Resection of the liver for colorectal carcinoma metastases. A multi-institutional study of long-term survivors. *Dis Colon Rectum* 1988; 31: 1–4

35. Wexler M, Olak J. Resection of the liver for metastatic disease. *Can J Surg* 1987; 30: 229

36. Northover J. The use of prognostic markers in surgery for colorectal cancer. *Eur J Cancer* 1995; 31: 1207–1209

37. Medical Research Council Rectal Cancer Working Party. Randomised trial of surgery alone versus radiotherapy followed by surgery for potentially operable locally advanced rectal cancer. *Lancet* 1996; 348: 1605–1610

38. Graf W, Dahlberg M, Ohlberg M *et al*. Short term preoperative radiotherapy results in down staging of rectal cancer: a study of 1316 patients. *Radiother Oncol* 1997; 43: 133–137

39. Swedish Rectal Cancer Group. Improved survival with preoperative radiotherapy in rectal cancer. *New Engl J Med* 1997; 336: 980–987

40. Moertel C, Fleming T, McDonald J. Fluorouracil plus levamisole as effective adjuvant therapy after resection of stage III colon carcinoma: a final report. *Ann Intern Med* 1995; 122: 321–326

41. Haller D, Catalano P, McDonald J. Fluorouracil (FU), leucovorin (LV) and levamisole (LEV) adjuvant therapy in colon cancer: preliminary results of INT-0089. *Proc Am Soc Clin Oncol* 1996; 15: A486

42. International-Multicentre-Pooled-Analysis-of-Colon-Cancer-Trials-(IMPACT)-Investigators. Efficacy of adjuvant fluorouracil and folinic acid in colon cancer. *Lancet* 1995; 345: 939–944

43. Krook J, Moertel C, Gunderson L *et al*. Effective adjuvant therapy for high-risk rectal carcinoma. *New Engl J Med* 1991; 324: 709–715

44. Roussouw J, Finnegan L, Harlan W. The evolution of the Women's Health Initiative: a perspective from the NIH. *J Am Med Wom Assoc* 1995; 50: 50–55

45. Greegor D. Occult blood testing for detection of asymptomatic colon cancer. *Cancer* 1971; 28: 131–133

46. Sidransky D, Tokino T, Hamilton S. Identification of ras oncogene mutations in the stool of patients with curable colorectal tumors. *Science* 1992; 256: 102–105

47. Bussey H. Familial polyposis coli. Family studies, histopathology, differential diagnosis, and results of treatment. Baltimore: The Johns Hopkins University Press, 1975

48. Leppert M, Dobbs M, Scambler P *et al*. The gene for familial polyposis coli maps to the long arm of chromosome 5. *Science* 1987; 238: 1411–1413

49. Lynch H, Kimberling W, Albano W *et al*. Hereditary nonpolyposis colorectal cancer (Lynch syndromes I and II). I. Clinical description of resource. *Cancer* 1985; 56: 934–938

50. Parsons R, Li G-M, Rao M. Hypermutability and mismatch repair deficiency in RER+ tumor cells. *Cell* 1993; 75: 1227

51. Hodgson SV, Bishop DT, Dunlop MG *et al*. Suggested screening guidelines for familial colorectal cancer. *J Med Screen* 1995; 2: 45–51

52. Lennard-Jones J, Morson B, Ritchie J, Williams C. Cancer surveillance in ulcerative colitis. Experience over 15 years. *Lancet* 1983; ii: 149–152

CHAPTER 8

Tobacco smoking, cancer and premature death in men

P. Boyle

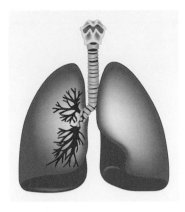

Introduction

The 20th century saw the greatest increase in life expectancy among the human population in such a short period of time. Increasing control of infection, improvements in surgical and anaesthetic techniques, the implementation of high sanitary standards and improving social circumstances have seen life expectancy soar around the world, particularly in the most developed countries. However, one downside has been the emergence of a group of chronic diseases that have come to be seen as the scourge of mankind — namely, cancer and cardiovascular disease. The real tragedy is that a large proportion of cases of cancer and cardiovascular disease have been caused by identifiable lifestyle factors, most notably tobacco smoking. Deaths caused by tobacco-related diseases are in large part premature and should be looked upon as avoidable.

Adverse effects associated with tobacco smoking

The first comment on tobacco smoking as a cause of cancer has been attributed to Samuel Thomas Sommering (1795), who wrote:

'Thus, carcinoma of the lip is most frequent where people indulge in (the use of) tobacco pipes. For the lower lip is particularly attacked by carcinoma, because it is compressed between the pipe and the teeth.' [1]

The association between tobacco smoking and the development of lung cancer appears to have been suggested in the UK in 1927 [2]. The rapid escalation in lung cancer incidence, which took place during the 1940s, reached a level that permitted a number of large studies to be con-

ducted. Between 1942 and 1944 at the Veterans Admini-stration Hospital in Illinois, 5003 male patients were interviewed with particular regard to their smoking habits [3]. Included in the group were 73 men with lung cancer and 69 with cancer of the larynx or pharynx, those with cancer at other sites acting as controls. A higher proportion of cigarette smokers was found among patients with cancers located in the lung and larynx. The authors concluded that there was a statistically and biologically significant association between the occurrence of cigarette smoking and cancer of the respiratory tract.

In Roswell Park Memorial Institute in Buffalo a scheme was introduced in 1938 whereby all patients were interviewed on admission regarding previous and present habits of smoking prior to diagnosis. This resource was to prove of great value in investigating the aetiology of many cancer sites during the 1950s and 1960s. Using this resource, a study was conducted comprising 263 patients with lung cancer and 605 patients without cancer (controls) [4]. This study revealed a prevalence rate of lung cancer of 8.6% among non-smokers compared with 20.9% for cigarette smokers. The authors concluded that, in their hospital population, cancer of the lung occurred more than twice as frequently among those who had smoked cigarettes for 25 years as among non-smokers of comparable age. This suggested, but did not establish, a causal relationship between the two.

Using only 'proved' cases of bronchogenic carcinoma, another 1950 study [5] conducted interviews in over 600 cases (605 male, 25 female). Smoking habits were classified into six categories (Table 8.1). Non-medically qualified investigators interviewed 780 unselected male patients and 552 women patients without lung cancer as controls. For those patients who had smoked for less than 20 years, the quantity of tobacco was adjusted to a 20-year period: a man who smoked 20 cigarettes a

Table 8.1. *Categorization of smokers in a 1950s lung cancer study [5]*

Group	Category
0	Non-smokers (< 1 cigarette*/day for > 20 years)
1	Light smokers (1–9 cigarettes/day for > 20 years)
2	Moderately heavy smokers (10–15 cigarettes/day for > 20 years)
3	Heavy smokers (16–20 cigarettes/day for > 20 years)
4	Excessive smokers (21–34 cigarettes/day for > 20 years)
5	Chain smokers (35+ cigarettes/day for > 20 years)

*1 cigar = 5 cigarettes; 1 pipeful = 2.5 cigarettes.

day for only 10 years was classified as smoking 10 cigarettes daily. Of the 605 men with lung cancer, 96.1% had smoked for 20 years or more and 50.2% for 40 years or more. Statistical analysis allowed the rejection of the null hypothesis that smoking has no effect on the induction of cancer of the lung. The data presented by Wynder and Graham [5] are capable of transformation to calculate the relative risks. Setting the risk among non-smokers to be 1.0, there is, to some extent or other, a dose–response relationship with increasing levels of smoking in all age groups. In the 30–39-year age group there were only moderate increases in risk with heavier smoking; the increase was much greater among the other groups (40–49, 50–59 and 60–69 years).

Another important epidemiological study was conducted between April 1948 and February 1952, involving 3446 patients with cancer of the lung, stomach or large bowel [6,7]. It was found that patients with cancer of the stomach and bowel gave smoking histories similar to those of non-cancer patients. It was then decided to expand the control group to include cancer at sites other than lip, tongue, mouth, pharynx, larynx, oesophagus and inside the chest. By the end of the study, 1488 patients with lung cancer (bronchial carcinoma, pleural endothelioma and alveolar cell carcinoma of the lung) had been interviewed, but 23 cases lacked controls. Results relate to 1465 cases and 1465 controls.

The strongest difference between cases and controls (for both men and women) was found to be the average amount smoked daily over the 10 years preceding the patient's illness. Qualitatively similar results were also obtained using the amount smoked immediately before the patient's illness;

the maximum amount ever smoked regularly; the total amount smoked since smoking began; and the average amount smoked daily over the 10 years preceding the patient's illness, over the penultimate 10 years and over the whole of the patient's life since the age of 15 (even after allowance had been made for recorded changes in the smoking habit). Patients who recognized that they inhaled were found no more frequently in the lung cancer group than in the control group, although those patients with growths of central origin inhaled less frequently than normal. It also appeared that lung cancer patients more frequently had a history of preceding pneumonia or chronic bronchitis, whereas other respiratory illnesses were referred to with approximately equal frequency by the two groups.

Doll and Hill's report [7] contained a remarkable amount of information but the fundamental finding in men was a highly significant difference between the proportions of non-smokers and of smokers in the disease group and in the control group. A less-marked series of differences was reported for women. Highly significant differences were also found between the proportions of both groups smoking different average amounts (i.e. between heavy and light smokers) and this result held for men and women. It is apparent from the raw data that a dose–response relationship exists. Less-marked, but nevertheless distinct, differences were found when the duration of smoking was considered. Lung cancer patients as a group began to smoke earlier, continued to smoke longer and gave up less often; when they did give up they did so for far shorter periods. In men, all these differences were statistically significant.

These studies, in particular the impact of two [5,6], alerted the medical and scientific community to the serious health hazards associated with cigarette smoking. Once alerted, the public response to these studies was a significant, but brief, drop in the per capita consumption of cigarettes in both the USA and the UK. Throughout the 1950s a mass of information was published, demonstrating the association between lung cancer and cigarette smoking, using data derived from retrospective studies. Many concentrated on inhalation: whereas some studies demonstrated a higher occurrence of inhalation among lung cancer patients than among controls, others failed to detect this association.

The US Surgeon General was moved by the weight of evidence associating smoking with cancer of the lung, as well as of the other sites, to produce an official statement on 'Smoking and Health' on behalf of the US Government [8]. This created a worldwide reaction as it implicated a frightening link between cigarette smoking and a variety of fatal diseases in a document of impeccable scientific authority. This report weighed the available evidence and considered that it had been established that cigarette smoking was causally related to lung cancer in men and judged cigarette smoking in the US a sufficiently important health hazard to warrant remedial action. In the 15 years that passed from that initial report, the body of evidence increased and extended to include women [9], in whom lung cancer had increased fivefold in two decades in the USA. The Secretary for Health of the time (Mr Joseph Califano) concluded that 'smoking is the largest preventable cause of death in America'.

An important factor in the causal relationship between smoking and lung cancer is the demonstrated dose–response relationship. In epidemiological studies, the dose has been estimated by the average number of cigarettes smoked per day, the maximum number of cigarettes smoked per day, age smoking commenced, degree of inhalation of tobacco smoke, total number of years smoked, total lifetime number of cigarettes smoked, tar and nicotine levels of the brand of cigarettes used, number of puffs per cigarette, length of the unburned portion of cigarette and a variety of combinations of these variables converted into 'dosage' scores. Lung cancer mortality ratios exhibit an inverse relationship with the age of initiation of the smoking habit. Those who develop the habit at school have a much higher risk of lung cancer than those who begin smoking at age 25+, in whom the risk is only four to five times that of non-smokers. Available data show a strong dose–response relationship between self-reported inhalation of cigarette smoke and lung cancer mortality: those who inhale deeply have risks double those of smokers who do not. The American Cancer Society 25 State Study [10] reported a mortality ratio among non-smokers of 1.0, a mortality ratio of 8.0 among smokers who stated that they did not inhale and elevations in this risk among those who inhaled slightly (8.9), moderately (13.1) and deeply (17.0). Similar results were reported from a Swedish study [11]: although the mortality ratios among non-smokers (1.0), non-inhalers (3.7), light inhalers (7.8) and deep inhalers (9.2) were smaller in magnitude, the same steady pattern was found.

It has been suggested for some time that the risk of developing lung cancer increases with the tar and nicotine content of cigarettes, although no substantial evidence exists to suggest that individuals who switch to cigarettes containing lower levels of tar and nicotine experience a lower lung cancer mortality [12]. It has been proposed that, if the tar and nicotine content of tobacco were to be reduced, smokers might increase the number of cigarettes smoked per day and effectively vitiate any benefit.

The relationship of tar and nicotine to lung cancer was carefully examined in a major study, in which 897 825 men and women were classified by levels of tar and nicotine smoked [13]. Brands were considered to be high in nicotine if they contained between 2.0 and 2.7 mg of nicotine and high in tar if they contained between 25.8 and 35.7 mg. The medium levels of tar and nicotine were set at 17.6–25.7 mg and 1.2–1.9 mg, respectively. Low tar and nicotine levels were all those below these limits. The risk in the high tar and nicotine group of men was set at 1.0 and the relative risks (RRs) in the medium group (RR = 0.95) and low group (RR = 0.81) were appreciably lower. Similar results were found for women: high (1.0), medium (RR = 0.79) and low (RR = 0.60). These results take into account the daily cigarette consumption. In other words, for men smoking the same number of cigarettes per day there appears to be an almost 20% reduction in risk of developing lung cancer with the use of cigarettes low in tar and nicotine. In women, keeping the number of cigarettes smoked per day constant, there was a 40% reduction in risk.

Cigarette smoking and cancer: the modern plague

At present, there is consistent evidence of a causal link between cigarette smoking, as well as other forms of tobacco use, and a variety of forms of cancer. It is widely held that around 30% of cancer deaths are attributable to tobacco smoking. Other causes of cancer have been identified and there is usually more than one cause of any particular form of cancer [14].

Cancer of the oral cavity

Oral cancer is a significant public health problem in many parts of the world. It is widely prevalent in India, several republics of the former Soviet Union, parts of South-East Asia and among men in certain regions of France. The risk among men appears to be increasing substantially in many countries [15], although the reasons for this increase are not completely understood. In the 19th century, its development had been associated with a number of factors in an anecdotal manner, including tobacco smoking.

Cancer of the lip

A qualitative association between pipe smoking and the development of lip cancer was made in central Europe in the mid-1800s [16]. Keller [17] analysed data on 314 men discharged from all Veterans Administration hospitals in the USA between 1958 and 1962. Two control groups were established — one with cancer of the mouth and pharynx and a second without a diagnosis of cancer at these sites. Keller concluded that the smoking of pipes alone was significantly associated with an increased risk of lip cancer.

Lindqvist [18] studied all cases of lip cancer in Finland diagnosed between 1972 and 1973. Using a control group drawn from patients with squamous-cell cancer of the skin of the head and neck, he concluded that, in men, tobacco smoking and an outdoor occupation combined to cause lip cancer (odds ratio [OR] = 15.4), but that neither factor alone had an effect (tobacco: OR = 2.0; outdoor work, OR = 1.4). Cigarette smoking accounted for almost all the tobacco use, with only 8% of male cases smoking a pipe.

In summary, it would appear that pipe smoking is a risk factor for lip cancer [19]. Whether this is an effect of the heat generated by the pipe or an effect of the tobacco content is not yet established. There is no evidence available to link lip cancer risk with cigarette smoking.

Cancer of the tongue, mouth and pharynx

An International Agency for Research on Cancer (IARC) Working Party concluded that there was sufficient evidence that tobacco was carcinogenic to humans and that the occurrence of malignant tumours of the upper digestive tract was causally related to the smoking of different forms of tobacco (cigarettes, cigars, pipes, bidis) [20]. Increased risk of cancers arising at these sites is also associated with alcohol consumption [21].

Merletti et al. [22] reported a case–control study of cancer of the oral cavity and oropharynx based on 122 cases (86 male, 36 female) and 606 controls (385 male, 221 female). The risk increased strongly with increasing tobacco consumption and there was a sharp reduction in risk following smoking cessation: in males, risk reduced to that compatible with non-smokers once 5 years had elapsed since smoking ceased. The effect of alcohol consumption was apparent and was independent of smoking. On the basis of their study findings, it was calculated that the attributable risks for alcohol and tobacco were 23 and 72%, respectively, in men and 34 and 54%, respectively, in women. These figures again emphasize the prospects that exist for prevention.

When the effect of stopping smoking was investigated, with the risk set to 1 among those who continued to smoke, the risk among those who stopped within 1 year of diagnosis (or interview in the case of controls) was 1.2; for those who quit between 1 and 9 years prior to diagnosis/interview, the risk decreased to 0.7 [95% confidence interval (CI) 0.5, 1.1]; and for those who had stopped for more than 9 years, the odds ratio fell to 0.5 (95% CI 0.3, 0.7). In other words, at 10 or more years after stopping smoking, the risk of developing an oral cancer had halved compared with the risk of those who continued to smoke.

Several other aspects of tobacco smoking have been investigated in epidemiological studies. There appears to be an increased risk of oral cancer associated with smoking cigarette brands that are high in tar content compared with low-tar cigarettes [23]. Although data are still relatively sparse, there does not appear to be any evidence of an extra risk associated with smoking mentholated cigarettes, which are commonly smoked by Afro-Americans in the USA, or the dark tobacco cigarettes that are smoked in some southern European countries and South America [24].

Tobacco is not only smoked and chewed: in some countries, the habit of snuff dipping (placing finely chopped tobacco in the cheek) is common. Vogler *et al.* observed that the male to female ratio of mouth cancer was lower in southern States in the USA and that a woman with a typical case of oral cancer had, as part of a description, 'admitted to the habitual use of (oral) snuff' [25]. It is considered that oral snuff is an avoidable carcinogenic hazard [26].

Cancer of the nose, nasal sinuses and nasal cavity

Nasal cancers are relatively rare, although they occur more frequently in residents of urban than rural areas among either sex. In addition, the disease appears slightly more common in Black residents of the same region compared with Whites. Nasal cancer is commoner in men than in women. Data are consistent with a moderate increase in risk of nasal cancer among smokers [14]. Six case–control studies have investigated the association between nasal cancer and cigarette smoking and five demonstrated an increased risk associated with cigarette smoking [27–32]. Fukada and Shibata [28] also reported a significantly increasing trend with the amount smoked, with a relative risk of 4.6 in those men smoking 40 or more cigarettes per day. In the other studies, with over 100 cases, small increases in risk of approximately 20% were evident [27–31]. Two studies have also reported a statistically significant association with exposure to environmental smoke [28,33]. In view of the consistency of the results, the biological gradients observed with amount smoked and time since smoking stopped, Doll concluded that cigarette smoking is a cause of some squamous cell carcinomas of the nasal cavity [19].

Cancer of the larynx

Tobacco smoking [20] and alcohol consumption [21] are the major established risk factors for laryngeal cancer. A recent study from Poland estimated that cigarette smoking alone accounted for an estimated 95% of cases of laryngeal cancer in that country [34]. There is little evidence that different types of alcohol have appreciably different effects on laryngeal cancer risk.

Cancer of the oesophagus

The most important risk factors for cancer of the oesophagus in developed countries are cigarette smoking [20] and alcohol consumption [21]. The highest rates of oesophageal cancer in European men are to be found in France [35–37], and findings from a series of studies conducted in the north-west of this country have led to the estimation that 85% of all oesophageal cancers could be attributable to the joint effects of cigarette smoking and alcohol consumption. Each of these factors is an independent carcinogen for the oesophageal epithelium [38]. This observation is particularly important, since alcohol is not thought to have any independent carcinogenic activity in animals although it may enhance the effects of other carcinogens [21]. Studies from France [39] and Italy [40] have reported relative risks of oesophageal cancer of between 5 and 10 for heavy smokers. All forms of tobacco smoking, including pipes and cigars, are associated with the increased risk of oesophageal cancer, but the risk is apparently less strong for the newer filter, lower-tar cigarettes than for the older, high-tar types.

Cancer of the stomach

Cancer of the stomach was the leading cause of cancer death on a global scale up to the early 1980s, and only recently has it been overtaken by the lung cancer epidemic. There are still areas of the world — notably China and Japan, but also Eastern European countries and northern Italy — where gastric cancer rates are notably high. There is no adequate explanation of the determinants of the declines. However, there is now consistent evidence, from descriptive as well as analytical epidemiology, that a more affluent diet and improved methods of food preservation including, specifically, refrigeration, are to some extent linked to these favourable trends, although the effects appear after a considerable time lag.

The IARC [20], in their review of the evidence available regarding the association between cigarette smoking and stomach cancer, concluded that: 'the data now available on tobacco smoking and stomach cancer do not permit a conclusion that the associations noted in some studies is causal.' During the decade which passed following that review, several case–control studies have been published on this topic. A significantly increased risk was found in most of the case–control studies [41–43], but not in all [44–46]. A series of prospective studies all demonstrated an increased risk of stomach cancer associated with cigarette smoking [47–50].

Cancer of the pancreas

Pancreatic cancer is consistently reported to occur more frequently in men than in women, in

Blacks than in Whites, and in urban compared with rural population groups. In some countries mortality rates continue to rise; in others, declining levels of disease can be seen among members of younger birth cohorts [51]. Although some of the patterns observed can be explained by variation in pancreatic cancer risk factors, many cannot.

Analytical studies based on patients with pancreatic cancer consistently demonstrate that cigarette smoking increases the risk of this cancer [20]. In the collaborative study conducted by the SEARCH programme of the IARC, a dose–response relationship was found with increasing pancreatic cancer risk and lifetime reported cigarette consumption [52]. The risk was found to be reduced among smokers to a level compatible with that of lifelong non-smokers, 15 years after quitting.

Cancer of the lung

Lung cancer rates in self-reported non-smokers from various studies are of the order of only 10–15/100 000. Estimates of the proportions of lung cancer deaths attributable to tobacco smoking in five developed countries (Canada, England and Wales, Japan, Sweden and the USA) range between 83 and 92% for men, and 57 and 80% for women [20]. In men in all European countries, except Portugal, lung cancer is now the leading cause of cancer death. In the USA (and in all except a few Scandinavian countries), it is the commonest tumour in terms of incidence as well, although prostate cancer in men is catching up. The range of geographical variation in lung cancer mortality in Europe is threefold in both sexes, the highest rates being observed in the UK, Belgium, the Netherlands and Czechoslovakia, and lowest rates reported in southern Europe and also in Norway and Sweden [35,37]. This overall pattern of age-standardized lung cancer mortality rates does not reveal the important and diverging cohort effects occurring in various countries: for instance, some of the countries in which there are now low rates, such as those in southern Europe and parts of Eastern Europe, experienced a later uptake and spread of tobacco use, and now have some of the most elevated rates in the younger age groups. This suggests that these same countries, including Italy, Greece, France, Spain and several countries in Eastern Europe, will have the highest lung cancer rates in men at the beginning of the 21st century, in the absence of rapid and effective intervention.

The importance of adequate intervention is shown by the low lung cancer rates in Scandinavian countries, which adopted integrated central and local policies and programmes against smoking in the early 1970s [53–54]. These policies may have been enabled by the limited influence of the tobacco lobby in these countries. The Scandinavian experience provides convincing evidence of the favourable impact, after a relatively short delay, of well-targeted, large-scale interventions on the most common cause of cancer death and of premature mortality in general.

In conclusion, the overwhelming role of tobacco smoking in the causation of lung cancer has been repeatedly demonstrated over the past 50 years [6–9,16]. Current lung cancer rates reflect cigarette smoking habits of men and women in the past decades, but not necessarily current smoking patterns, since there is an interval of several decades between the change in smoking habits in a population and its consequences regarding lung cancer rates. Over 90% of cases of lung cancer may be avoidable simply through avoidance of cigarette smoking. Many solutions have been attempted to reduce cigarette smoking and, increasingly, many countries are enacting legislation to curb this habit [55].

Cancer of the bladder

There is overwhelming evidence for an association between bladder cancer and cigarette smoking [20]; the only remaining question surrounds the strength of the association. The large majority of studies find relationships between bladder cancer risk and 'dose' of cigarettes smoked. Furthermore, smokers of black tobacco appear to be at higher risk than smokers of blond cigarettes [56].

The predominant role of cigarette smoking is reflected in the geographical distribution of the disease, with high rates in predominantly urban areas of Europe and North America, although areas with extensive chemical industry and endemic *Schistosomiasis haematobium* also tend to have high rates. In developed countries, cigarette smoking is by far the most important single determinant of the disease: the RR is of the order of 3–5, and the population attributable risk has been estimated to be from around 50% to as high as 85% in British males. Duration of cigarette smoking shows a direct relationship with RR values of bladder cancer, with the risk rising to between 3 and 5 for 40 years of cigarette smoking and over [57–59].

Several studies have examined the association between smoking, type of tumour and disease progression. A case–control study conducted in the Boston Metropolitan Area has demonstrated different risks for superficial and invasive bladder cancers: the tobacco-associated risk was 2.6 for superficial bladder cancer and 1.7 for invasive tumours; only for patients younger than 60 years was the risk greater for invasive tumours [60]. Another study found higher risk (5.2) for invasive than for superficial tumours (3.0). After adjustment for stage, cigarette smoking was associated with higher risk of low-grade than high-grade tumours [61]. There is also some evidence that smoking may influence the natural history of bladder cancer [62]: in a follow-up study of 252 consecutive patients with histologically verified transitional cell cancer of the bladder, 27% of the non-smokers and 40% of the smokers had died during the first 10 years after diagnosis, suggesting that smoking may be associated with higher mortality from the disease in the longer term [63].

Several recent studies have found a significant impact of smoking on the mutation of the *p17* and *p53* genes in bladder cancer, leading to the suggestion that certain carcinogens in tobacco may cause DNA damage and may produce specific mutations [64–66]. One of these studies demonstrated a significant association between the number of cigarettes smoked per day and *p53* nuclear overexpression, with a 2.3 times higher risk for those smoking one to two packs per day and 8.4 times higher for smoking more than two packs per day [65].

Cancer of the kidney

Cancer of the kidney is a relatively common cancer in many Western countries, and occurs more frequently among men than women, at a ratio of around 2:1. Very little is known about the causes of kidney cancer. The single established risk factor is cigarette smoking, but the RR is approximately a factor of two in current smokers versus those who have never smoked, and is lower than for bladder and most other tobacco-related neoplasms [20]. The risk associated with cigarette smoking is higher for cancer of the renal pelvis [67].

Leukaemia

Although not definitive, the evidence implicating cigarette smoking in the aetiology of leukaemia, particularly acute myeloid leukaemia, is quite suggestive. The elevated risks of leukaemia among smokers were virtually all observed in epidemiological investigations of the hypothesis, although most studies (but by no means all) where the relationship has been evaluated have demonstrated a positive association. Three overviews (critical analysis or meta-analysis) have concluded that most of the data support

an association, particularly among men [68–70]. Attributable risks for smoking and deaths from myeloid leukaemia (24%) [71] and acute myeloid leukaemia incidence (31%) [72] have been estimated.

Tobacco smoking and other causes of death

There are a number of very common diseases other than cancer that are also linked to tobacco smoking. Among many studies in this field of research, a group of male doctors in the UK has been assembled and followed up for 40 years to investigate the differences in disease occurrence and death among smokers and non-smokers [50]. The results of this study are summarized in Table 8.2, which contains, for a variety of different diseases, the RR and the absolute excess risk in cigarette smokers, together with the attributable fraction — the proportion of all deaths for each specified disease that is due to smoking [73].

Apart from cancer, there are six other diseases that are caused by smoking, including the extremely common ischaemic heart disease (IHD). IHD is the commonest cause of death in industrialized countries and smoking causes more deaths from IHD than any other disease. Smokers are also more likely to die from respiratory heart disease, aortic aneurysm and chronic obstructive lung disease [50,73]. Overall, the death rate in cigarette smokers from all the specified diseases is double that in lifelong non-smokers.

There are also some instances in which the increased risk is associated with some other external influence. Fatal diseases that fall into this category include cirrhosis of the liver, cancer of the liver, suicide and poisoning [50,73].

Tobacco smoking and non-fatal diseases

Wald and Hackshaw [73] determined from a number of different sources that there were several other diseases that were non-fatal but for which the risk was increased among smokers: these include peripheral vascular disease, cataracts, Crohn's disease, gastric ulcer, duodenal ulcer, hip fracture and periodontitis (Table 8.3).

Table 8.2. *Fatal diseases positively associated with smoking: results of 40-year follow-up of UK doctors [73]*

Disease	Relative risk	Attributable proportion* (%)
A. Increased risk largely or entirely caused by smoking		
Cancer of the lung	15.0	81
Cancer of the upper respiratory tract	24.0	87
Cancer of the bladder	2.3	28
Cancer of the pancreas	2.2	26
Ischaemic heart disease	1.6	15
Respiratory heart disease	†	100
Aortic aneurysm	4.1	48
Chronic obstructive lung disease	12.7	78
B. Increased risk partly caused by smoking		
Cancer of the oesophagus	7.5	66
Cancer of the stomach	1.7	17
Cancer of the kidney	2.1	25
Leukaemia	1.8	19
Stroke	1.3	8
Pneumonia	1.9	21
C. Increased risk due to confounding		
Cirrhosis of the liver	5.3	–
Cancer of the liver	1.6	–
Suicide	1.6	–
Poisoning	2.7	–
All disease excluding part C	2.0	23
All disease excluding parts B and C	2.2	26

*The attributable proportion was calculated assuming 30% of the population are current smokers and that all excess risk is due to smoking.
†Could not be calculated since there were no deaths among non-smokers and 10 among current smokers.

Tobacco smoking and deaths in Europe

Peto *et al.* [74] have estimated the numbers of deaths attributable to smoking in each country (Tables 8.4 and 8.5). The number of deaths estimated to occur as a result of smoking is enormous. In 1990, it amounted to 24% of all deaths in developed countries combined and 35% of all deaths occurring in middle age (defined as death occurring between 35 and 69 years of age).

It has been estimated that the average loss of life for those killed by tobacco in developed countries is about 16 years. Since about half of all regular smokers in developed countries are eventually killed by the smoking habit, teenagers or

Table 8.3. *Non-fatal diseases positively associated with smoking: results of 40-year follow-up of UK doctors [73]*

Disease or condition	Relative risk	Attributable proportion* (%)
A. Increased risk largely or entirely caused by smoking		
Peripheral vascular disease (age 45–74 years)	2.0	23
B. Increased risk partly caused by smoking		
Cataract (men aged 40–84 years)	2.2	26
Crohn's disease	2.1	25
Gastric ulcer (age 20–61 years)	3.4	42
Duodenal ulcer (age 20–61 years)	4.1	48
Hip fracture (aged > 65 years)	1.3	8
Periodontitis (age 19–40 years)	3.0	38

*The attributable proportion was calculated assuming 30% of the population are current smokers and that all excess risk is due to smoking.

Table 8.4. *Number* of deaths in 1990 attributable to smoking in EC countries in men; the USA and Japan have been added for comparison purposes [74]*

Country	Age (years)		
	35–69	**> 70**	**All**
Austria	4 000 (28)	3 600 (16)	7 500 (20)
Belgium	7 900 (41)	8 600 (28)	16 500 (31)
Denmark	3 300 (32)	4 300 (22)	7 600 (25)
Finland	2 600 (25)	2 700 (21)	5 300 (21)
France	32 600 (32)	24 500 (16)	57 100 (21)
Germany	52 000 (32)	43 300 (18)	95 300 (22)
Greece	5 200 (33)	5 200 (17)	10 400 (21)
Ireland	1 700 (31)	2 500 (24)	4 200 (25)
Italy	37 800 (37)	34 900 (21)	72 700 (26)
Luxembourg	200 (34)	300 (25)	500 (27)
The Netherlands	8 600 (38)	13 000 (32)	21 600 (32)
Portugal	4 000 (21)	2 800 (09)	6 800 (13)
Spain	20 500 (33)	19 400 (19)	40 000 (23)
Sweden	2 100 (16)	3 200 (09)	5 300 (11)
UK	37 200 (35)	52 100 (27)	89 400 (28)
USA	150 000 (36)	136 200 (23)	286 300 (26)
Japan	26 800 (16)	41 500 (16)	68 300 (15)

*Percentages in parentheses.

Table 8.5. *Number* of deaths in 1990 attributable to smoking in countries of central and Eastern Europe, including the former USSR, in men [74]*

Country	Age (years) 35–69	> 70
Armenia	2 200 (38)	500 (13)
Azerbaijan	2 700 (24)	500 (8)
Belarus	11 000 (39)	3100 (16)
Bulgaria	8200 (30)	2200 (7)
Czech Republic	13 300 (42)	6100 (19)
Estonia	1900 (38)	500 (15)
Georgia	2800 (24)	700 (9)
Hungary	16 000 (41)	6500 (19)
Kazakhstan	15 200 (43)	3700 (22)
Kyrgyzstan	2000 (28)	700 (17)
Latvia	3300 (38)	1000 (15)
Lithuania	3800 (38)	1400 (17)
Moldavia	3500 (31)	700 (10)
Poland	44 600 (42)	15 300 (18)
Romania	19 600 (32)	4200 (8)
Russia	191 900 (42)	48 600 (20)
Slovakia	5800 (38)	1900 (15)
Tajikstan	700 (14)	200 (6)
Turkmenistan	1100 (22)	200 (6)
Ukraine	64 400 (40)	19 500 (17)
Uzbekistan	4700 (20)	900 (5)
Yugoslavia (former)	19 400 (36)	6300 (13)
All above countries	441 200 (39)	126 300 (17)

*Percentages in parentheses.

young adults who become regular cigarette smokers must be reducing their life expectancy by about 8 years [74].

Every part of society is responsible

It has been demonstrated that changes in cigarette consumption are affected mainly at a sociological level rather than by actions, such as individual smoking-cessation programmes targeted at individuals. Actions such as advertising bans and increases in the price of cigarettes influence cigarette sales, particularly among adolescents. This suggests the necessity of a tobacco policy to reduce the health consequences of tobacco. Experience shows that this should be targeted through a variety of actions aimed to prevent young people from starting smoking and to help smokers to stop. To be efficient and successful, a tobacco policy has to be comprehensive and maintained over a long period. Increased taxes on tobacco, total bans on direct and indirect advertising, smoke-free enclosed public areas, education, effective health-warning labels on tobacco products, a policy of low maximum tar and nicotine levels in cigarettes, encouragement of stopping smoking and individual health interventions have to be implemented.

There is no real alternative at present to the creation of effective programmes in tobacco control. There are a number of agreed elements to the core strategies of a comprehensive tobacco-control strategy which have the support of the International Union Against Cancer (UICC), the World Health Organization (WHO), the 'Europe Against Cancer' programme of the European Community and the European Institute of Oncology. These include the following:

1. A ban on all advertising and promotion of tobacco products;
2. Effective Government health warnings on all tobacco products;
3. A low tar/nicotine policy;
4. Tax and pricing policies;
5. Alternative economic policies;
6. Policies to protect young people from tobacco promotion and sales to prevent the onset of tobacco use;
7. Policies to protect the rights of non-smokers and establish in law the right to smoke-free environments, including the workplace;
8. Policies to control smokeless tobacco and prohibit other new methods of nicotine delivery;
9. Policies to ensure the wide availability of help for tobacco users who wish to stop.

The importance of adequate intervention is demonstrated by the low lung cancer rates in Scandinavian countries which, since the early 1970s, have adopted integrated policies and programmes against smoking. In the UK, tobacco consumption has declined by 30% since 1970, and lung cancer mortality among men has been decreasing since 1980, although the rate remains high. In France, between 1992 and 1993 there was a 3% reduction in tobacco consumption due to the implementation of anti-tobacco measures.

There have been some steps taken to reduce the impact of smoking that have had some surprising results. The move towards smoking brands of cigarettes that were lower in tar and nicotine content was assumed to be leading to a reduction of the risk of lung cancer. However, marked changes in the rates of the major histological cell types of lung cancer can now be seen to be compatible with increased risk of adenocarcinoma due to increasing levels of smoking of light cigarettes ('low tar, low nicotine') [75,76]. It appears that although abandoning high-tar cigarettes (15–45 mg tar) may have had some impact on reducing the risk of squamous cell carcinoma, there is now a 'balancing' effect in that light cigarettes increase the risk of adenocarcinoma.

Attempts to reduce the impact of the effects of cigarette smoking have revolved around attempts at chemoprevention. High consumption of fruits and vegetables is associated with a reduced risk of a number of forms of cancer, including those of the lung, mouth, pancreas, larynx, oesophagus, bladder and stomach: the major exceptions have been the lack of strong association with hormonally related forms of cancer such as those of the prostate, breast, ovary and endometrium [77]. The relationship appears to be a general effect and is consistently found with many different groups of fruits and vegetables. Although many candidate mechanisms (and molecules) have been put forward, there is little real evidence to suggest that it is one particular component of diet as opposed to another that is responsible. Chemoprevention for lung cancer has not been effective in three randomized studies [78–80].

Conclusions

In Europe at present, tobacco smoking is a major cause of premature death. Throughout Europe in 1990, tobacco smoking caused three-quarters of a million deaths in middle age (between the ages of 35 and 69). In the Member States of the European Union in 1990, there were over one-quarter of a million deaths in middle age directly caused by tobacco smoking — 219 700 in men and 31 900 in women; many more deaths at older ages were caused by tobacco. In countries of central and Eastern Europe, including the former USSR, there were 441 200 deaths in middle-aged men and 42 100 deaths in women. There is a need for urgent action to help contain this important and unnecessary loss of life. The individual has actions which he or she can take: the important message is that cancer can be avoided and that three items with regard to cigarette smoking should be respected: (1) do not smoke; (2) smokers, stop as quickly as possible and do not smoke in the presence of others; and (3) if you do not smoke, do not experiment with tobacco.

Acknowledgements

This work was prepared within the framework of support from AIRC (Italian Association for Cancer Research).

References

1. Sommering ST. De morbis vasorum absorbentium corporis humani. Frankfurt: Varentrapp and Wenner, 1795

2. Tylecote FE. Cancer of the lung. *Lancet* 1927; 2: 256–257

3. Schrek R, Baker LA, Ballard GP, Dolgoff S. Tobacco smoking as an etiologic factor in disease. *Cancer Res* 1950; 10: 49–58

4. Levin ML, Goldstein H, Gerhardt PR. Cancer and tobacco smoking. *JAMA* 1950; 143: 336–338

5. Wynder EL, Graham EA. Tobacco smoking as a possible etiologic factor in bronchiogenic carcinoma. *JAMA* 1950; 143: 329–336

6. Doll R, Hill AB. Smoking and carcinoma of the lung. *Br Med J* 1950; 2: 739–748

7. Doll R, Hill AB. A study of the aetiology of carcinoma of the lung. *Br Med J* 1952; 2: 1271–1286

8. United States Public Health Service. Smoking and health. Report of the Advisory Committee to the Surgeon General of the Public Health Service. DHEW Publication no. 1103. Bethesda, Maryland: US Department of Health, Education and Welfare, Public Health Service, Centers for Disease Control and Prevention, 1964

9. United States Surgeon General. Smoking and health. A report of the Surgeon General. DHEW Publication number (PHS) 79-50066. Bethesda, Maryland: United States Department of Health, Education and Welfare, Public Health Service, Washington DC, 1979

10. Hammond EC. Smoking in relation to death rates of one million men and women. *NCI Monogr* 1966; 19: 127–204

11. Cederlof R, Friberg L, Hrubec Z, Lorich U. The relationship of smoking and some social covariates to mortality and cancer morbidity. A ten year follow-up in a probability sample of 55,000 Swedish subjects age 18–69, Part 1 and Part 2. Stockholm: The Karolinska Institute, 1975

12. Bross IDJ, Gibson R. Risks of lung cancer in smokers who switch to filter cigarettes. *Am J Public Health* 1968; 58: 1396–1403

13. Hammond EC, Garfinkel L, Seidman H, Lew EA. Some recent findings concerning cigarette smoking. In: Hiatt HH, Watson JD, Winsten JA (eds) Origins of human cancer. Book A: Incidence of cancer in humans. New York: Cold Spring Harbor Laboratory, 1977: 101–112

14. Boyle P, La Vecchia C, Maisonneuve P *et al.* Cancer epidemiology and prevention. In: MJ Peckam, H Pinedo, U Veronesi (eds) Oxford textbook of oncology. Oxford: Oxford Medical Publications, 1995: 199–273

15. Macfarlane GJ, Boyle P, Evstifeeva TV *et al.* Rising trends of oral cancer mortality among males worldwide: the return of an old public health problem. *Cancer Causes Control* 1994; 5: 259–265

16. Clemmesen J. Statistical studies in malignant neoplasms. I. Review and results. Copenhagen: Munksgaard, 1965

17. Keller AZ. Cellular types, survival race, nativity, occupation, habits and associated diseases in the pathogenesis of lip cancers. *Am J Epidemiol* 1970; 91: 486–499

18. Lindqvist C. Risk factors for lip cancer. A questionnaire survey. *Am J Epidemiol* 1979; 109: 521–530

19. Doll R. Cancers weakly related to smoking. *Br Med Bull* 1996; 52: 35–49

20. IARC Monographs on the Evaluation of Carcinogenic Risk to Humans. Vol 38. Tobacco smoking. Lyon: International Agency for Research on Cancer, 1986

21. IARC Monographs on the Evaluation of Carcinogenic Risk to Humans. Vol 44. Alcohol drinking. Lyon: International Agency for Research on Cancer, 1988

22. Merletti F, Boffetta P, Ciccone G *et al.* Role of tobacco and alcoholic beverages in the aetiology of cancer of the oral cavity/oropharynx in Torino, Italy. *Cancer Res* 1989; 49: 4919–4924

23. La Vecchia C, Bidoli E, Barra S *et al.* Type of cigarettes and cancers of the upper digestive and respiratory tract. *Cancer Causes Control* 1990; 1: 69–74

24. Boffetta P. Black (air-cured) and blond (flue-cured) tobacco and cancer risk. V: Oral cavity cancer. *Eur J Cancer* 1993; 29: 1331–1335

25. Vogler WR, Lloyd JW, Millmore BK. A retrospective study of etiological factors in cancer of the mouth, pharynx and larynx. *Cancer* 1962; 15: 246–248

26. Lancet (Editorial). Oral snuff: a preventable carcinogenic hazard. *Lancet* 1986; i: 198–201

27. Brinton LA, Blot WJ, Becker JA *et al.* A case–control study of cancers of the nasal cavity and paranasal sinuses. *Am J Epidemiol* 1984: 119; 896–906

28. Fukuda K, Shibata A. Exposure–response relationships between woodworking, smoking or passive smoking, and squamous cell neoplasms of the maxillary sinus. *Cancer Causes Control* 1990; 1: 165–168

29. Hayes RB, Kardaun JWPE, de Bruyn J. Tobacco use and sinonasal cancers: a case–control study. *Br J Cancer* 1987; 56: 843–846

30. Strader CH, Vaughan TL, Stergachii A. Use of nasal preparations and the incidence of sinonasal cancer. *J Epidemiol Community Health* 1983; 42: 243–248

31. Zheng W, Blot WJ, Diamond EL *et al.* A population-based case–control study of cancers of the nasal cavity and paranasal sinuses in Shanghai. *Int J Cancer* 1992; 52: 557–561

32. Zheng W, McLaughlin JK, Chow WH *et al.* Risk factors for cancers of the nasal cavity and paranasal sinuses among white men in the United States. *Am J Epidemiol* 1993; 138: 965–972

33. Hirayama T. Cancer mortality in non-smoking women with smoking husbands based on a large-scale cohort study in Japan. *Prev Med* 1984; 13: 680–690

34. Zatonski W, Becker H, Lissowska J, Wahrendorf J. Tobacco, alcohol, and diet in the etiology of laryngeal cancer: a population-based case–control study. *Cancer Causes Control* 1991; 2: 3–11

35. Levi F, Maisonneuve P, Filiberti R *et al.* Cancer incidence and mortality in Europe. *Soz Praventivmed* 1989; 34: 1–84

36. Smans M, Muir CS, Boyle P. Atlas of cancer mortality in the European Economic Community. IARC Publication Series 107. Oxford: Oxford University Press, 1992

37. Levi F, Lucchini F, Boyle P *et al.* Cancer incidence and mortality in Europe, 1988–92. *J Epidemiol Biostat* 1998; 3

38. La Vecchia C, Negri E. The role of alcohol in oesophageal cancer in non-smokers and of tobacco in non-drinkers. *Int J Cancer* 1989; 43: 784–785

39. Tuyns AJ, Pequinot G, Jensen OM. Le cancer de l'oesophage en Ille-et-Villaine en fonction des niveaux de consommation d'alcool et de tabac. Des risques qui se multiplient. *Bull Cancer* (Paris) 1977; 64: 45–60

40. La Vecchia C, Bidoli E, Barra S *et al.* Type of cigarettes and cancers of the upper digestive and respiratory tract. *Cancer Causes Control* 1990; 1: 69–74

41. You WC, Blot WJ, Chang YS *et al.* Diet and high risk of stomach cancer in Shandong, China. *Cancer Res* 1988; 48: 3518–3535

42. Correa P, Fontham E, Pickle L *et al.* Dietary determinants of gastric cancer in South Louisiana inhabitants. *J Natl Cancer Inst* 1985; 75: 645–654

43. Tominga K, Koyama Y, Sasagawa M *et al.* A case–control study of stomach cancer and its genesis in relation to alcohol consumption, smoking and familial cancer history. *Jpn J Cancer Res* 1991; 82: 974–979

44. Jedrychowski W, Wahrendorf J, Popiela T, Rachtan J. A case–control study of dietary factors and stomach cancer risk in Poland. *Int J Cancer* 1986; 37: 837–842

45. Boeing H, Frentzel-Beyme R, Berger M et al. Case–control study of stomach cancer in Germany. Int J Cancer 1991; 47: 858–864

46. Marshall JR, Boyle P. Nutrition and oral cancer. Cancer Causes Control 1996; 7: 101–111

47. Nomura A, Grove JS, Stemmerman GN, Severson RK. A prospective study of stomach cancer and its relation to diet, cigarettes and alcohol consumption. Cancer Res 1990; 50: 627–631

48. Kato I, Tominga S, Matsumoto KA. Prospective study of stomach cancer among rural Japanese population: a six-year survey. Jpn J Cancer Res 1992; 83: 568–575

49. Kato I, Tominga S, Ito Y et al. A prospective study of atrophic gastritis and stomach cancer risk. Jpn J Cancer Res 1992; 83: 1137–1142

50. Doll R, Peto R, Wheatley K et al. Mortality in relation to smoking: 40 years' observations on male British doctors. Br Med J 1994; 309: 901–911

51. Boyle P, Hsieh CC, Maisonneuve P et al. Epidemiology of pancreas cancer (1988). Int J Pancreatol 1989; 5: 327–346

52. Boyle P, Maisonneuve P, Bueno de Mesquita B et al. Cigarette smoking and pancreas cancer risk: a case–control study of the SEARCH Programme of the IARC. Int J Cancer 1996; 67: 63–71

53. Bjartveit K. Legislation and political activity. In: DG Zaridze and R Peto (eds) Tobacco: a major international health hazard. Lyon: IARC, 1986: 285–298

54. Della-Vorgia P, Sasco AJ, Skalkidis Y et al. An evaluation of the effectiveness of tobacco-control legislative policies in European Community countries. Scand J Soc Med 1990; 18: 81–89

55. Roemer R. Legislative action to combat the world tobacco epidemic. Geneva: WHO, 1993

56. D'Avanzo B, Negri E, la Vecchia C et al. Cigarette smoking and bladder cancer. Eur J Cancer 1990; 26: 714–718

57. Howe GR, Burch JD, Miller AB et al. Tobacco use, occupation, coffee, various nutrients, and bladder cancer. J Natl Cancer Inst 1980; 64: 701–713

58. Wynder EL, Goldsmith R. The epidemiology of bladder cancer. A second look. Cancer 1977; 40: 1246–1268

59. Tyrrell AB, MacAirt JG, McCaughey WTE. Occupational and non-occupational factors associated with vesical neoplasms in Ireland. J Irish Med Assoc 1971; 64: 213–217

60. Hayes RB, Friedell GH, Zahm SH, Cole P. Are the known bladder cancer risk-factors associated with more advanced bladder cancer? Cancer Causes Control 1993; 4: 157–162

61. Sturgeon SR, Hartge P, Silverman DT et al. Associations between bladder cancer risk factors and tumor stage and grade at diagnosis. Epidemiology 1994; 5: 218–225

62. Fitzpatrick JM. Superficial bladder carcinoma. Factors affecting the natural history. World J Urol 1993; 11: 142–147

63. Raitanen MP, Nieminen P, Tammela TL. Impact of tumour grade, stage, number and size, and smoking and sex, on survival in patients with transitional cell carcinoma of the bladder. Br J Urol 1995; 76: 470–474

64. Habuchi T, Takahashi R, Yamada H et al. Influence of cigarette smoking and schistosomiasis on p53 gene mutation in urological cancer. Cancer Res 1993; 53: 3795–3799

65. Zhang ZF, Sarkis AS, Cordon Cardo C et al. Tobacco smoking, occupation, and p53 nuclear overexpression in early stage bladder cancer. Cancer Epidemiol Biomarkers Prev 1994; 3: 19–24

66. Uchida T, Wada C, Ishida H et al. p53 mutations and prognosis in bladder tumors. J Urol 1995; 153: 1097–1104

67. Jensen OM, Wahrendorf J, Blettner M et al. The Copenhagen case–control study of bladder cancer: role of smoking in invasive and non-invasive bladder tumours. J Epidemiol Community Health 1987; 41: 30–36

68. Brown LM, Gibson R, Blair A et al. Smoking and risk of leukaemia. Am J Epidemiol 1992; 135: 763–768

69. Wald N. Smoking and leukaemia. Br Med J 1988: 297–638

70. Siegel M. Smoking and leukemia: evaluation of a causal hypothesis. Am J Epidemiol 1993; 138: 1–9

71. McLaughlin JK, Hrubec Z, Linet MS et al. Cigarette smoking and leukaemia. J Natl Cancer Inst 1989; 81: 1262–1263

72. Severson RK. Cigarette smoking and leukemia. Cancer 1987; 60: 141–144

73. Wald NJ, Hackshaw AK. Cigarette smoking: an epidemiological overview. Br Med Bull 1996; 52: 3–11

74. Peto R, Lopez AD, Boreham J et al. Mortality from smoking world-wide. Br Med Bull 1996; 52: 12–21

75. Zheng T, Holford TR, Boyle P et al. Time trend and the age–period–cohort effect on the incidence of histologic types of lung cancer in Connecticut, 1960–1989. Cancer 1994; 74(5): 1556–1567

76. Levi F, Franceschi S, La Vecchia C et al. Lung cancer trends by histological type in Vaud and Neuchatel, Switzerland, 1974–1994. Cancer 1997; 79: 906–914

77. Steinmetz KA, Potter JD. Vegetables, fruit, and cancer. I. Epidemiology. Cancer Causes Control 1991; 2: 325–358

78. The Alpha-Tocopherol, Beta-Carotene Cancer Prevention Study Group: the effect of vitamin E and beta carotene on the incidence of lung cancer and other cancers in male smokers. N Engl J Med 1994; 330: 1029–1035

79. Omenn GS, Goodman GE, Thornquist MD et al. Effects of combination of beta-carotene and vitamin A on lung cancer and cardiovascular disease. N Engl J Med 1996; 334: 1150–1155

80. Hennekens CH, Buring JE, Manson JE et al. Lack of effect of long-term supplementation with beta-carotene on the incidence of malignant neoplasms and cardiovascular disease. N Engl J Med 1996; 334: 1145–1149

CHAPTER 9

Lumps, lesions and skin cancer

G. R. Mikhail, S. D. Shetty and R. N. Farah

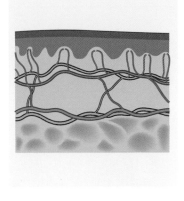

Scrotal masses of surgical significance

A number of conditions extend the normal appearance of the scrotum (Fig. 9.1a). Those of surgical significance are discussed in this chapter.

Hydrocele

Hydroceles are soft cystic swellings that can reach enormous proportions. They result from the collection of fluid around the testis in the cavity of tunica vaginalis (Fig. 9.1b). Testicular function is maintained despite the potential long-standing nature of the swelling. Most hydroceles are idiopathic and are thought to arise from failure of absorption of fluid secreted by the visceral layer of the tunica vaginalis. Secondary causes include trauma, epididymo-orchitis, filariasis, testicular tumours, or surgery (e.g. hernia or varicocele repair). The majority of hydroceles are soft and contain clear, transparent fluid; they are therefore transilluminable with a penlight. Exceptions are tense hydroceles (which may feel hard and can be mistaken for a tumour), and chronic hydroceles (which have a thick sac and may not be transilluminable). Hydroceles in the newborn and infants are usually communicating hydroceles caused by patent processus vaginalis. Most of these communicating hydroceles close by 1 year of age and do not need treatment; however, the presence of bowel in the hernial sac requires repair.

All males with a scrotal swelling should be evaluated with scrotal ultrasonography at the earliest opportunity, in order to rule out testicular tumour. Surgical repair, usually carried out for cosmetic reasons, involves drainage of the hydrocele fluid and inversion of the parietal layer of the tunica vaginalis. This allows the testis to be exposed to the rich lymphatics of the scrotal layers so that any future fluid would be absorbed quickly. If the sac is thin, a Lord's plication of the parietal layer can be performed. If the sac is thick, a subtotal excision of the parietal layer is recommended. Post-operative complications include scrotal haematoma, infection and scrotal oedema. Patients should be advised that the scrotum will not return to its normal size until 4–6 weeks after surgery.

Inguinoscrotal hernia

Large hernias may extend to the bottom of the scrotal sac, but swelling is usually reducible unless incarcerated. Large incarcerated hernias may contain sizeable sections of omentum, sigmoid colon, or loops of the bowel (Fig. 9.1c) and require surgical correction. If not corrected promptly, obstruction and strangulation may result. Reducible hernias should therefore be surgically repaired electively, but incarcerated hernia at the earliest opportunity. Complications following surgery include hydrocele formation, spermatic cord haematoma and, occasionally, testicular atrophy due to injury to the testicular artery.

Epididymal cyst

Cystic swellings from the head of the epididymis are a common cause of scrotal swelling. Spermatoceles are solitary unilocular cysts within the epididymal head, containing turbid fluid (Fig. 9.1d). Spermatoceles may not exceed 2–3 cm in size. Epididymal cysts are often multilocular, larger and easily mistaken for hydroceles. The head of the epididymis is usually the site for both spermatoceles and epididymal cysts. Although these structures are benign, they can be excised for cosmetic reasons. However, caution is necessary when operating on young men who need to maintain fertility.

Varicocele

Varicoceles are large, dilated, tortuous veins in the pampiniform plexus of the spermatic cord (Fig. 9.1e). They are present in 15% of the general population and 40% of infertile men.

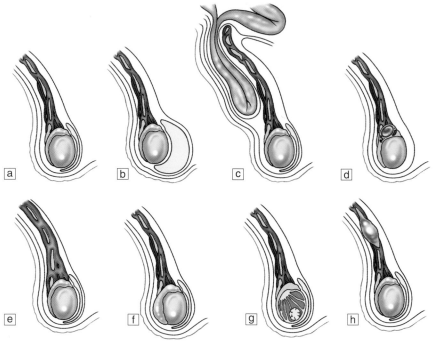

Figure 9.1. *Normal testicular anatomy (a) and a range of conditions involving swelling of the scrotum: (b) hydrocele; (c) inguinoscrotal hernia; (d) epididymal cyst; (e) varicocele; (f) epididymo-orchitis; (g) testicular tumour; (h) encysted hydrocele of the cord.*

Although varicoceles usually occur on the left side, bilateral and right-sided varicoceles are not unusual. They usually present as a painless mass with a dragging sensation and there is increased distention of the veins on Valsalva manoeuvre. Sudden onset of varicocele in an adult may represent a renal tumour. Varicoceles in children may result in decreased testicular size.

Varicoceles lead to increase in the scrotal temperature, which can affect spermatogenesis. In adults, a stress pattern is seen on semen analysis (decreased motility, decreased count and increased abnormal forms); surgical correction improves the semen parameters. Repair of adolescent varicocele is said to improve testicular growth [1]. Repair of varicocele for testicular pain is usually fraught with recurrence of the pain in the postoperative period and patients should be counselled carefully. Varicocele surgery is an ambulatory surgery procedure. Percutaneous embolization of the testicular vein has been recommended in recurrent varicoceles.

Varicoceles have been repaired with an inguinal (Ivanesevich), retroperitoneal (Palomo) or scrotal approach. Microscopic repair has also been advocated. Laparoscopic varicocele ligation has not become widely accepted.

Epididymo-orchitis
Epididymo-orchitis is one of the very painful conditions that may affect men from pubertal age. It is associated with acute inflammation of epididymis and the testis (Fig. 9.1f). There is usually a significant swelling of the scrotal skin with oedema. Occasionally, there may be inflammation of the spermatic cord (funiculitis) and an associated hydrocele. *Chlamydia trachomatis* has been isolated in 60% of patients over 35 years of age; in men under 35 years of age, *Escherichia coli*, *Klebsiella* spp. and other Gram-negative uropathogens have been isolated. Bladder outflow problems are more likely to be present in older men. Epididymo-orchitis in prepubertal children is debatable. Testicular torsion should be the primary diagnosis in these children and exploration should be considered. Ultrasonography is used to evaluate testicular blood flow in order to rule out torsion, even in older men. If the response to antibiotics is slow or if the patient continues to be febrile, drainage of scrotal abscess or orchiectomy may be required. The urinary tract should be evaluated in older men to detect other problems, such as an outflow obstruction. The sequelae of acute epididymitis include hydrocele, scrotal abscess, epididymal tubular obstruction leading to infertility and, occasionally, testicular atrophy. Even after acute inflammatory features resolve, an indurated scrotal swelling may persist for 4–6 weeks, and often may be mistaken for a testicular tumour owing to its firm to hard nature.

Testicular tumour
Germ cell tumour (Fig. 9.1g) is the most life-threatening condition arising from the testis and

therefore all scrotal swellings deserve early evaluation to rule out malignancy. An undescended testis is a definite risk factor. Although testicular tumours can occur at any age, there are three peaks of incidence: birth to 10 years; 20–40 years; and older than 60 years. Caucasians are four times more likely than Blacks to develop testicular tumours. Testicular tumour has been reported in fathers and sons, but a definite inheritance pattern has not been established. Seminoma and mixed germ cell tumour are common in postpubertal men up to the age of 40 years. Yolk sac tumours and pure teratoma are common in infancy; in men over 50 years, spermatocytic seminoma and lymphoma are more frequent.

Testicular tumours are painless and may present with heaviness. Occasionally, minor testicular trauma brings attention to a slow-growing testicular mass. There is evidence to suggest that delay in diagnosis occurs in this population and leads to advanced clinical stage and higher morbidity. Scrotal ultrasonography may demonstrate characteristic hypoechoic shadows within the testis, although these appearances are not specific. Levels of tumour markers, such as alpha-fetoprotein and beta human chorionic gonadotrophin (βhCG), may be raised in men with these tumours. Abdominal examination may reveal para-aortic nodal masses. Detailed evaluation and treatment of testicular tumours is discussed in Chapter 4.

Encysted hydrocele of the cord
Occasionally, a cystic swelling is felt along the upper part of the scrotum separate from the testis, the epididymis and the vas deferens (Fig. 9.1h). This is the remnant of the processus vaginalis, which contains a clear fluid and is transilluminable. Surgical excision is recommended.

Genital lesions

Cutaneous genital lesions encountered in men include those caused by infections, trauma, some skin diseases, benign tumours, premalignant lesions and malignancies. Changes in sexual attitudes and practices have contributed to the resurgence of venereal disease infections and the spread of the human immunodeficiency virus (HIV) infection, many lesions of which may mimic other skin diseases and even neoplasms. Hence, the importance of acute awareness by the physician confronted with a genital lesion.

Infections

Herpes genitalis
Herpes genitalis is due to infection with herpes simplex virus (HSV) type 2 and is estimated to affect 20% of sexually active adults [2]. The primary lesion has an incubation period of 2–7 days, is vesicular and is associated with tender lymphadenopathy and mild fever. History of exposure, the Tzanck smear and tissue culture establish the diagnosis. The acute episode lasts for 7–14 days. Recurrent lesions are also vesicular and painful, but unattended with adenopathy; Tzanck smear and tissue culture are positive. The treatment of both conditions is oral acyclovir, 200 mg five times daily.

Syphilis
Treponema pallidum is the causative agent in syphilis. The primary lesion may be a papule, an erosion or an ulcer, usually on the penis, and the incubation period is 10–90 days. The lesion and bilateral adenopathy are indurated and non-tender. The lesion heals spontaneously in about 3–6 weeks, leaving an atrophic scar. Diagnosis is established by darkfield microscopy and/or serological tests. Penicillin is the treatment of choice.

Chancroid
Chancroid is caused by *Haemophilus ducreyi* and presents as a vesicle, papule or pustule, 3–5 days after exposure. Suppurative adenopathy develops 1 week later. Diagnosis is made by Gram stain of purulent secretion from the sore or lymph node aspirate. The treatment is ceftriaxone, 250 mg once intramuscularly, or ciprofloxacin, 500 mg orally twice a day for 3 days.

Lymphogranuloma venereum
Lymphogranuloma venereum lesions are due to infection with *Chlamydia trachomatis*; the incubation period is 5–21 days. The primary lesion — which may be a papule, vesicle or ulcer — lasts for only 2–3 days and is noted in only 10–40% of cases. Shortly thereafter, bilateral, tender, matted adenopathy appears; ultimately, abscess, fistula and ulceration develop. Fever, arthritis, pericarditis, proctitis, meningoencephalitis and keratoconjunctivitis are serious sequelae. The diagnosis may be made by positive complement fixation test, rheumatoid factor and cryoglobulins. The treatment of choice is doxycycline, 100 mg twice daily for 7 days.

Condylomata acuminata

Condylomata acuminata (genital warts) are common and are due to infection with the human papilloma virus (HPV). Two prognostically related lesions have been identified: those caused by HPV 6 have a benign course [3], whereas those caused by HPV 16, 18, 31, 33, or 51, which are oncogenic, are associated with a high cancer risk [4–6]. The lesions are characteristically large, fleshy, cauliflower-like excrescences around the glans, urethral orifice or perineum (Fig. 9.2). At times, the lesions, even the non-cancerous type, acquire huge proportions and invade tissues in a manner strongly suggestive of squamous cell carcinoma, particularly when the urethra is involved [7]. Genito-anal condylomata acuminata are common among heterosexual and homosexual men, but intra-anal warts are more common among the latter [3]. Treatment is by means of topical podophyllin or, preferably, by surgery.

Acquired immmunodeficiency syndrome

Acquired immmunodeficiency syndrome (AIDS) is a spectrum of disorders that may mimic or complicate other diseases and may predispose to infections by pathogens or opportunistic organisms. Many of these conditions have cutaneous manifestations. It is only by keeping in mind this possibility that the physician can achieve the best results in treatment and prevention. The scope of the problem has become so extensive that a multidisciplinary approach is mandatory. The most common genital dermatological conditions in HIV infection are herpes genitalis, staphylococcal folliculitis, molluscum contagiosum, seborrhoeic dermatitis, psoriasis and *Candida balanitis*.

Organ transplant recipients

Although anogenital lesions in organ transplant recipients are rare, they may represent a marker of immunosuppression. The presence of dysplastic histological aspects and oncogenic human papilloma virus (HPV) types may pave the way towards malignant transformation [8]. It has been shown that, of 291 renal allograft recipients, 172 had cutaneous warts and 64 had non-melanoma skin cancers [9].

Trauma-related lesions

Trauma-related lesions are usually skin tears or ulcers with irregular margins and are easily recognized by history and by the lack of features which, to the dermatologist, would fit the pattern of a skin disease. The determination of the nature of the presenting lesion is in itself adequate therapy; psychiatry may be helpful in some cases.

Skin diseases

Skin diseases affecting the genitalia are almost invariably part and parcel of the entity in question. However, some nonconforming conditions have been encountered: lichen planus of the glans, a mucosal surface, can exist without overt cutaneous lesions; the same applies to Behçet's disease (aphthosis), which is a symptom complex of oral and genital ulceration. The importance of

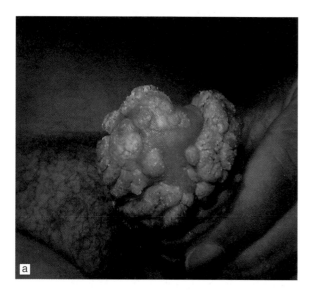

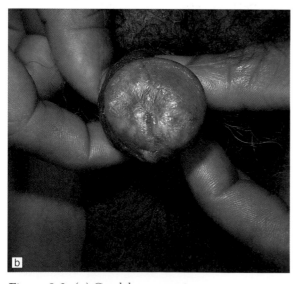

Figure 9.2. *(a) Condyloma acuminatum: verrucous growth on the glans, encroaching on the meatus; (b) following excision.*

obtaining a detailed history and undertaking careful examination of the entire body surface, when confronted with any type of cutaneous lesion, cannot be overemphasized, however trivial that lesion may appear to be.

Benign tumours

Benign tumours of the genitalia are relatively uncommon and usually not much of a problem. They include epithelial cysts, angiomas, angiokeratoma (Fordyce), fibromas, neuromas, myomas and lipomas. Although condyloma acuminatum (venereal wart) is generally considered to be a benign lesion that presents little difficulty in diagnosis, its eradication can prove problematic [3]. In addition, some authors have found a relationship to verrucous carcinoma of the Buschke– Lowenstein type [10,11].

Premalignant lesions and carcinoma in situ

Clinicopathological considerations

The clinical features of premalignant and malignant lesions of the external genitalia can be protean. Lesions may appear banal or may simulate benign conditions, often resulting in incorrect diagnosis. Furthermore, many skin diseases, including malignancies, in the genital region can closely mimic one another. It is, therefore, imperative to identify the true nature of the lesion under consideration so that a malignancy is treated as early as possible. This is best achieved by histopathological examination. Biopsy material is most adequate and informative when obtained by excision or through an incision. Deep shave and punch biopsies are satisfactory if subcutaneous tissue is included in the material.

The techniques of administering anaesthesia for surgical procedures on the male genitalia depend on the diagnosis, the size and site of the lesion, and the type of surgery. Local infiltration or field block are recommended for excision of lesions on the scrotum or in the skin of the shaft of the penis. Regional block of the penis is required when the lesions are numerous and when the glans, corpus spongiosum, corpora cavernosa or fraenulum are involved.

Erythroplasia of Queyrat (EQ)

EQ is a squamous cell carcinoma in situ that affects genital mucosae of men and women, but is more common in men. In the latter, it occurs almost exclusively on the inner surface of the prepuce and on the glans [11]. Although the aetiology of EQ remains unclear, the condition appears to be related to irritation by an agent in smegma inside the preputial sac; it is not seen in individuals who have been circumcized during infancy. The normal age range for occurrence is 20–80 years [12].

Lesions present as reddish, shiny, velvety plaques (Fig. 9.3), which may be asymptomatic but are usually pruritic. In many cases such lesions have been mistaken for inflammatory conditions, notably eczema, contact dermatitis and candidiasis. The development of ulceration signifies the development of invasive epidermoid (squamous cell) carcinoma. It has been estimated that about 10% of EQ cases have evidence of squamous cell carcinoma, and 2% have lymph node metastasis by the time that the patients present for treatment [12]. A recent study found the oncogenic HPV 16 present in 92% (23/25) of lesions of carcinoma in situ [13].

The histopathology of EQ is similar to that of Bowen's precancerous dermatosis (Bowen's disease). However, it differs from it with regard to aetiology, course and prognosis. Unlike Bowen's disease, EQ is not associated with an increased incidence of internal malignancies nor is it related to the ingestion of arsenic, but it has a greater propensity towards invasiveness and metastasis. In one series of 42 cases of EQ, invasive carcinoma had developed in 14 (33%); of 21 cases of carcinoma, 30% had EQ [14]. The importance of obtaining biopsy material from any recalcitrant lesion cannot be overemphasized. A urological consultation is mandatory in all cases, as lesions have been known to extend proximally along the urethral mucosa.

Topical chemotherapy with 5-fluorouracil (5-FU), applied as a 5% cream preparation twice daily for a minimum of 3–4 weeks, has been used [15,16], but this modality is more suited to small, non-ulcerated lesions if the patient declines surgery. An inflammatory reaction may result, taking 1–5 months to subside. This treatment is apparently effective in some cases, but several courses may be necessary to achieve cure; unsatisfactory results have been reported [17–19].

Because EQ is unresponsive to radiotherapy [12], ablation is the treatment of choice. Surgery is effective and the morbidity is short. The type of surgical approach depends upon the site of the lesion and its extent: circumcision is curative when the disease is limited to the prepuce; lesions on the glans can be adequately excised by Mohs' micrographic surgery. The base of the resulting wound is usually electrocoagulated to control bleeding and is left to heal by granula-

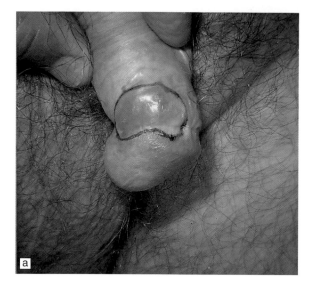

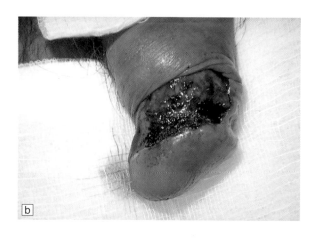

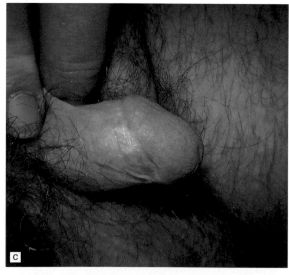

Figure 9.3. *Erythroplasia of Queyrat: (a) velvety erythematous plaque in the coronal sulcus; (b) wound after Mohs' fresh tissue excision; (c) 6 weeks after healing by second intention.*

tion. Healing is excellent, even when the wound is large (Fig. 9.4). When foreskin is available, the defect on the glans may be covered with a graft from the preputial skin; when the site is in the coronal sulcus, the wound may be repaired by simple approximating suture of the margins.

Bowen's disease

Bowen's disease is a squamous cell carcinoma in situ of the skin of middle-aged or elderly people. It may be encountered on the shaft of the penis, the inguinal and suprapubic areas, the scrotum and the perineum (i.e. sites that contain pilosebaceous follicles and sweat glands). The lesion usually presents as a solitary, crusted, dull-red plaque that may simulate psoriasis, dermatophytosis, or other inflammatory conditions (Fig. 9.5). As in EQ, histopathology is the clue to the diagnosis. Unlike EQ, which involves the mucosae, Bowen's disease affects the epithelium of the skin and its adnexa. This attribute renders topical 5-FU inadequate because the drug lacks deep penetration. This is especially important as invasive carcinoma is likely to have developed in 50% of cases by the time that patients present themselves for treatment [12]. The standard recommended treatment is excision with a surgical margin of 0.5 cm. The excised tissue should include subcutaneous fat to ensure removal of any underlying carcinoma. It has been reported that Bowen's disease, especially when it occurs on covered areas of the body, may be associated with internal malignancies [12]; however, Bowen's disease should not be considered a skin marker for internal malignancy.

Bowenoid papulosis

Bowenoid papulosis of the genitalia is a recently documented lesion that occurs in sexually active young men and women [20]. The lesions of bowenoid papulosis are multiple and appear as small, hyperpigmented papules that resemble venereal warts (Fig. 9.6). The aetiological agent is the HPV group, which contains as many as 67 recognized types. Of these, the oncogenic HPV 16, 18, 31, 33 and 51 have been encountered in bowenoid papulosis [5]. Without doubt, the disease is sexually transmitted. Diagnosis is made by histological examination and the pathology is identical to that of Bowen's disease, but the lesions are smaller. In a series of 12 men, nine of their consorts were also infected, and six of the women had squamous cell carcinoma in situ of the cervix uteri. It is, therefore, important carefully to examine

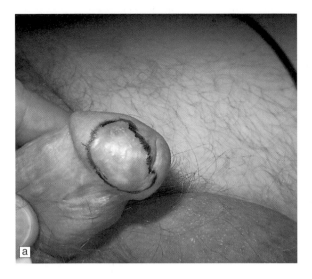

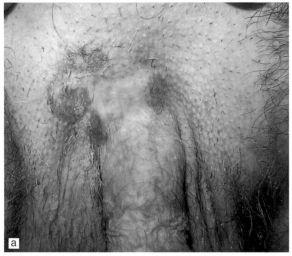

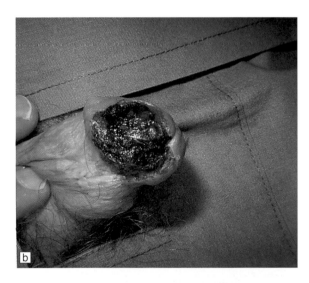

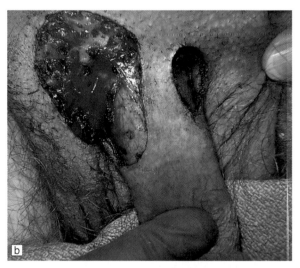

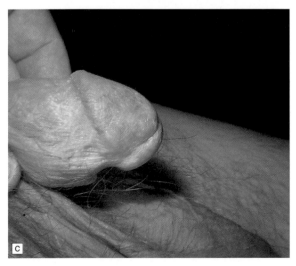

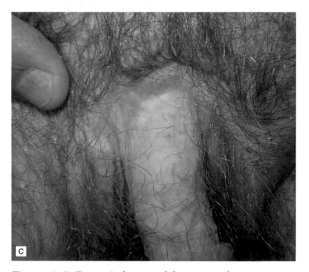

Figure 9.4. *Erythroplasia of Queyrat: (a) smooth plaque on glans; (b) wound after Mohs' fresh tissue excision; (c) 6 months after surgery.*

Figure 9.5. *Bowen's disease of the suprapubic area: (a) crusted, erythematous plaques; (b) after Mohs' fresh tissue excision; (c) after healing by second intention.*

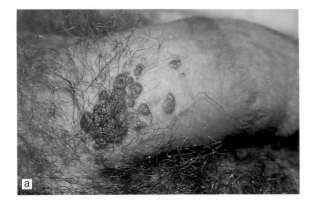

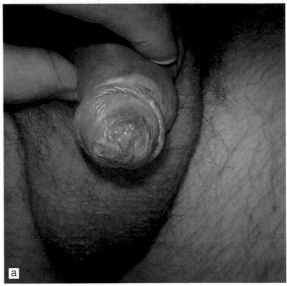

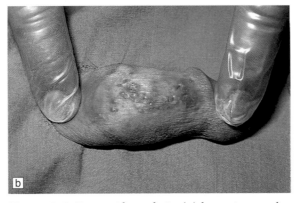

Figure 9.6. *Bowenoid papulosis: (a) hyperpigmented verrucous papules; (b) multiple, small erythematous papules.*

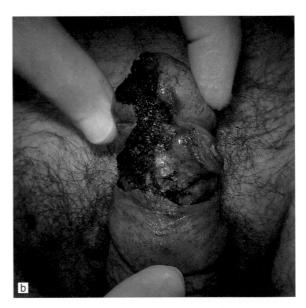

all sexual contacts. Subclinical penile HPV infection and dysplasias in consorts of women with cervical neoplasia have also been reported [21]. Although lesions may regress spontaneously, extirpation is recommended by simple excision or by destruction with fulgurating current.

Leukoplakia

Leukoplakia of the mucosal surface of the glans is rare and appears to occur with greater frequency in diabetic patients. The condition is precancerous and is even considered an epidermoid carcinoma in situ by some pathologists [10]. The lesion presents as a scaly, greyish-white patch, usually with surrounding erythema (Fig. 9.7). The urethral meatus is commonly involved, and this may eventually result in stricture. The condition is often diagnosed as lichen sclerosus et atrophicus in men and kraurosis vulvae in women. The real identity of the lesion is usually recognized in retrospect after the development of a frank carcinoma. The histology is identical with that of leukoplakia of

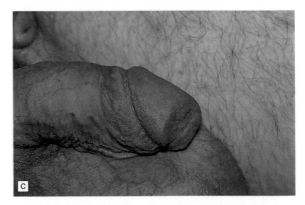

Figure 9.7. *Leukoplakia: (a) scaly, greyish plaque on the glans with an erythematous base; (b) extent of the disease after Mohs' excision; (c) healed lesion.*

the oral mucosa. Mohs' micrographic surgery is the usual treatment.

Verrucous carcinoma of the penis

Verrucous carcinoma, also called giant condyloma acuminatum or Buschke–Lowenstein tumour, is believed by some to be an invasive variant of condyloma acuminatum; similarly, it is caused by the non-oncogenic HPV 6 [3,5]. Other workers consider the lesion to be a low-grade malignancy that has a protracted course, is locally aggressive but does not have the tendency to metastasize [10,22]. The neoplasm develops and grows to a large, exophytic, fungating mass on the glans and prepuce (Fig. 9.2). When the meatus is involved, there is marked tendency of proximal extension along the urethra. The histopathology is similar to that of condyloma acuminatum. The only satisfactory treatment is surgical ablation. Mohs' technique gives excellent results by extirpating the tumour while maximally preserving normal

tissues and function, especially when there is proximal extension along the urethra [23].

Epidermoid (squamous cell) carcinoma of the penis

Although relatively rare, squamous (epidermoid) carcinoma is the most frequent form of penile cancer, second only to squamous cell carcinoma in situ (EQ and Bowen's disease). Many patients have advanced disease by the time they seek treatment, because of either the fear of phallectomy or failure of recognition of an early lesion beneath a phimotic prepuce. Hence the importance of adopting a high index of suspicion and performing biopsies on any recalcitrant lesion to ensure early treatment.

The clinical presentation of epidermoid carcinoma of the penis can be quite protean. It may be a papule, a nodule, a plaque, an erosion or an ulcer (Fig. 9.8). The histopathology is characteristic and the staging system devised by Jackson is

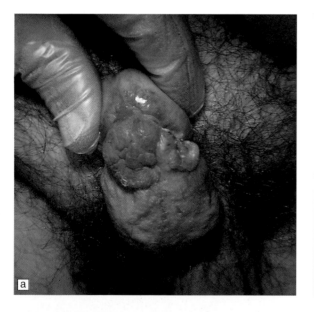

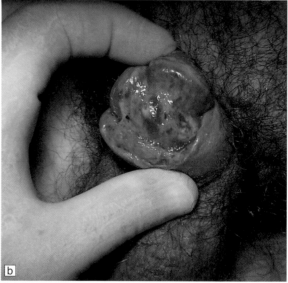

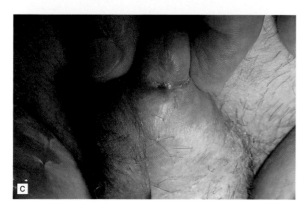

Figure 9.8. *Stage II squamous cell carcinoma of the glans and the coronal sulcus: (a) large ulcerated nodule; (b) granulating wound after excision by Mohs' fixed tissue technique; (c) small urethral fistula that resulted (lesion later classified stage III because of a positive inguinal node).*

Table 9.1. *Jackson staging for carcinoma of the penis [24]*

Stage	Description
I	Tumour limited to glans and/or prepuce
II	Involvement of shaft or corpora cavernosa with absence of lymph node or distant metastases
III	Tumour in shaft with biopsy-proven regional node metastasis
IV	Inoperable regional node involvement or distant metastasis

universally recognized (Table 9.1) [24]. Prognosis has proved to correlate well with tumour stage [10,24].

The standard surgical practice among most urologists has been circumcision when the tumour is limited to the prepuce, amputation at 2–2.5 cm proximal to visible or palpable neoplasm when the lesion is on the glans or coronal sulcus, and radical phallectomy when the tumour site is higher up on the shaft. As the majority of lesions occur on the glans, amputation at 2.5 cm beyond the clinical limits is rather mutilating. Conservative excision employing the Mohs' technique maximally preserves normal tissue [14,19,25].

Epidermoid (squamous cell) carcinoma of the perineum

Although rare, cancer of the perineum and anal region is often mistaken for benign skin diseases or inflammatory conditions, resulting in delayed diagnosis and treatment. Pathologically, the majority are of the epidermoid (squamous cell carcinoma) type and usually arise in the cloacogenic zone (anorectal junction), which is lined with transitional epithelium, or in the anal orifice, which is lined with squamous epithelium. The peak frequency is at age 55–60, with the greater occurrence in women than in men [26]. The most common presenting symptom is bleeding and the sensation of an obstructive mass, which is often ulcerated and draining; anal fistulas may be present. These complications render the prognosis ominous. Radical surgery and/or radiotherapy are the recommended treatment modalities.

Extramammary Paget's disease

Extramammary Paget's disease (EMPD) is a rare intra-epidermal apocrine sweat gland carcinoma, which most commonly affects the vulva in post-menopausal women and, less frequently, in the anogenital area of elderly men [27]. The disease presents clinically as one or more slowly enlarging, inflammatory, erythematous plaques on the genital, perigenital or perineal skin. The lesions resemble, among other conditions, psoriasis, intertrigo, dermatophytosis and candidiasis (Fig. 9.9), accounting for the delay in initiating treatment. More than 50% of the patients complain of pruritus and some experience pain or bleeding. The histopathology of EMPD is characteristic and is the clue to the diagnosis. The epidermis contains distinctive clear cells which are large, have a pale cytoplasm and are replete with neutral and sulphonated mucopolysaccharides. Paget's cells can be traced from the epidermis to deeper tissues along cutaneous appendages. Invasion of the corium and lymph node metastasis may thus result. In rare instances, EMPD is a secondary event caused by extension of an adenocarcinoma either of the rectum to the perianal region [28], or from the urinary bladder to the urethra and glans penis [29] or to the inguinal region [30]. All patients should be submitted to a careful search for concomitant rectal or colonic carcinoma.

Like Bowen's disease, EMPD can involve the epithelium of hair follicles and sweat ducts. Consequently, topical chemotherapy with 5-FU or bleomycin is not effective; the disease is also recalcitrant to radiotherapy [28], the only effective treatment being surgical excision. Because of the characteristic histology, which is easily recognized in frozen sections, Mohs' surgery is well

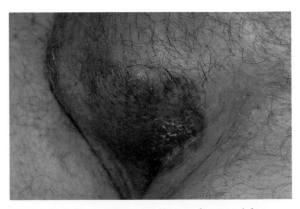

Figure 9.9. *Extramammary Paget's disease of the scrotum and perineum, showing close resemblance to Bowen's disease and inflammatory skin conditions.*

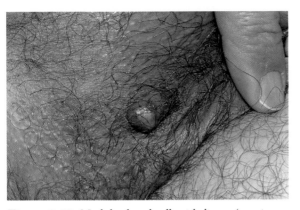

Figure 9.10. *Nodular basal cell epithelioma (carcinoma) on the scrotum.*

suited. Mohs and Blanchard have reported five cases of EMPD treated successfully by microscopically controlled surgery [31]: patients remained free of disease for periods ranging from 4 months to 9 years. However, recurrences may appear beyond 10 years because the disease is usually multifocal [26].

Basal cell carcinoma

Basal cell carcinomas are only rarely seen on the genitals. A large number of cases are of the nodular pigmented type (Fig. 9.10). They can be 0.5–2.0 cm in diameter and appear to be equally divided between men and women. Of note is the case of a woman with the naevoid basal cell carcinoma syndrome: in addition to a multitude of face, scalp and trunk lesions, she had about 15 lesions on the vulva. Again, the clue to the diagnosis is the histopathology; treatment is surgical.

Malignant melanoma

Malignant melanoma of the genitalia is rare and amounts to less than 1% of all primary carcinomas of the penis. The prognosis is poor, even with radical surgery, owing to the frequency of early metastases.

References

1. Kass EJ, Freitas JE, Bour JB. Adolescent varicocele: objective indication for treatment. *J Urol* 1989; 142: 579–582
2. Sparling PF, Hook EW. Sexually transmitted diseases. In: Bennett JC, Plum F (eds) Cecil textbook of medicine, 20th edn. Philadelphia: Saunders, 1995: 1696–1713
3. Wikstrom A. Clinical and serological manifestations of genital human papillomavirus infection. *Acta Derm Venereol Suppl* (Stockh) 1995; 75(193): 1–85
4. Della Torre G, Donghi R, Longoni A *et al.* HPV DNA in intraepithelial neoplasia and carcinoma of the vulva and penis. *Diagn Mol Pathol* 1992; 1: 25–31
5. Pennys N. Diseases caused by viruses. In: Elder D (ed) Lever's histopathology of the skin, 8th edn. Philadelphia: Lippincott–Raven 1997: 569–589
6. Obalek S, Jablonska S, Beaudenon S *et al.* Bowenoid papulosis of the male and female genitalia: risk of cervical neoplasia. *J Am Acad Dermatol* 1986; 14: 433–437
7. Kaplinsky RS, Pranikoff K, Chasan S, DeBerry JL. Indications for urethroscopy in male patients with penile condylomata. *J Urol* 1995; 153(4): 1120–1121
8. Euvrard S, Kanitakis J, Chardonnet Y *et al.* External anogenital lesions in organ transplant recipients. *Arch Dermatol* 1997; 133: 175–178
9. Glover MT, Niranjan N, Kwan JTC, Leigh IM. Non-melanoma skin cancer in renal transplant recipients: the extent of the problem and a strategy for management. *Br J Plast Surg* 1994; 47: 86–89
10. Schellhamer PE, Grabstaldt H. Tumors of the penis. In: Campbell's urology, 4th edn. Philadelphia: Saunders, 1979; 1175–1188
11. Sanderson KV. Erythroplasia of Queyrat. In: Rook A, Wilkinson D, Ebling F (eds) Textbook of dermatology, 3rd edn. Oxford: Blackwell Scientific, 1979; 1963–1964
12. Graham JH, Helwig EB. Erythroplasia of Queyrat: a clinicopathologic and histochemical study. *Cancer* 1973; 32: 1396–1414
13. Cupp ED, Malek RS, Goellner JR *et al.* The detection of human papillomavirus desoxyribonucleic acid in intraepithelial, in situ, verrucous and invasive carcinoma of the penis. *J Urol* 1995; 154(3): 1024–1029
14. Mikhail GR. Cancers, precancers, and pseudocancers on the male genitalia. *J Dermatol Surg Oncol* 1980; 6: 1027–1035
15. Goette DK, Carson TE. Erythroplasia of Queyrat. *Cancer* 1976; 38: 1498–1502
16. Goette DK, Elgart M, De Villez RL. Erythroplasia of Queyrat: treatment with topically applied fluorouracil. *JAMA* 1975; 232: 934–937
17. Kopf AW, Bart RS. Skin tumor conference No. 5: Erythematous plaque of the penis. *J Dermatol Surg* 1976; 2: 14
18. Lifshit S, Roberts JA. Treatment of carcinoma in situ of the vulva with topical 5-fluorouracil. *Obstet Gynecol* 1980; 56: 242–244
19. Mikhail GR. Cancers of the genitalia and the perineum. In: Mikhail GR (ed) Mohs micrographic surgery. Philadelphia: Saunders, 1991: 234–260
20. Turner MLC. Human papilloma virus infection of the genital tract. *Prog Dermatol* 1989; 23(2): 1–12
21. Campion MJ, McCane DJ, Mitchell HS *et al.* Subclinical penile human papilloma virus infection and dysplasia in consorts of women with cervical neoplasia. *Genitourin Med* 1988; 64: 90–99
22. Hotchkiss RS. Cancer of the skin of the male genitalia. In: Andrade R, Gumport SL, Popkin GL *et al.* (eds) Cancer of the skin. Philadelphia: Saunders, 1976: 1409–1432

23. Mohs FE. Chemosurgery: microscopically controlled surgery for skin cancer, 2nd edn. Springfield, IL: Charles C. Thomas, 1978: 210–214

24. Jackson SM. The treatment of carcinoma of the penis. *Br J Surg* 1966; 53: 33–35

25. Snow SN. Techniques and indications for Mohs micrographic surgery. In: Mikhail GR (ed) Mohs micrographic surgery. Philadelphia: Saunders, 1991: 11–60

26. Taylor PT, Stenwig JT, Clausen H. Paget's disease of the vulva. *Gynecol Oncol* 1975; 3: 46–50

27. Murrell TW Jr, McCullan FH. Extramammary Paget's disease. *Arch Dermatol* 1962; 85: 600–601

28. Helwig EB, Graham JH. Anogenital (extramammary) Paget's disease: a clinicopathological study. *Cancer* 1963; 16: 387–395

29. Metcalf JS, Lee RE, Maise JC. Epidermotropic urothelial carcinoma involving the glans penis. *Arch Dermatol* 1985; 121: 532–533

30. Ojeda VJ, Heenan PJ, Watson SH. Paget's disease of the groin associated with adenocarcinoma of the urinary bladder. *J Cutan Pathol* 1987; 14: 227–229

31. Mohs FE, Blanchard L. Microscopically controlled surgery for extramammary Paget's disease. *Arch Dermatol* 1979; 115: 706–708

Heart disease: lipids and hypertension

A. F. Winder and I. James

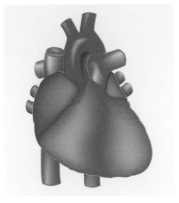

LIPIDS

Introduction

Atherosclerosis-related diseases, and particularly ischaemic heart disease (IHD), are now the commonest cause of death worldwide, especially among men [1]. There are many associations with risk of premature IHD [2], the primary ones being hypertension, cigarette smoking and lipid profile (i.e. levels of blood fats, such as cholesterol, triglycerides and lipoproteins). Levels of cholesterol in the UK are high by world standards, as are deaths from IHD. This is particularly so for Scotland and Northern Ireland, where heavier cigarette smoking may explain the relative lack of improvement in recent years compared with England and Wales [3]. Comparisons between and within different countries suggest that risk of IHD increases with cholesterol level.

Average levels of cholesterol in the UK are currently 12% above those in North America, where a desirable level of 5.2 mmol/l suggested for adults is exceeded by some 80% of adults in the UK [3]. Epidemiological data suggest that risk of a first heart attack increases sharply above 5.2 mmol/l, and even lower levels are now recommended in the USA, Europe and the UK for secondary prevention in patients with established angina or infarction [4]. Such patients with evident atherosclerotic disease have an approximate 90% chance of death through a cardiac event, and recent lipid-lowering trials have shown clear benefits in such secondary prevention. Primary prevention through treatment of patients who are clinically well has potential [5], but individuals who might benefit cannot yet be clearly defined.

Establishing a single recommended lipid level is difficult, as levels increase with age and are different in men and women. Furthermore, the contribution of individual lipoproteins to total cholesterol needs to be considered, as well as other factors, such as blood pressure (BP). This whole-patient approach has been favoured in the UK and Europe, where treatment decisions are based on a perception of overall (i.e. absolute) risk. Raised cholesterol increases cholesterol-related relative risk but, in the absence of other influences, the overall risk can still be low [6,7].

The female:male ratio

Average levels of total cholesterol for the UK population steadily increase with age until beyond the age of 75 years [3,8]. Levels in adult men slow down at 5.9–6.0 mmol/l by about 45 years of age, when they are overtaken by levels in women, which increase steadily to mean levels of about 7.0 mmol/l by 72 years of age. The general increase with age is seen worldwide for industrialized countries and may well relate to lifestyle, weight gain in particular. Triglyceride level also increases with age, but there is little effect on high-density lipoprotein (HDL), for which levels are uniform in children, but in boys fall by some 20% at puberty. The higher HDL levels in females are presumed to be oestrogen dependent but, oddly, do not fall to male levels at the menopause. IHD is the commonest single cause of death in men and women, but develops a decade earlier in men.

Aetiology

The main fats in the blood are cholesterol, cholesterol derivatives (esters) and triglycerides, carried as complexes with proteins — the lipoproteins. Lipoproteins contain different proportions of fat and protein and can be usefully classified and separated on the basis of density (i.e.

higher levels of protein result in higher density). Some 70% of the total cholesterol in plasma is carried as low-density lipoprotein (LDL), so the levels of the two are closely related. LDL level is also closely related to the development of atheroma. Of the remaining lipoproteins, approximately 25% is HDL (of which high levels seem advantageous) and very-low-density lipoprotein (VLDL). Population studies show that above-mean levels of HDL can be associated with a below-mean incidence of premature IHD. Mean levels of HDL are about 1.25 mmol/l in men and 1.55 mmol/l in women. High values above 1.6 or 2.0 mmol/l, respectively, can be reassuring and show that a moderately raised cholesterol is not associated with LDL excess. Levels below 1.0 mmol/l in women and 0.9 mmol/l in men are of concern. Weight loss and aerobic exercise through lifestyle is generally associated with an increase in HDL and some reduction in LDL, cholesterol and triglycerides, although individual responses vary. As well as lifestyle, many other metabolic disorders can secondarily affect lipid profiles, notably hypothyroidism with raised cholesterol and LDL, alcoholism, diabetes, glucose intolerance and chronic liver or renal impairment, all with excess of cholesterol and triglycerides and reduced HDL [9,10]. VLDL is the main carrier of triglycerides in the fasting state. Triglyceride-rich chylomicrons are also produced by the intestine in response to a fat-rich meal, but are normally cleared in a few hours. Excess levels of VLDL and triglycerides can be associated with increased cardiovascular risk, but the mechanisms involved are not yet clearly defined.

Studies of settled populations, and of those which migrate and change their dietary habits, show that diets, particularly the intake of total fat, have strong associations with lipid profiles and particularly levels of cholesterol and LDL. Incidental medication may also adversely affect lipid profiles, such as some beta blockers or diuretics for hypertension (see below) and, in occasional patients, retinoids prescribed for psoriasis. Many single-gene defects have been identified with effects on lipid profiles [11]; these include variant or defective proteins and enzymes affecting the assembly or turnover of chylomicrons and HDL and of LDL clearance through defects in the LDL cell-surface receptors, or the LDL apoB protein to which it binds, all collectively forming the clinical syndrome of heterozygous familial hypercholesterolaemia (FH). FH affects around 1 in 500 in the UK, but over 400 different gene defects are known with essentially the same end result. Less rare

influences, perhaps affecting a few per cent of the population, include structurally incomplete low-activity variants of the enzyme lipoprotein lipase (LPL), which is released into plasma and contributes to clearance of triglyceride-rich lipoproteins and the generation of HDL.

The fifth set of proteins defined in the lipoproteins, the apolipoprotein E family, has three common forms (E-2, E-3, E-4) differing by one amino acid, and many other collectively rare genetic variants. For populations the common patterns have some influence on lipid profiles and also responses to diets. Both parental genes are expressed, occasional individuals from the 1 in 70 with the E-2/E-2 profile may show major delay in chylomicron and VLDL clearance and associated arterial disease if another provoking lipid disorder such as diabetes or alcoholism is also present, showing the interaction between genes and environment, nature and nurture. The impact of hypercholesterolaemia and LDL excess may also be increased in the presence of high levels of lipoprotein [Lp(a)]. Lp(a) is LDL linked to a further protein designated apolipoprotein(a) and has some structural similarity to plasminogen, active in clot breakdown. Lp(a) may bind to clots in place of plasminogen and high levels may therefore be antithrombolytic. Each parent transmits a gene for one of at least 40 molecular forms of Lp(a). Forms with a shorter chain length produce higher levels of Lp(a) in plasma, which can act as a conditional risk factor in the presence of LDL excess. Very high levels in excess of 10 times the normal value are found in young survivors of myocardial infarcts and may therefore constitute a direct risk of premature clinical events. These uncommon-to-rare specific defects are probably the tip of a genetic iceberg [11].

Investigation

Targeted lipid screening is an attractive approach to risk assessment and wider issues, such as blood pressure and lifestyle, should also be considered [6,9,10,12]. Lipid screening is recommended for patients and families with (a) premature coronary or other arterial disease, (b) other known cardiovascular risks, particularly hypertension, (c) a known family lipid problem, and (d) physical signs consistent with lipid problems, such as corneal arcus before the age of 50 years, xanthelasmata or other rarer lipid deposits such as tendon xanthomata. Lipaemic cigarette smokers are also at increased cardiovascular risk until about 5 years after they stop, but opinion as to whether they merit priority lipid screening and potential lipid medication is divided: greater short-term benefit comes from persuading patients to give up smoking. Recent trials have shown benefits from lipid medication in diabetic patients [13], but less than 10% of such patients are treated.

The basic lipid profile involves determination of total cholesterol, triglycerides and HDL as HDL-cholesterol [10]. The HDL contribution to risk can be expressed as the HDL:cholesterol or HDL:LDL ratios. The value of these terms in patient management can be overemphasized, however: they are produced from two measurements, each subject to error, and most of the variation in ratios within populations is actually from LDL. Triglycerides are not of particular concern if fasting levels are below approximately 1.3 mmol/l.

Some cardiac units have a special interest in levels and isoforms (size patterns) of Lp(a). ApoE patterns may help in defining cause of unusual mixed lipaemia, particularly if the spectacular physical sign of yellow palmar creases is present. Studies of apoE and LPL variants are also recommended if parents could be distantly related and thus, through consanguinity, increasing the chance of a double dose of an adverse gene.

Serious attention to the underlying cause of a lipid abnormality is important, as approximately half of the patients referred have a contributory disorder, such as diabetes. Family screening of all available first-degree relatives is particularly recommended under two circumstances: (1) when a familial disorder is suspected from the history and clinical findings, and (2) when no apparent cause has emerged.

Treatment

The majority of treatment guidelines are based on calculations from the Framingham study [7]. The first priority for treatment goes to patients with former infarcts, angina or other atherosclerotic disease, or severe genetic lipaemias. Next priority is to patients with additional risk factors, notably hypertension, family history of early heart disease and diabetes. Lowest priority goes to the elderly without symptoms who are incidentally found to have some lipid abnormality, often mild in comparison with age-related means [8]. All the large lipid-lowering trials have shown that treatment benefits can take about 2 years to develop, so for elderly patients otherwise at priority, a life expectancy of at least 2 high-quality years may influence a decision to treat.

Diet

Dietary change is the initial approach to all lipaemic patients. Patients with mixed lipaemia and raised triglycerides are usually overweight. A reduced-fat diet can help, as fat provides more calories per gram than protein or carbohydrate. A switch from stable saturated lardy fats and foods to lower-fat products and unsaturated oils, such as olive oil, can also be of benefit; nevertheless, the 'good fats' are also calorie rich and must be used sparingly or weight will be hard to control. Green vegetables in the diet can help, as they provide some bulk to meals and reduce appetite without much increase in the calorie load. Eating is one of the pleasures of life, and patients are not well served by daunting regimens with wholemeal bread, lentils and sunflower margarine; it is better to be less hostile to some favourite foods but to cut down on quantity. The same applies to alcohol, which can be a major source of excess calories. Changes in behaviour and attitude to food are important and can be helped by group sessions.

An undervalued effect of diet change is that lipaemic patients who lose weight have a greater response to any subsequent lipid medication. National surveys show that average calorie intakes have fallen in recent years, but activity levels have fallen even more [14]. So, nationally, the case for more exercise and activity is clear.

Statins and fibrates

The main drugs in current use are the statins and the fibrates. Statins reversibly inhibit a key enzyme in the cholesterol synthetic pathway, which is predominantly active in the liver. Recent statin trials have shown very clear benefits in terms of reduction in deaths and cardiovascular events, including stroke, in secondary prevention for patients with existing heart disease [15,16] and less clear, but still definite, benefits in primary prevention [5]. There are some differences between the six statins now available in the extent and time course of their body distribution, effects on blood coagulation, pathways of metabolic inactivation and maximum potency. Statins are generally well tolerated and complications are uncommon, but can include hypersensitivity with rashes, muscle and joint aches and, very rarely, extreme muscle breakdown (rhabdomyolysis), particularly when given in combination with other drugs, notably cyclosporin;

hence, any combination therapy must be approached with extreme caution. Statins mainly affect cholesterol and LDL levels, so hypercholesterolaemic patients are targeted.

Fibrates have a quite different effect, indirectly increasing activity of the enzyme LPL, which is released into plasma and promotes the breakdown of triglyceride lipoproteins and the generation of HDL [17]. Some fibrates reduce fibrinogen by up to 30%. Although this effect has not been proved to benefit patients, a major reduction can influence choice of fibrate. Fibrates may be considered for patients with mixed lipaemia and low HDL. A brief 3-week trial can also be informative, as a lack of response may show that the problem is not of triglyceride–lipoprotein processing. A statin may then be considered if there is an excess of LDL. As with statins, patients are occasionally hypersensitive with rashes and muscle cramps; warfarin effects are increased through displacement from plasma protein binding and prothrombin times should be monitored.

There is increasing interest in statin/fibrate combination therapy for patients with refractory mixed lipaemia, although clear guidelines and benefits have not yet been defined. Cholesterol levels have a close association with large-vessel disease and early death in type II diabetic patients. This may be due to modification of the LDL fraction to smaller, denser triglyceride-rich material sensitive to minor chemical change through oxidation and which accumulates in artery walls. Although statins have been shown to have clear clinical benefits for diabetic patients [13], perhaps because LDL is lowered, the composition is little changed, whereas it can revert towards normal with fibrates. Trials of combination therapy in type II diabetes are now in progress.

Other agents in occasional use include resins, which combine with bile acids in the small intestine and induce their loss in stools. This necessitates the synthesis of new bile acids via diversion of cholesterol in the liver. Resins can alter bowel habits, cause gastritis and interfere with the absorption of other medications. Concerns that absorption of vitamins and other essential nutrients might be impaired have been allayed. Nicotinates can suppress tissue lipolysis and release of fatty acids for lipoprotein production, but are not effective until doses are in the grams/day range. They may cause major flushing and sometimes dermatitis and liver toxicity. Low-dose aspirin (generally 75 mg/day) is also recommended as an antiplatelet agent for all those with established vascular disease, and for those regarded to be at increased risk of stroke [18]. It is also possible that non-insulin dependent diabetic patients without vascular symptoms may benefit, but a place in general primary prevention is not yet defined.

Shared care and evidence-based guidelines

Lipids are only one aspect of cardiac risk and their significance depends on the overall risk to the patient. The development of systems to evaluate overall risk from all available information continues, generally based on the calculations from the Framingham study [7]. The Sheffield table (and its later versions) [19,20] is one such development, heavily influencing the Standing Medical Advisory Committee (SMAC) in the production of their own guidelines. These guidelines are considered too absolute, however: they are expressed, for example, as whether hypertension is present or not, with no light or shade to account for severity in individuals rather than populations.

Within the spectrum of cardiovascular disease, some GPs are reluctant to manage lipidaemic patients, in spite of the relative simplicity of this area of medicine today and the considerable postgraduate support with seminars and clinic attachments available. Costs, and the continuing development of new agents, are a part of this concern, but these pressures also apply to clinics. Existing guidelines, such as those of the joint British recommendations [9] and the SMAC [4], apply to prioritization as well as to targets. The issue of whether there is a target level of cholesterol or other lipid marker beyond which few, if any, further benefits arise forms the basis of the SMAC guidelines for secondary prevention and the targets of 4.8 and 5.5 mmol/l of total cholesterol in patients with infarction or angina. For such secondary prevention, there are clear benefits from lowering LDL to below 3 mmol/l. However, greater reduction will probably not provide a proportionally greater benefit.

The ASPIRE (Action on Secondary Prevention through Intervention to Reduce Events) study showed that lipid profile and other risk factors identified in postinfarct patients are not well managed in the hospital ward and clinic [21]. One difficulty is that the acute circumstances of the coronary care unit are not well suited to detailed investigation of any metabolic disorder or family background, which is best addressed in the calmer circumstances of the 6–12-week follow-up. However, if lipid management is not initiated at the admission, then the family practitioner and patient may not see this as important. Thus, at least in secondary prevention, lipid medication from admission and based on levels of total cholesterol only may be a necessary compromise, with agreement on when patients are to be followed up, what is to be done and by whom. Opportunities for clear-cut benefits, including the use of aspirin, are also missed in primary care [22]. These observations are being developed into widely based protocols for management of cardiovascular risk in primary care [22,23]. Shared care and a more cooperative approach are obviously appropriate, but present arrangements need both more commitment and more attention [22].

HYPERTENSION

Introduction

Between 10 and 20% of people develop abnormally high arterial pressure, which poses a threat to their health and life [24,25]: the higher the arterial pressure, the greater the risk. This applies both to systolic pressure (the pressure immediately after heart contraction) and the diastolic pressure (the pressure just prior to the next heart contraction). Hypertensive patients are at greater risk from strokes (both cerebral thrombosis and cerebral haemorrhage), from coronary artery disease, and from heart and renal failure. There is now good evidence that reducing BP lowers the incidence of both kinds of stroke, of heart failure and of renal failure. The incidence of coronary artery disease is also lowered, the extent of which depends on other coexisting factors, such as hyperlipidaemia, diabetes and smoking. These risk factors are multiplicative in nature, so that if a person has a threefold risk from hypertension, a threefold risk from a lipid abnormality and a threefold risk from smoking, then the risk is not ninefold (3+3+3) but 27-fold (3×3×3). Since very many hypertensive patients have these abnormalities, it is important that all hypertensive patients be adequately investigated.

The female:male ratio

The incidence of hypertension is defined by relationships between pressure and outcome in population studies. On that basis, it rises with age in both sexes, but it does so more steeply in females. Hypertension is more common in men below the age of 50, after which the incidence in women rapidly catches up and surpasses that of men. Cardiovascular morbidity and mortality is much higher in men below the age of 50 than in women: it is rare, for example, to see a coronary thrombosis in a woman below the age of 55. It has been argued that female hormones are cardioprotective and this is why problems do not occur until well after the menopause. This concept fits in well with the fact that there may be as much as a 50% reduction in cardiovascular mortality in women between the ages of 50 and 60 if they are receiving hormone replacement therapy, although these studies have mainly involved professional women at low overall risk.

Aetiology

Essential hypertension
Essential hypertension is the term used for the 90–95% of cases where no definite cause can be identified. Undoubtedly, both genetic and environmental factors have an important role.

Genetic factors
Specific genetic disorders associated with hypertension are very rarely identified, but hypertension often runs in families, consistent with genetic as well as environmental influences. New developments in insulin resistance, which can run in families and populations, are of particular interest [26]. After food, insulin secretion by the beta cells of the pancreas increases in response to the rise in blood glucose. Insulin increases the passage of glucose into the cells of the body and increases the transference of glucose into the liver for storage as glycogen. The resulting fall in blood glucose switches off the release of insulin. In late-onset diabetes, in obese people and in many hypertensive patients, insulin resistance is found. The term insulin resistance is slightly misleading as the only action that is resisted is the passage of glucose into cells (i.e. insulin-mediated disposal of glucose is impaired). Blood glucose remains high and insulin secretion is not switched off, leading to higher levels of insulin. The hyperinsulin state may be dangerous in that insulin has many other actions: it can cause sodium retention, which increases the blood volume, which in turn may raise BP. It may also cause an increase in the activity of the sympathetic nerv-

ous system, leading to blood vessel constriction and a rise in cardiac output and thereby a rise in BP. Insulin has an effect on the sodium/potassium pump of all cells, leading to an increase in intracellular sodium. The rise in sodium inside vascular smooth muscle cells enhances their constriction to naturally released substances, such as noradrenaline and angiotensin. Increased insulin secretion also provokes lipid abnormalities, such as an increase in levels of LDL and a fall in HDL, changes that can promote atherosclerosis. British Asian men are particularly prone to the impact of the metabolic effects associated with insulin resistance, amplified by central obesity, on the risk of premature coronary heart disease [27].

Environmental factors

It should first be explained that BP does not remain constant throughout the day and night: nocturnal BP is much lower than daytime BP (Fig. 10a.1). The pressure rises fairly abruptly on wakening and is usually higher in the morning, gradually settling to lower levels in the afternoon and early evening. In addition, any stressful event may cause a very large increase in BP. There is evidence that adverse cardiovascular events are associated with these pressure rises, particularly the early morning pressure rise, but also those related to stressful events.

Secondary hypertension
Renal causes

Renal causes of secondary hypertension include glomerular nephritis, congenital polycystic kidneys, chronic pyelonephritis and damage induced by diabetes. Renal vascular disease, such as renal artery stenosis, is not uncommon. This is often unilateral and may be correctable by vascular surgery.

Endocrine causes

Endocrine causes include diseases of the adrenal cortex, such as primary hyperaldosteronism. This is usually due to a hormone-secreting tumour and can be surgically corrected. Similarly, Cushing's syndrome is amenable to treatment. Tumours of the adrenal medulla releasing either adrenaline or noradrenaline may also present as hypertension and are usually surgically amenable.

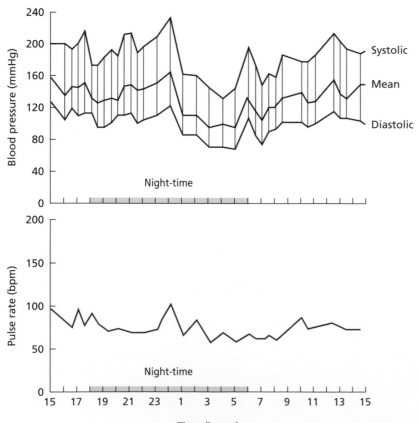

Figure 10a.1. *Ambulatory blood pressure monitoring over a 24-hour period showing systolic, diastolic and mean blood pressures with matching pulse rates: bpm, beats/min. Patient has moderate hypertension, but with a definite night-time dip.*

Other causes

Other rarer causes of hypertension include coarctation of the aorta. In this congenital narrowing of the aorta, the pressure above the structure is high, while below the structure it is low. Such cases are usually spotted in childhood, but they can be detected in people in their 50s and 60s on rare occasions.

Effect of hypertension on the body

Hypertension does not cause any symptoms or any signs in the early stages. These occur only later, when there is established damage to the supplied organs (i.e. end-organ failure). Visual disturbance can be indicative of retinal artery thrombosis or swelling of the optic nerve; retinal haemorrhages also disturb vision. Cerebral thrombosis and haemorrhage cause severe neurological disturbance and loss of consciousness. Heart failure leads to breathlessness. The increased demands on the heart in pumping at higher pressure may also cause angina or myocardial infarction. Renal impairment usually causes frequent micturition, particularly at night.

Blood vessels

The arterial wall comprises three layers (Fig. 10a.2): the intima is the internal layer of endothelial cells; there is then an elastic layer between the intima and the media, which is composed of a layer of muscle cells and elastic fibres; the outside lining is called the adventitial layer. In hypertension, the muscular layer increases in size and the cells of the endothelial layer become enlarged and more numerous; the net effect is a marked narrowing of the lumen. Atheroma may occur in certain vessels, owing to a certain type of cholesterol-rich LDL being laid down in the subintima (Fig. 10a.3). This deposit distorts the vessel and eventually ulceration occurs, exposing the lipid to blood vessels and platelets; this leads, in turn, to thrombosis and occlusion of the vessel. The tissue to which the blood supply is obstructed can become ischaemic with poor function or death of cells — an infarct. Factors other than hypertension are involved in coronary artery thrombosis and cerebral arterial thrombosis.

The heart

Hypertension causes the muscle fibres of the heart to increase in size and number so that the left

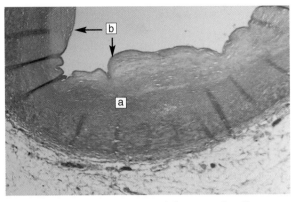

Figure 10a.2. *Cross-section of the arterial wall: (a) media; (b) intima.*

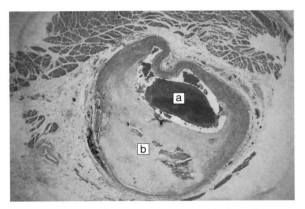

Figure 10a.3. *Atheromatous artery with thrombus: (a) overlying thrombus; (b) cholesterol-rich athermatous plague.*

ventricle of the heart becomes hypertrophied. The increase in muscle bulk leads to a demand for an even greater oxygen supply. If there is any coronary arterial disease, coronary artery insufficiency occurs (angina) and, eventually, myocardial infarction.

The brain

Cerebral thrombosis or cerebral haemorrhage are associated with hypertension. In the first instance, thrombosis occurs and blocks a cerebral vessel. One of the small micro-aneurysms may then burst into the surrounding brain, resulting in a cerebral haemorrhage.

The kidney

The kidney is very susceptible to hypertension. The first sign is micro-albuminuria — traces of protein in the urine — and then more severe proteinuria. Many glomeruli are damaged by becoming hyalinized, with fibrosis between the cells. Ischaemia to renal tubules results. There is a malignant phase where fibrinoid necrosis of the glomerular arterioles occurs: the structure and function of the arteriolar wall are destroyed. Renal failure is a not uncommon result of poorly controlled hypertension.

The eye

The first change in the eye due to hypertension is an increased tortuosity of the retinal arterioles. The second stage is arteriovenous nipping, where the calibre of the retinal veins appears to be occluded where they are crossed by arterioles. The third stage is leakage of blood and plasma from vessels with haemorrhages and exudates. The fourth is a swelling of the optic disc with haemorrhages, termed papilloedema.

Investigation

Measurement of blood pressure

Normotensive and hypertensive BP values are shown in Table 10a.1. The most accurate way of measuring BP is still by the mercury sphygmomanometer. Unfortunately, this gives only a 'snapshot' picture at one moment in time, and measurements over a 24-hour period are needed to determine how the patient responds to stressful circumstances. This can be done only through 24-hour ambulatory blood pressure monitoring (ABPM) (Fig. 10a.1) [28]. The ABPM result gives a much more reproducible mean value than that obtained on three separate occasions with the sphygmomanometer — the technique used in most clinical trials. This means that smaller numbers of patients are required for clinical trials and that new, more effective treatments, or ones with fewer side effects, can be brought onto the market more quickly. The main advantage of ABPM is that it is not subject to the 'white coat effect' (i.e. an increase in BP when the patient sees a doctor). Without ABPM, there is a very real risk that patients, especially the elderly, can be started on lifelong therapy when it is unneces-

sary or may even be doing harm. ABPM also correlates better with hypertensive organ damage, such as left ventricular hypertrophy, lacunar brain infarcts, micro-albuminuria (a sign of renal involvement) and the fundal eye changes of hypertension. It has also shown itself to be a better predictor of cardiovascular events. Obviously, all 24-hour ABPM machines need to be properly validated. In terms of cost, the outlay on such a machine by an average GP practice is recouped within 2 years from the saving on unnecessary medication alone, but some investment in time and education is necessary.

Other useful investigations are shown in Table 10a.2.

Non-drug treatment of hypertension

The British Hypertension Society has particularly emphasized that non-pharmacological measures should be used in all cases of hypertension [29]: these include weight reduction and lower intake of both alcohol and salt [30]. Non-extreme exercise should also be increased and any identified associated risk factors addressed, notably continued cigarette smoking and lipid abnormalities.

Drug treatment of hypertension
Diuretics

Thiazides (not loop diuretics such as frusemide) are effective in lowering pressure at low doses. They reduce intracellular sodium levels, which diminishes the response of vascular smooth muscle to noradrenaline and angiotensin. Side effects include loss of potassium, promotion of gout, exacerbation of any diabetes and, rarely, impotence.

Beta-adrenoceptor-blocking drugs

Beta blockers decrease cardiac output, but the main BP-lowering effect is through decreased

Table 10a.1. *Normotensive and hypertensive blood pressure (BP) values according to age*

Age (years)	Normotensive BP (mmHg)	Hypertensive BP (mmHg)
17–40	<140/90	>160/100
41–60	<150/90	>160/100
>60	<160/90	>175/100

Table 10a.2. *Investigations used in diagnosing hypertension*

Investigation	Objective/circumstances
Electrocardiogram, chest radiography and echocardiogram	To detect cardiac pathology and overgrowth of the heart muscle wall (ventricular hypertrophy)
Simple renal function tests	To assess renal function as a contributory cause of hypertension and to review safety of ACE therapy
Special investigations, e.g. of renal arteries or hormone release	When the initial screening tests are abnormal and if there is some clinical suspicion from the history or examination
Lipid profile, markers of alcohol excess	Risk assessment

ACE = angiotensin-converting enzyme.

renin release, leading to decreased brain-driven sympathetic vascular tone with resetting of baroceptors. The sympathetic effect occurs through prejunctional reduction of noradrenaline release. Potential side effects include promotion of heart failure, asthma, worsening of the lipid profile, tiredness and impotence. Newer, more cardioselective agents, such as atenolol, may be less likely to cause asthma; however, beta blockers should never be used by asthmatic patients.

Calcium antagonists

Calcium antagonists decrease the force of heart contraction and the ability of vessels to constrict. Diltiazem and verapamil also have an effect on cardiac conducting tissue and may cause slowing of the heart; this does not occur with nifedipine or amlodipine. Other occasional side effects include constipation, ankle swelling, flushing of the face and headaches. Calcium antagonists are lipid neutral, with no particular effect on lipid profile.

Angiotensin-converting enzyme (ACE) inhibitors

ACE inhibitors work on the renin–angiotensin system by blocking the conversion of inactive angiotensin I to angiotensin II, the active agent in vascular tone and aldosterone release, thus causing a fall in BP. They also block the degradation of the endogenous agent bradykinin, which may also have an antihypertensive effect. Unfortunately, bradykinin produces cough, which is a serious disadvantage. ACE inhibitors are dangerous in renal artery stenosis as their use

can promote loss of renal artery blood flow and renal infarction. Other complications include a marked response to the first dose (especially if diuretics have been given), angioneurotic oedema and skin rashes. ACE inhibitors are also lipid neutral.

Alpha-1-adrenoceptor antagonists

Alpha-1 blockers block the effect of noradrenaline on the vasculature; however, the antihypertensive effect tends to wear off. Many regard them as useful ancillary drugs where there is a lipid disorder, as they can improve the lipid profile. They do not provoke heart failure or asthma, but may cause tiredness and headaches.

Sartans

The sartans are a new group of drugs that act on the angiotensin II type 1 receptor, blocking the effect of angiotensin. They are lipid neutral and either do not or only rarely cause cough. Not all sartans are necessarily equally effective and they must be used with great care in the presence of renal artery stenosis.

Prevention

Prevention of hypertension is difficult as there are familial influences. Attention to lifestyle is important and effective. Avoidance of becoming overweight, not drinking too much alcohol, regulating salt intake and periodic checks of BP are useful measures.

Shared care and evidence-based guidelines

Most cases of hypertension can be well managed in general practice with the support of an ABPM device. However, as with cholesterol and other aspects of risk, opportunities to achieve appropriate control continue to be missed in both the hospital clinic and general practice setting. The good sense of combined approaches to cardiovascular risk continues to be demonstrated. Statins prescribed for hyperlipidaemia can reduce the risk of thrombotic stroke [31]. Survival of patients on long-term medication for hypertension is related, not to the level of control of BP but to other risk associations, particularly blood cholesterol and smoking habits [32].

References

1. Murray CL, Lopez AD. Mortality by cause for eight regions of the world: global burden of disease study. *Lancet* 1997; 349: 1269–1286

2. Hopkins PN, Williams RR. A survey of 246 suggested coronary risk factors. *Atherosclerosis* 1981; 40: 1–52

3. Mann JI, Lewis B, Shepherd J *et al.* Blood lipids and other cardiovascular risk factors; their prevalence in Britain. *Br Med J* 1988; 296: 1702–1706

4. NHS Executive. SMAC statement on use of statins. Executive letter EL(97)41. Wetherby (West Yorkshire). Department of Health, 1997

5. Shepherd J, Cobbe SM, Ford I *et al.* Prevention of coronary heart disease with pravastatin in men with hypercholesterolaemia. *N Engl J Med* 1995; 333: 1301–1307

6. Pyorala K, De Backer G, Poole-Wilson P, Wood D. Prevention of heart disease in clinical practice. Recommendations of the task force of the European Society of Cardiology, European Atherosclerosis Society and European Society of Hypertension. *Eur Heart J* 1994; 15: 1300–1331

7. Levy D, Wilson PWF, Anderson KM, Castelli WP. Stratifying the patient at risk from coronary disease: new insights from Framingham. *Am Heart J* 1990; 119: 712–717

8. Winder AF. Management of lipids in the elderly. *J Roy Soc Med* 1998; 91: 189–191

9. Wood D, Durington P, Poulter N *et al.* Joint British recommendations on prevention of coronary heart disease in clinical practice. *Heart* 1998; 80(Suppl. 2): 51–529

10. Winder AF, Vallance DT, Richmond W. Investigation of dyslipidaemias. *J Clin Pathol* 1997; 50: 721–734

11. Galton DJ. Genetic determinants of atherosclerosis-related dyslipidemias and their clinical implications. *Clin Chim Acta* 1997; 257: 181–197

12. The Expert Panel: summary of the second report of the National Cholesterol Education Program (NCEP) Expert Panel on detection, evaluation and treatment of high blood cholesterol in adults (Adult Treatment Panel II). *JAMA* 1993; 269: 3015–3123

13. Pyörälä K, Olsson AG, Pedersen TJ *et al.* Cholesterol lowering with simvastatin improves prognosis of diabetic patients with coronary heart disease. A subgroup analysis of the Scandinavian Simvastatin Survival Study (4S). *Diabetes Care* 1997; 20: 614–620

14. Prentice AM, Jebb S. Obesity in Britain: gluttony or sloth? *Br Med J* 1995; 311: 437–439

15. Scandinavian Simvastatin Survival Group. Randomised trial of cholesterol lowering in 4444 patients with coronary heart disease: the Scandinavian Simvastatin Survival Study 4S. *Lancet* 1994; 344: 1383–1389

16. Sacks FM, Pfeffer MA, Moye LA *et al.* The effect of pravastatin on coronary events after myocardial infarction in patients with average cholesterol levels. *N Engl J Med* 1996; 335: 1001–1009

17. Fruchart JC, Brewer HB Jr, Leitersdorf E. Consensus for the use of fibrates in the treatment of dyslipoproteinaemia and coronary heart disease. *Am J Cardiol* 1998; 81: 912–917

18. Antiplatelet Trialists Collaboration. Collaborative overview of randomised trials of antiplatelet therapy — I. Prevention of death, myocardial infarction and stroke by prolonged platelet therapy in various categories of patients. *Br Med J* 1994; 308: 81–106

19. Ramsey LE, Haq U, Jackson PR *et al.* Targeting lipid-lowering drug therapy for primary prevention of coronary heart disease: an updated Sheffield table. *Lancet* 1996; 348: 387–388

20. Haq IU, Ramsay LE, Pickin D *et al.* Lipid-lowering for the prevention of coronary heart disease: what policy now? *Clin Sci* 1996; 91: 399–413

21. Aspire Steering Group. A British Cardiac Society survey of the potential for the secondary prevention of coronary disease: ASPIRE (Action on Secondary Prevention through Intervention to Reduce Events). Principal results. *Heart* 1996; 75: 334–342

22. Campbell NC, Thain J, Deans HD *et al.* Secondary prevention in coronary heart disease: baseline survey of provision in general practice. *Br Med J* 1998; 316: 1430–1434

23. Giles PD, Ramachandran S, Whitaker AJ *et al.* The one-stop cholesterol clinic: a multidisciplinary approach to implementing evidence-based treatment. *Postgrad Med J* 1996; 77: 744–748

24. Reid J, Swales JD. Hypertension in theory and practice. *Br Med Bull* 1994; 50: 255–314

25. Joint National Committee on Prevention, Detection and Treatment of High Blood Pressure. Sixth report. NIH Publication 98-4080. Bethesda, MD: National Institutes of Health, 1997

26. Reaven GM. Role of insulin resistance in human disease (syndrome X): an expanded definition. *Annu Rev Med* 1993; 44: 121–131

27. Bhatnagar D, Anand IS, Durrington PN *et al.* Coronary risk factors in people from the Indian sub-continent living in West London and their siblings in India. *Lancet* 1995; 345: 405–409

28. Taylor RS, Stockman J, Kernick D *et al.* Ambulatory blood pressure monitoring for hypertension in general practice. *J R Soc Med* 1998; 91: 301–304

29. Sever P, Beevers G, Bulpitt HC *et al.* Management guidelines in essential hypertension: report of the second working party of the British Hypertension Society. *Br Med J* 1993; 306: 983–987

30. Elliott P. Lower sodium for all. *Lancet* 1997; 350: 825–826

31. Rosendorff C. Statins for prevention of stroke. *Lancet* 1998; 351: 1002–1003

32. Andersson OK, Almgren T, Persson B *et al.* Survival in treated hypertension: follow up study after two decades. *Br Med J* 1998; 317: 167–171

Heart disease: interventional cardiology

A. E. Abdelmeguid

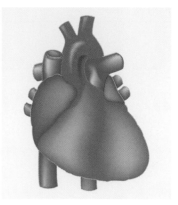

Introduction

It is well established that men have a higher incidence of coronary artery disease than women. On average, it has been estimated that women live 5 to 8 years longer than men, and that 40% of the excess male mortality is caused by coronary artery disease. In addition, men under the age of 45 are up to 10 times more likely to develop myocardial infarction (MI) than women.

Coronary revascularization has been shown to have a significant impact on survival and relief of anginal symptoms in many patients with coronary artery disease. Until recently, open heart surgery (coronary artery bypass grafting; CABG) was the only option available for coronary revascularization, and has been accepted as the revascularization 'gold standard'. The overwhelming attractiveness of a percutaneous coronary revascularization procedure did not materialize until Andreas Gruentizig performed the first coronary angioplasty in 1977. The initial system used was a coaxial catheter system consisting of an outer guide catheter to deliver the dilating catheter system to the coronary orifice and an inner balloon-bearing dilating catheter that could be manipulated into position within the stenosis to be dilated. Later, the balloon catheter itself was modified by John Simpson to allow the passage of the dilating catheter over a guidewire (over-the-wire system), which is introduced first across the stenosis. The balloon is then advanced over the wire to the stenosis site to be dilated. Initially, coronary angioplasty was believed to have relatively limited clinical applicability; however, a prodigious effort on the part of industry and physicians to refine the instrumentation and to develop techniques to address more complex situations resulted in a great increase in the number of percutaneous coronary procedures. Indeed, the technology of angioplasty has undergone revolutionary changes since the introduction of the procedure more than a decade ago. None of the guiding or dilatation catheters or guidewires used today were clinically available a decade ago. Balloon catheters are 30–50% lower in profile and more trackable than earlier prototypes. Balloon material has improved, and monorail long balloons and perfusion balloons have become available.

In response to the striking improvement in the success rate of coronary angioplasty, there has also been a dramatic increase in the number of procedures. The US National Center for Health Statistics estimated that 331 000 coronary angioplasty procedures were performed in the USA in 1991. In the same year, 300 000 coronary bypass operations were performed [1]. Thus, in the USA, coronary angioplasty is now a widely used technique for coronary revascularization and is performed at a frequency comparable to that of coronary bypass surgery.

Acute results of PTCA

The standard definition of acute success for percutaneous transluminal coronary angioplasty (PTCA) is reduction of the diameter stenosis to less than 50% without any cardiac ischaemic complications. Using this definition, success rates greater than 90% have been reported (Table 10b.1). Success rates are heavily influenced by case selection and operator's skill. The principal case-selection variable is the location and geometric complexity of the stenosis. A classification of stenosis complexity has been developed, and correlations between increasing complexity and decreasing success rate have been documented (Table 10b.2).

Acute complications of PTCA

The complications of PTCA can be divided into major and minor complications. The major com-

Table 10b.1. *Success and major complications of percutaneous transluminal coronary angioplasty*

	Complications				
Study	Major (%)	MI (%)	CABG (%)	Death (%)	Success (%)
NHLBI 1977–81	NR	4.9	5.8	1.2	67
NHLBI 1985–86	NR	4.3	3.4	1.0	88
Bredlau 1985	4.1	2.6	2.7	0.1	91
MAPS-I 1986–87*	8.0	2.0	5.5	1.0	84
Nobuyoshi 1991	NR	2.1	0.5	0.6	85
MAPS-II 1991*	3.5	1.5	0.5	1.0	90
Myler 1992	3.0	0.8	1.3	0.0	92

NR, not reported; NHLBI, National Heart, Lung and Blood Institute; MAPS, Multivessel Angioplasty Prognosis Study; MI, myocardial infarction; CABG, coronary artery bypass grafting.

*Multivessel disease patients only.

(From ref. 2 with permission.)

Table 10b.2. *AHA/ACC classification* of lesion type*

Type A lesions (high success: > 85%; low risk)

- Discrete (< 10 mm length)
- Concentric
- Readily accessible
- Non-angulated segment, < 45°
- Smooth contour
- Little or no calcification
- Less than totally occlusive
- Non-ostial location
- No major branch involvement
- Absence of thrombus

Type B lesions (moderate success: 60–85%; moderate risk)

- Tubular (10–20 mm length)
- Eccentric
- Moderate tortuosity of proximal segment
- Moderately angulated segment, > 45°, < 90°
- Irregular contour
- Moderate to heavy calcification
- Total occlusions < 3 months old
- Ostial in location
- Bifurcation lesions requiring double guidewires
- Some thrombus present

Type C lesions (low success, < 60%; high risk)

- Diffuse (> 2 cm length)
- Excessive tortuosity of proximal segment
- Extremely angulated segments > 90°
- Total occlusions > 3 months old
- Inability to protect major side branches
- Degenerated vein grafts with friable lesions

*The modified classification suggested by Ellis *et al.* [3] subdivides B lesions into lesions with only one B parameter (B1), or lesions with more than one B parameter (B2).

(From ref. 38 with permission.)

plications are death, MI and emergency CABG (E-CABG). The incidence of these complications has not increased despite the application of PTCA to a higher-risk population, including the elderly and patients with multivessel disease, poor left ventricular function and prior CABG. This is probably related to increased operator experience, improved balloon and catheter technology and better patient selection [2].

The most frequent sequence of events leading to myocardial ischaemia with PTCA is intimal and medial disruption (coronary dissection), superimposed on a significant plaque burden, which causes blood flow reduction by itself or precipitates obstructive thrombus formation. Primary thrombus propagation may be more important when PTCA is performed in the setting of unstable angina or MI. Secondary increases in coronary vasomotor tone (coronary spasm) may also contribute to ischaemia.

Coronary dissection

Intimal dissections usually occur as a result of vessel–balloon interactions. Less commonly, dissections are caused by guide catheter or guidewire manipulation. Dissection of the left main (LM) coronary artery by the guide catheter is an infrequent but serious complication of PTCA. Similarly, dissection of the proximal right coronary artery (RCA) can also result from guide catheter manipulation. In one study, LM dissections accounted for 13% of deaths after PTCA [3]. If adequate coronary blood flow cannot be restored, this complication carries with it more than 50% mortality, even with rapid transportation to the operating room. To avoid this complication, a guide catheter should be chosen to allow atraumatic coaxial intubation of the coronary ostium and to provide adequate backup.

Plaque disruption from guidewire-induced trauma is a well-recognized complication of PTCA, which is more likely with the use of relatively stiff guidewires, particularly in eccentric stenoses. Common sense dictates that forceful probing with stiff guidewires should be avoided at all times and, in particular, in the presence of eccentric and long stenoses. Intimal splitting and plaque fracture are frequently associated with PTCA. Indeed, plaque and intimal disruption with or without localized medial dissection are components of the major mechanism of successful PTCA. The likelihood of dissection has been related to a number of angiographic features, including plaque eccentricity, lesion length, vessel tortuosity or branching, balloon:artery ratio

and calcification. Indeed, many features included in the American College of Cardiology/American Heart Association (ACC/AHA) classification of coronary stenoses (Table 10b.2) play a major part in the vessel–balloon interactions, stress distribution and the occurrence of major dissections. Proper sizing of the balloon to the arterial segment to be dilated is also extremely important. Use of larger balloons may be fraught with risk of extensive dissection or even vessel rupture [4].

In the pre-stent era, the presence of coronary dissection has been associated with a more than sixfold increase in the risk of ischaemic complications (death, MI, CABG). However, the term 'dissection' has been used freely for various luminographic appearances. Small dissections in the form of intimal tears are near-ubiquitous results of angioplasty, and the frequency of this finding suggests that limited dissection by angiography does not represent a complication of PTCA in the majority of patients, but probably represents the most common mechanism of successful PTCA. Lesions with only minimal flow disruption and no persistent staining of the vessel wall or extravasation will probably remain open and be associated with clinical success; conversely, complex dissections and those with persistence of dye outside the lumen are associated with low success rates and a high incidence of in-hospital complications.

Management

The management of coronary dissections is guided by clinical parameters, such as the presence of pain after the procedure, haemodynamic stability and evolving electrocardiographic changes, in addition to the angiographic parameters previously described. The experienced operator will use all available data and observe all dissections in the laboratory to assure that flow and lumen size remain stable. Short non-occlusive dissections (< 30% residual narrowing) with no evidence of ongoing ischaemia can be managed medically; although some cardiologists use prolonged (12–24 h) heparin infusion in this situation, the utility of such therapy is somewhat controversial [2]. Dissections that compromise blood flow and induce ischaemia require more than medical management, and should be dealt with as outlined under 'abrupt closure'.

Coronary thrombus

Coronary thrombosis can be superimposed on PTCA-induced dissections; however, extensive coronary thrombosis can be the main aetiological factor in abrupt closure complicating PTCA independent of the presence of dissection. Angioplasty of thrombus-containing lesions is associated with an increased risk of acute thrombotic coronary occlusion with subsequent increased incidence of death, MI and emergency CABG [5].

Management

For routine PTCA, aspirin and heparin are universally used. The role of aspirin in reducing the ischaemic complications of PTCA is clearly established. In a study randomizing patients to aspirin and dipyridamole or placebo, the incidence of periprocedural Q-wave MI was significantly lower among patients receiving antiplatelet agents (7% in the placebo group vs 2% in the aspirin group) [6]. Low aspirin dose (80 mg) seems to be adequate, and the addition of dipyridamole to aspirin does not significantly reduce acute complications compared with aspirin alone. It is the author's practice to administer 325 mg of aspirin at least 1 day prior to PTCA. The use of heparin during PTCA is also universally accepted. Low rates of periprocedural ischaemic complications have been associated with activated partial thromboplastin times (aPTTs) more than three times those of controls, or activated clotting times (ACT) of more than 300 s. The author usually administers 10 000 units at the beginning of the procedure and subsequently determines an ACT. Further boluses are given as needed to obtain an ACT of more than 300 s; the ACT is then determined at 30-minute intervals throughout the procedure.

There is a twofold increase in the risk of ischaemic complications when PTCA is performed in the presence of thrombus-containing lesions [7]. When an intracoronary thrombus is present prior to PTCA, the author's traditional approach has been to administer heparin to the patient for a few days before performing balloon dilatation. This approach stems from the rationale that the risk of PTCA-related complications appears to be reduced when a period of pharmacological stabilization with heparin and aspirin precedes PTCA, not only in patients with an angiographically evident clot but also in those with unstable angina [2]. Recently, the author has been using Abciximab, the c7E3 monoclonal antibody directed against the glycoprotein (GP) integrin receptor IIb/IIIa, which has been shown to reduce thrombotic complications significantly in cases of PTCA with intracoronary thrombus, unless there is a contraindication to administer this drug [8]. This strategy does not require prolonged preheparinization and obviates unnecessary delay in performing the procedure.

Abrupt vessel closure

Abrupt closure is the most common cause of major PTCA-related complications, with an incidence of death of 0–8%, of MI 20–54% and of E-CABG 20–72% in the pre-stent era [2]. Depending on the definition and the patient population, abrupt closure has been reported in 2–9% of cases of elective PTCA. The majority of these closures occur within 6 hours of the procedure, with 50–90% occurring in the catheterization laboratory. Abrupt closure usually occurs in the setting of coronary dissections (35–80% of reported closures), but it can also follow the formation of intracoronary thrombus without dissection, or can rarely be caused exclusively by spasm.

Management

The first two steps in the management of acute ischaemia during PTCA are a brief evaluation of its haemodynamic consequences and an assessment and treatment of its cause; the first step will determine the pace of the second. The most common causes of prolonged ischaemia during PTCA are, in approximate order of frequency: (1) coronary dissection; (2) intracoronary thrombus formation; (3) guide catheter damping; and (4) coronary spasm. The last two causes are usually readily identifiable and treatable, with catheter withdrawal and intracoronary nitroglycerine (i.c. NTG) or, rarely, sublingual nifedipine, respectively. Although the appearance of a large dissection or globular filling defect is usually conclusive for the cause of ischaemia, smaller defects or poor imaging may make this distinction difficult. All patients should receive i.c. NTG to exclude contributory coronary spasm, and further i.v. heparin if there is any question as to the adequacy of anticoagulation. Thereafter, treatment is dependent on the presumed cause, the initial response to therapy and the level of haemodynamic compromise. If the vessel is found to be occluded, the decision has to be made whether to open it or to treat the patient medically. Medical management is appropriate if the vessel supplies a small amount of viable myocardium, it is well collateralized, the patient is haemodynamically stable, and the chances of delivering a stent are not very high. The decision to manage an abrupt occlusion medically should be made only after ensuring that the abrupt closure is limited to the PTCA site and has not propagated proximally to involve vessels other than the target vessel. E-CABG is usually reserved for patients who cannot be managed successfully by percutaneous techniques, or if the results of these techniques are felt to be suboptimal and unstable.

Percutaneous management of abrupt closure

Following treatment with i.c. NTG and adequate heparinization, the occlusion is crossed with a guidewire and balloon dilatation performed. If a dissection is present or suspected, repeat dilatation with long inflations, perhaps best achieved with low inflation pressure and slightly oversized balloons, can yield an adequate result and obviate the need for bypass surgery in 44–85% of cases of coronary occlusion [9]. Prolonged balloon inflation is performed until a stable final result is achieved (thrombolysis in myocardial infarction [TIMI] grade III flow, < 30% residual stenosis, no chest pain and stable haemodynamics). A perfusion balloon catheter may allow prolonged balloon inflation, while maintaining distal perfusion, and may improve the angiographic outcome and complication rates.

Since redilatation is successful in only 40–85% of cases, a variety of management strategies, including directional coronary atherectomy (DCA) [10] and stenting [11], have been used to reverse abrupt closure in the laboratory with variable degrees of success. DCA has been used to treat abrupt occlusion by a debulking effect — excising an occluding intraluminal dissection or intraluminal defect superimposed on atheromatous tissue [10]. However, this 'bail-out atherectomy' is limited to proximal lesions in large vessels, and should not be used in cases of spiral dissections because of the risk of vessel perforation. The procedure also requires exchanging the guide catheter with a larger size to accommodate the bulky device and, in many instances, this requires re-wiring of the occlusion. Stenting has the greatest impact on the percutaneous management of abrupt closure that fails repeat of PTCA. In the author's opinion, abrupt closure following PTCA should prompt immediate stent placement (with or without the use of Abciximab) if substantial amounts of viable myocardium are at risk. The availability of endoluminal stents for bail-out use has further altered the assessment of the high-risk patient: an assessment of the likelihood of being able to deliver such a device rapidly in the event of coronary closure, especially as it relates to guide catheter choice, has become of paramount importance in the assessment of risk. It is important to know when to stop and not waste valuable time by repeatedly attempting to redilate a lesion that has not responded to prolonged dilatation, since rapid delivery of the stent is an important factor. Stenting for threatened closure with persistent TIMI grade III flow is also extremely important and may, in fact, avoid abrupt closure.

E-CABG When percutaneous revascularization is not successful and the decision is made to pursue E-CABG, all possible interventions to minimize myocardial ischaemia should be employed: these include i.v. NTG, calcium-channel blockers and heparin. An intra-aortic balloon pump (IABP) should be inserted and a perfusion balloon (or bail-out catheter) should be placed across the abrupt occlusion.

In-hospital mortality after E-CABG ranges from 0 to 16.6% (average 6%) [12]. Surgical results in this setting vary widely, depending on the experience of the angioplasty operator and surgical team, as well as the patient population. However, when compared with patients operated on electively or semi-electively, it is clear that, within a single institution, the results of E-CABG are clearly inferior to elective procedures, and even experienced surgeons may find it difficult to use internal mammary arteries (IMAs) as conduits in this setting.

Death

The largest and most comprehensive analysis of death after PTCA showed an incidence of 0.4% (32 deaths with 8052 PTCAs) [3]. Death was directly related to coronary artery closure precipitating left ventricular failure in 82% of cases (Table 10b.3). Other causes of death include right ventricular failure, LM coronary artery dissection and arrhythmias. Other causes of death that are not related to acute vessel closure include pulmonary embolism, intracranial haemorrhage, sepsis and anaphylaxis.

Non-Q-wave infarction after PTCA

MI, as diagnosed by modest elevations of cardiac enzymes following percutaneous coronary interventions, are relatively common following PCTA (15–29% of cases of successful PTCA) [13]. In part, because of this common occurrence following 'apparently' successful coronary interventions, it has been assumed that these 'infarctlets' are relatively benign and that they do not have any adverse impact on long-term outcome. Another related controversial issue is the threshold at which post-procedural cardiac enzyme elevations should be considered abnormal. At present, the 'definition' of non-Q-wave MI after percutaneous coronary interventions requires an elevation of creatine kinase (CK) ranging in various studies from twice to over five times the laboratory's upper limit of normal (ULN). This wide range is due to the absence of any systematic evaluation of the prognostic implications of cardiac enzyme elevation in this setting [13].

Table 10b.3. *Causes of death in 32 patients after percutaneous transluminal coronary angioplasty*

Cause	Patients	
	No.	%
Abrupt closure		
LV failure	13	41
RV failure	5	16
LM dissection	4	13
LV failure (post-CABG)	3	9
Sudden cardiac death	1	3
Not related to vessel closure		
Pulmonary embolus	2	6
Intracranial haemorrhage	2	6
Sepsis	1	3
Anaphylaxis	1	3

LV, left ventricular; RV, right ventricular; LM, left main; CABG, coronary artery bypass grafting.

(From ref. 2 with permission.)

In an attempt to define the appropriate threshold of CK elevation following successful PTCA, the author's group undertook a study of 4664 consecutive patients with successful PTCA or DCA [14]. The patients were divided into three groups according to post-procedural peak CK: group I (4480 patients) had peak CK levels following the procedure of less than twice the ULN (i.e. < 360 IU/l); group II (123 patients) had a peak CK level between two and five times the ULN (i.e. 361–900 IU/l), with positive myocardial band (MB) isoenzymes (CK-MB > 4%); group III (61 patients) had a peak level of more than 900 IU/l with positive CK-MB.

Clinical follow-up extending up to 8.5 years revealed a striking difference in survival among the three groups (88.54, 77.81 and 77.05% for groups I, II and III, respectively; $p < 0.0001$). This difference in survival was totally accounted for by a difference in cardiac survival (92.26 vs 81.15 vs 77.05%; $p < 0.0001$), with no difference among the three groups in the incidence of non-cardiac death ($p = 0.699$). Adding all major complications on follow-up together (death, MI, CABG and repeat angioplasty), the event survival rate was significantly higher in the group with no infarct (group I): 61.55 vs. 48.90 vs. 52.72%; $p = 0.002$.

The author's group have also studied the effects of even smaller increases in CK in the largest series reported to date [15]. The study comprised 4484 patients who underwent successful PTCA or DCA at the Cleveland Clinic between 1984 and 1991, and whose post-procedural peak CK levels did not exceed twice the ULN (i.e. 2×180 IU/l). Patients were divided into three groups according to peak CK and MB isoenzyme levels after the procedure. Group I (3776 patients) had no CK or MB elevation following the procedure (i.e. CK ≤ 180 IU/l, with MB fraction ≤ 4%); group II (450 patients) had a peak CK level between 100 and 180 IU/l, with MB fraction greater than 4%; and group III (258 patients) had a peak CK level between 181 and 360 IU/l, with MB fraction > 4%. Long-term clinical follow-up revealed results comparable to the author's previous analysis. Freedom from cardiac death was lower in the groups with elevated CK-MB (groups I vs II vs III: 92.95 vs 88.25 vs 88.66%; $p = 0.036$). As a composite, the event survival rate was significantly higher in the group with no myocardial necrosis (group I): 62.71, 57.71 and 52.10% for groups I, II and III, respectively; $p = 0.009$. These results substantiate the finding that minor elevations of CK are associated with adverse long-term outcome (Fig. 10b.1). The interaction between the level of post-procedural CK-MB and the risk of cardiac death is shown in Figure 10b.2 and shows that a modest increase of CK-MB to 40 IU/l is associated with more than doubling of the risk of cardiac death. Further increases in myocardial isoenzymes are associated with further increase in risk, albeit not directly proportional. The plot shows a continuous relation between increased CK-MB and long-term outcome, pointing to the fact that any degree of necrosis is 'harmful' and that attempting to conclude that a certain amount of necrosis is not significant, by setting the threshold at an arbitrary level, is simply not accurate.

In summary, a growing body of evidence is accumulating linking the small non-Q-wave MIs after 'apparently successful' coronary interventions to an adverse long-term prognosis.

Other complications

Other complications include vascular sequelae, such as pseudoaneurysm formation, large haematoma requiring surgical repair, atrioventricular fistulas, coronary perforation and coronary embo-

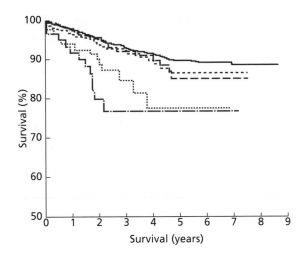

Figure 10b.1. *Plot showing long-term survival for patients undergoing percutaneous transluminal coronary angioplasty grouped according to peak creatine kinase (CK) values (IU/l):* (——— 180, MB ≤ 4%; ---- 101–179, MB > 4%; ——180–359, MB > 4%; ······· 360–899, MB > 4%; —·— ≥ 900, MB > 4%); *MB, myocardial band. (From ref. 13 with permission.)*

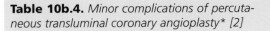

Table 10b.4. *Minor complications of percutaneous transluminal coronary angioplasty* [2]*

Complication	Episodes	(%)
Side branch closure	59	(1.7)
Ventricular arrhythmias (DC shock)	54	(1.5)
New conduction defects	31	(0.9)
Emergency recatheterization	27	(0.8)
Repair of femoral artery	22	(0.6)
Atrial fibrillation/flutter	14	(0.4)
Excessive blood loss requiring transfusion	9	(0.3)
Coronary embolus	5	(0.1)
Tamponade	3	(0.1)
Stroke	1	(0.03)
Miscellaneous	19	(0.5)
Total episodes	244	(7.0)
Total patients	241	(6.9)

*n = 3500.

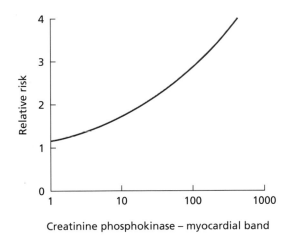

Figure 10b.2. *Plot showing the relation between risk of cardiac death on follow-up and peak creatine kinase–myocardial band after the procedure. [14]*

lus. Table 10b.4 lists other complications that result from PTCA.

Late results

The major deficiency of coronary angioplasty as a treatment for coronary artery disease is the high incidence of restenosis. Although there are several definitions of restenosis in active use, most are similar to the commonly used criterion of a 50% diameter stenosis on follow-up. The predominant cause of restenosis is neointimal proliferation, in which media-derived smooth muscle cells proliferate and migrate into the intimal layer of the vessel, reducing the diameter of the lumen [1]. The cause of this process is not understood, but current concepts regard it as a non-specific response to the physical trauma of the angioplasty process. However, recent studies have demonstrated that the contribution of neointimal hyperplasia to restenosis after balloon angioplasty is relatively limited and that lumen renarrowing is, in fact, mostly related to vessel remodelling (chronic sclerosis with vessel constriction) [16]. Immediate recoil also appears to have an important role. Further studies are needed, however, to address this issue directly.

Reported angiographic coronary restenosis rates range between 30 and 45% [1]. Several correlates of restenosis probability have been identified. Most describe the lesion and the quality of the angioplasty result rather than the characteristics of the patient. However, a greater frequency of restenosis has also been reported in diabetic patients [17].

Limitations of PTCA

Despite the advanced technology, PTCA continues to exhibit two major limitations — abrupt closure and restenosis. In addition, the treatment of complex lesions (such as calcified lesions, long lesions, ulcerated lesions and vein grafts) has a low success rate and a high incidence of complications. New modalities of therapeutic percutaneous interventions (such as atherectomy, laser and stents) have been developed to overcome many of the limitations of PTCA with the objectives of maintaining a high success rate with reduction of residual stenosis, minimizing dissection and abrupt closure, expanding the treatment of lesions currently unfavourable for PTCA and potentially reducing the incidence of restenosis.

New antiplatelet agents

Recently, new antiplatelet agents, far more powerful than aspirin, have undergone testing in the setting of angioplasty. As previously mentioned, Abciximab, the c7E3 monoclonal antibody directed against the platelet GP IIb/IIIa receptor, has been shown to reduce significantly any thrombotic complications occurring after PTCA in high-risk populations [8]: Abciximab reduced the composite incidence of death, MI, emergency CABG or stent implantation by 35% at both 2 and 30 days. It is the author's practice to use Abciximab in the majority of cases of high-risk PTCA, particularly in the presence of intracoronary thrombus, post-MI angina and multivessel PTCA.

Coronary stenting

The single most important advance in the field of interventional cardiology since the introduction of the balloon has been the use of coronary stenting. Stenting consists of deploying an expandable endovascular prosthesis at an angioplasty site to attempt to solve the three principal dilemmas of coronary angioplasty — (1) inadequate lumen enlargement of the target site, (2) acute occlusion due to dissection flaps and (3) restenosis. The

concept of stenting was developed to oppose elastic recoil, to 'scaffold' dissection flaps away from the vascular lumen and to decrease restenosis. Stents seem to address these problems [1].

Stent designs
There are several stent designs currently in various stages of clinical evaluation. The stents differ in one or more of their specifications, including material composition, metallic surface area, strut design and thickness, longitudinal flexibility and mechanisms of deployment. These specifications affect the characteristics of each stent (such as its flexibility, trackability, symmetry, degree of radial strength, visualization and side branch access) and therefore its use in specific clinical and anatomical situations.

Acute results
All the currently available designs perform well acutely, and delivery success rates of more than 90% have been reported [18,19]. The principal short-term problem is subacute thrombosis which — depending on the stent used and the circumstances of deployment — occurred in 3–13% of patients within the first 14 days in the early stent experience, with a maximal incidence on the fifth day after stent deployment in the earlier series. Subacute thrombosis was two to three times more common in stents deployed for acute occlusion complicating conventional PTCA than in those for elective placement in stable patients. The conventional strategy has been to maintain anticoagulation with i.v. heparin until full warfarin anticoagulation (international normalized ratio 2.5–3.0) has been established. Warfarin anticoagulation with concomitant aspirin therapy was conventionally maintained for at least 1 month after stent deployment. Recently reported observations with the Palmaz–Schatz stent suggest that optimal deployment using high-pressure balloons (12–18 atm; ≈ 1.2–1.8 MPa), to ensure uniform expansion and to complete stent–vessel wall contact, minimizes the likelihood of stent thrombosis. Indeed, the incidence of this problem has decreased to less than 1% with the use of high-pressure balloon dilatation of the stent [20]. Intravascular ultrasound (IVUS) can also be an adjunctive tool to stent deployment. IVUS allows the visualization of the stent and artery 'from within', to ensure adequate stent expansion. With this technique, anticoagulation with warfarin is no longer standard, and the patients are maintained only on a combination of aspirin and ticlopidine [21].

Late results

The effectiveness of the Palmaz–Schatz stent in reducing restenosis has been examined in two prospective randomized trials [18,19]. Both have shown that, compared with conventional balloon angioplasty, stenting provides a larger lumen diameter acutely. At the 6-month follow-up, the average amount of lumen dimension lost is greater in stented lesions than in lesions treated with conventional balloon angioplasty. However, because the dimension achieved acutely is considerably greater, the net effect is a slightly greater lumen diameter in stented lesions at 6-month angiographic follow-up. In the Stent Restenosis Study, stented lesions had a mean minimal lumen diameter at follow-up of 1.75 ± 0.60 mm, whereas lesions treated with conventional balloon angioplasty had a mean minimal lumen diameter of 1.55 ± 0.56 mm. There was a statistically significantly lower categorical restenosis rate (29.1 vs 42.7%) in the stented group [18].

In summary, stenting has been the single most important addition since the introduction of conventional balloon angioplasty. It is clearly effective at improving the acute angiographic outcome of conventional balloon coronary angioplasty and at salvaging threatened and abrupt closure after conventional coronary angioplasty. At this time, limitations of stenting are the difficulties of deploying the device and its expense.

Atherectomy

New modalities for plaque removal and ablation have been developed to improve success, reduce residual stenosis, minimize dissection and abrupt closure, expand the treatment of lesions currently unfavourable for PTCA, and potentially reduce the incidence of restenosis [22]. The roles of directional, rotational and extraction atherectomy devices in addressing these problems are examined below.

Directional coronary atherectomy

DCA involves the selective excision and removal of obstructive atheromatous or abnormally proliferating lesions from the vessel wall. The DCA catheter (Devices for Vascular Intervention, Inc., Redwood City, CA, USA) (Fig. 10b.3) consists of a metal housing with an affixed balloon and a flexible nose cone collection chamber at the distal end of a hollow rigid tube. Within the housing there is a retractable cup-shaped cutter, which is activated by an external hand-held motor drive

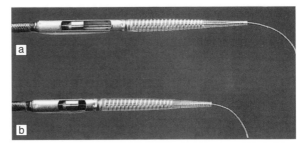

Figure 10b.3. *Directional coronary atherectomy catheter: (a) 9 mm window; (b) the modified short cutter (5 mm window) can negotiate tortuosity with a tighter radius of curvature. (Courtesy of Guidant Corp., Santa Clara, CA, USA.)*

unit connected by a torque cable. After a guidewire has been placed distal to the target stenosis, the atherectomy catheter is advanced into the lesion and oriented so that the cutting window faces the bulk of the atheroma. The balloon is inflated, the cutter is retracted and the motor drive unit is then activated. A lever allows the operator to advance the cutter slowly through the lesion as it rotates at 2000 rpm. The balloon is then deflated, the catheter reoriented and the procedure repeated until the desired result is achieved. The excised atheroma is stored in the distal nose cone, which is emptied at the end of the procedure (or whenever it becomes full and prevents free movement of the guidewire). Appropriate sizing of the device, a sufficient number of cuts and adequate balloon inflation pressure are necessary for optimal tissue removal. Post-DCA angioplasty is performed if a significant stenosis remains after the atherectomy, with a target residual stenosis of 0–10% [23].

Acute results

The extent of luminal improvement after DCA appears to be due to a combination of Dotter effect, PTCA effect and tissue removal. Compared with conventional balloon angioplasty, DCA results in a larger lumen with less incidence of dissection. Recent studies reviewing the procedural outcome of DCA have shown success and complication rates comparable to those associated with PTCA (Table 10b.5) [24–27]. Similar to PTCA, DCA is very effective in treating focal, non-calcified lesions, but is less effective in treating lesions associated with diffuse disease, calcification, proximal vessel tortuosity or degenerated saphenous vein grafts (SVG). The Coronary Angioplasty Versus Excisional Atherectomy Trial (CAVEAT) was the first prospective randomized

Table 10b.5. *Directional atherectomy: acute procedural results*

| Study | n | Result | | | |
		Success (%)	MI (%)	CABG (%)	Death (%)
Hinohara 1991 [25]	382	94	5.0	4.6	0.3
Ellis 1991 [24]	378	88	1.8	5.5	1.0
Fishman 1992 [26]	190	98	0.0	0.5	0.0
CAVEAT 1993 [27]	1012	89	6.0*	3.0	0.0

MI, myocardial infarction; CABG, coronary artery bypass grafting.

*Detected clinically by site.

comparison of DCA versus PTCA. The recently published results showed that DCA has a higher success rate (89 vs 80%, $p < 0.001$) at the expense of a higher rate of early complications [11 vs 5%, $p < 0.001$ (death: 0 vs 0.4%; clinically detected MI: 6 vs 3%; emergency CABG: 3 vs 2%; abrupt closure: 7 vs 3%)] [27].

Restenosis

Despite a better acute angiographic result compared with PTCA, the incidence of restenosis has been only mildly reduced by the use of DCA. The CAVEAT demonstrated an acute luminal gain of 1.04 mm for DCA compared with 0.85 mm for PTCA ($p <0.0001$). However, late loss was also more prominent in the DCA group (−0.54 vs −0.41 mm for PTCA; $p = 0.003$), resulting in a similar final net gain (0.47 mm for DCA vs. 0.40 mm for PTCA; $p = 0.30$) [27]. The CAVEAT also showed a 6-month angiographic restenosis rate of 50% for DCA versus 57% for PTCA ($p = 0.06$) [27]. Table 10b.6 shows the indications and contraindications of DCA.

Rotational atherectomy

Rotational atherectomy involves the use of a Rotablator (SciMed, Maple Grove, MI, USA), which consists of an elliptically shaped brass burr coated with 5–10 μm diamond chips bonded to a flexible drive shaft (Fig. 10b.4). The drive shaft and the burr rotate at 140 000–180 000 rpm as they are advanced over a 0.009-inch stainless steel guidewire. After wiring the stenosis, the Rotablator is tracked just proximal to the lesion and subsequently activated. The operator uses a control knob to advance the rotating burr slowly over the guidewire and through the

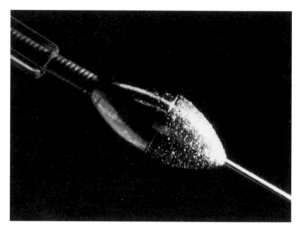

Figure 10b.4. *Magnified view of the Rotablator burr, sheath and drive shaft over a 0.009 in guidewire. (Courtesy of SciMed, Maple Grove, MI, USA.)*

lesion, resulting in a micro-ablation of the obstructing atheroma. If adjunctive intervention is required (which is frequently the case), the Rotablator can be exchanged over the guidewire for a larger burr or another definitive device. Because of its high rotational speed, the Rotablator preferentially ablates inelastic, non-compliant, atheromatous tissue. Plaque-free wall segments are spared from mechanical trauma because their visco-elastic properties make them deflect around the rotating burr. Thus, rotational atherectomy is particularly suited for calcified lesions.

Acute results

In reviewing the results of rotational atherectomy, it should be noted that most rotational atherectomy patients have lesions of complex morphology (type B or C) that are known to have an adverse

Table 10b.6. *Indications and contraindications for directional coronary atherectomy (DCA)*

Indications

▪ Stenosis in proximal or mid segments of large vessel in the absence of contraindications

▪ Saphenous vein graft lesions

▪ Bifurcation lesions

▪ Selected lesions failing angioplasty

Contraindications

▪ Large thrombi

▪ Excessive proximal tortuosity

▪ Diffuse disease (> 20 mm)

▪ Small vessel (< 2.5 mm)

▪ Degenerated saphenous vein grafts

▪ Moderate to heavy calcification

▪ Extensive or spiral dissections

▪ Recurrent restenosis, especially in saphenous vein grafts after repeated PTCA procedures, unless the final minimal residual diameter achieved can be improved by DCA compared with previous procedures

PCTA, percutaneous transluminal coronary angioplasty.

(From ref. 22 with permission.)

effect on the results of PTCA. Nevertheless, the angiographic success, complication profile and restenosis associated with this procedure appear to compare favourably with PTCA (Table 10b.7) [28–31]. Whitlow *et al.* reported on 874 lesions in 745 patients treated with the Rotablator and found that lesion calcification, eccentricity, lesion length of more than 10 mm and vessel tortuosity did not have an adverse effect on angiographic success [32]. Moreover, unlike PTCA, cumulative effects of angiographic risk factors on success were not apparent; in fact, type A, B1, B2 and C lesions had comparable angiographic success rates (97, 94, 95 and 95%, respectively). However, major complications (death, MI and bypass surgery) were increased with more complex lesion morphology: 0% for type A lesions, 7% for type B1, 8% for type B2 and 15% for type C lesions.

Restenosis

Popma *et al.* studied restenosis after rotational atherectomy in 210 patients, and showed that symptoms recurred in 46% of patients [33]. Angiographic restenosis (> 50% stenosis) was present in 52% of lesions with angiographic follow-up, with no clear advantage over PTCA. A randomized comparison of PTCA and rotational atherectomy also showed no restenosis advantage for using the Rotablator in complex coronary lesions [34]. Table 10b.8 shows the indications and contraindications for Rotablator use.

Transluminal extraction catheter atherectomy

The transluminal extraction catheter (TEC) atherectomy device (Interventional Technologies Inc., San Diego, CA, USA) consists of two stainless steel blades at the distal end of a rotating hollow flexible tube (Fig. 10b.5). A pressurized flush solution is infused into the guide catheter and around the activated TEC device. When activated, the device functions as a cutting and aspiration system, removing the occluding atherothrombotic plaque inside the blood vessel to an attached vacuum bottle. During the procedure, a special exchange length guidewire (0.014 inch) with an enlarged olive tip is positioned beyond the stenosis, and the TEC cutter is advanced just proximal to the lesion. With the cutter and vacuum system activated, the rotating cutter (750 rpm) is slowly advanced over the guidewire through the lesion. Several passes are performed until there is little or no resistance. If further intervention is required, the TEC device can be exchanged for a larger cutter or another definitive device.

Results

Unlike standard balloon angioplasty, which improves coronary dimension by splitting and tearing the obstructive atheroma, TEC exerts its beneficial effect on coronary stenoses by excising the atherosclerotic plaque and extracting the debris by continuous vacuum suction, thus avoiding the potential risks of vascular barotrauma and distal particulate embolization. This technique has potential applications in lesions within SVGs, lesions with thrombus, or lesions with marked luminal irregularities.

It was hoped that the TEC would find a niche in treating the high-risk subgroup of patients with diseased SVGs. Indeed, TEC has been proposed as a treatment of choice for diseased, degenerated SVGs, since its cutting–aspirating technique is thought to be particularly well suited for the treat-

Table 10b.7. *Rotational atherectomy: acute results*

| Study | n | Result | | | | |
		Success (%)	Q-MI (%)	non Q-MI (%)	CABG (%)	Death (%)
Buchbinder 1991 [29]	745	94	0.8	4.6	1.4	0.0
Bertrand 1992 [31]	129	86	2.3	5.5	1.6	0.0
Stertzer 1993 [28]	302	95	3.3	11.0	1.2	0.0
Cowley 1993 [30]	1362	95	0.9	4.6	2.1	0.8

Q-MI, Q-wave myocardial infarction; CABG, coronary artery bypass grafting.

Table 10b.8. *Indications and contraindications for rotational atherectomy*

Indications

- Ostial stenosis
- Calcified lesions
- Elastic lesions
- Undilatable lesions
- Restenotic lesions

Contraindications

- Thrombus-containing lesions
- Degenerated saphenous vein grafts
- Diffuse disease with large plaque load and limited distal runoff
- Angulation > 45°*
- Branch point disease*

*Relative contraindication.

(From ref. 22 with permission.)

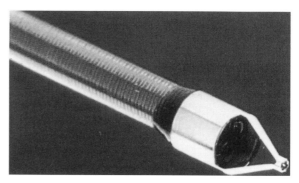

Figure 10b.5. *The transluminal extraction catheter: front cutting blades with aspiration channel effectively remove atherosclerotic debris. (Courtesy of InterVentional Technologies Inc., San Diego, CA, USA.)*

< 0.05) and a higher residual stenosis (24 vs 12%; *p* < 0.05). There were no major acute ischaemic complications in the young SVG group, whereas the group with old SVGs showed an 8% incidence of death, 1% of E-CABG, and 1% Q-wave myocardial infarction (Q-MI). Follow-up at 6 months revealed a 14% combined incidence of death, MI and CABG for the old SVG group versus 0% for the group with young SVGs.

These significant complication rates have led to utilization of the TEC in older, degenerated SVGs with unfavourable morphology only in patients who fail medical therapy and who are poor reoperative candidates. Instead, a period of prolonged heparinization or graft thrombolysis may be preferred, with the possible use of new antithrombotic agents (Hirudin) or new antiplatelet agents (7E3), followed by TEC, DCA or stenting after resolution of the thrombus angiographically. It is possible, although yet untested, that the use of potent antithrombotic or

ment of saphenous graft stenosis. However, recent studies indicate that the TEC procedure performed on old degenerated SVGs that contain thrombus is associated with lower success and higher complication rates than TEC in discrete lesions. Abdelmeguid *et al.* analysed 104 lesions in SVGs treated with TEC and compared the results of the procedure in old (> 36 months) and young (< 36 months) grafts [35]: they found that old SVGs were associated with a lower success rate (86 vs 93%; *p*

Table 10b.9. *Indications and contraindications for extraction atherectomy*

Indications

- Thrombus-containing lesions

- Focal saphenous vein graft lesions

- Medically refractory degenerated saphenous grafts in poor operative candidates

Contraindications

- Heavily calcified lesions

- Severely angled stenoses

- Small vessels

- Bifurcated lesions

- Dissections

(From ref. 28 with permission.)

antiplatelet agents before TEC might decrease the complication rate. It is also possible that stenting after TEC might have a better result than adjunctive balloon angioplasty. Obviously, this is an area of great controversy and advances in interventional cardiology have yet to provide a safe, definitive answer for this high-risk group with degenerated vein graft disease. Table 10b.9 lists the indications and contraindications of TEC atherectomy.

Laser ablation techniques

The rationale that debulking of the atheromatous plaque would improve the success of PTCA was the initial stimulus for the development of mechanical atherectomy and laser systems. Initial laser systems used continuous-wave energy delivered through a bare fibre-optic wire, but they conveyed a high degree of thermal energy to adjacent tissue, stimulating a strong hyperplastic response. Current systems use pulsed high-energy waves to ablate plaque with minimal thermal damage. The success of laser angioplasty is still limited by the small size of channel created and the high cost of laser systems and catheters [1].

Although several different types of lasers are currently used, only one is Food and Drug Administration (FDA)-approved for coronary use in the USA (Advanced Interventional Systems Inc. [Irvine, CA, USA] excimer laser). This device uses pulsed-wave energy in the ultraviolet (308 nm xenon chloride excimer) spectrum. This device delivers high energy via multiple fibres concentrically (or eccentrically) arranged around a central lumen, and can thus be advanced over a guidewire to minimize the risk of perforation.

Results

Most of the experience of laser ablation in the coronary arteries in the USA has been accumulated with the AIS excimer device. The holmium YAG laser is relatively new, is somewhat bulkier, and has fewer optical fibres, possibly accounting for a lower success rate in early trials. In the multicentre US experience with excimer coronary angioplasty, acute success rates of 84–90% have been achieved; however, adjunctive balloon angioplasty was used in 70–95% of procedures [1,36]. Complication rates have been relatively low and resemble those of conventional PTCA. However, vessel perforation with major clinical events has occurred in 1% of procedures [37]. Most procedures require adjunctive balloon angioplasty to achieve satisfactory results. Restenosis rates in selected series of excimer laser angioplasty have remained above 50% [34]. In view of the high frequency of adjunctive balloon angioplasty, it is difficult to determine how the laser procedure contributes to either the long-term outcome or the short-term success rate.

In summary, laser coronary angioplasty remains at an early investigational stage of development. The ability to use laser energy to ablate coronary atherosclerotic plaque in a reasonably safe fashion has been clearly demonstrated. However, no convincing evidence that lasers can improve the success rate and predictability of PTCA, or lower the complication and restenosis rates, has been presented [34].

Conclusions

Balloon angioplasty remains the mainstay of percutaneous revascularization techniques for the treatment of obstructive coronary artery disease. Success rates generally exceed 90%, despite trends in recent years to attempt more complex and distal lesions in patients with multivessel disease.

The safety of this procedure is well established, with major complication rates of less than 5%. Major complications of balloon angioplasty are primarily due to periprocedural abrupt vessel occlusion and frequently result in acute MI or the need for emergency bypass surgery. Coronary stenting has largely decreased the incidence of this complication and is also being used effectively to treat it when it occurs (bail-out stenting).

The efficacy of balloon angioplasty in patients with medically refractory unstable angina and acute MI has been conclusively demonstrated. Its efficacy in symptomatic patients with chronic stable angina is also well documented [1].

Despite the high safety and efficacy of PTCA, the major limitation of the procedure is restenosis. Unlike acute occlusion, which occurs in a small minority of procedures, restenosis may occur in up to 45% of dilated lesions. Its occurrence has been a major stimulus to the development of the newer interventional technologies. Among these, stents hold the most promise and are the only devices shown so far to affect the restenosis rate after percutaneous coronary interventions.

References

1. Herrmann HC, Hirshfield JW, Jr. Coronary angioplasty and related techniques. In: Baum S (ed) Abrams' angiography. Boston: Little, Brown and Company, 1997: 366–385

2. Abdelmeguid AE, Ellis SG. Complications of PTCA. In: Vliestra RE, Holmes DR, Jr (eds) Coronary balloon angioplasty. Cambridge, Mass.: Blackwell Scientific Publications, 1994: 399–451

3. Ellis SG, Myler RK, King SB et al. Causes and correlates of death after unsuccessful coronary angioplasty: implications for use of angioplasty and advanced support strategies in high risk settings. Am J Cardiol 1991; 68: 1447–1451

4. Nichols AB, Smith R, Berke AD et al. Importance of balloon size in coronary angioplasty. J Am Coll Cardiol 1989; 13: 1094–1100

5. Ellis SG, Roubin GS, King SB et al. Angiographic and clinical predictors of acute closure after native vessel coronary angioplasty. Circulation 1988; 77: 372–379

6. Schwartz L, Bourassa MG, Lesperance J et al. Aspirin and dipyridamole in the prevention of re-stenosis after percutaneous transluminal coronary angioplasty. N Engl J Med 1988; 318: 1714–1719

7. Deligonul O, Gabliani GI, Caroles DG et al. Percutaneous transluminal coronary angioplasty in patients with intracoronary thrombus. Am J Cardiol 1988; 62: 474–476

8. The EPIC Investigators. Use of monoclonal antibody directed against the platelet glycoprotein IIb/IIIa receptor in high risk coronary angioplasty. N Engl J Med 1994; 330: 956–961

9. Sinclair IN, McCabe GH, Sipperly ME et al. Predictors, therapeutic options, and long term outcome of abrupt reclosure. Am J Cardiol 1988; 61: 61G–66G

10. Hofling B, Gonschior P, Simpson L et al. Efficacy of directional coronary atherectomy in cases unsuitable for percutaneous transluminal coronary angioplasty (PTCA) and after unsuccessful percutaneous transluminal coronary angioplasty. Am Heart J 1992; 124: 341–348

11. Roubin GS, Cannon AD, Agrawal SK et al. Intracoronary stenting for acute and threatened closure complicating percutaneous transluminal coronary angioplasty. Circulation 1992; 85: 916–927

12. Greene MA, Gray LA Jr, Slater AD et al. Emergency aortocoronary bypass after failed angioplasty. Ann Thorac Surg 1991; 51: 194–199

13. Abdelmeguid AE, Topol EJ. The myth of the myocardial 'infarctlet' during percutaneous coronary revascularization procedures. Circulation 1996; 94: 3369–3375

14. Abdelmeguid AE, Ellis SG, Sapp SK et al. Defining the appropriate threshold of creatine kinase elevation after percutaneous coronary interventions. Am Heart J 1996; 131: 1097–1105

15. Abdelmeguid AE, Topol EJ, Whitlow PL et al. Significance of mild transient release of creatine kinase-MB fraction after percutaneous coronary interventions. Circulation 1996; 94: 1528–1536

16. Mintz GS, Popma JJ, Pichard AD et al. Arterial remodeling after coronary angioplasty: a serial intravascular ultrasound study. Circulation 1996; 94: 35–43

17. Van Belle E, Bauters C, Hubert E et al. Restenosis rates in diabetic patients. A comparison of coronary stenting and balloon angioplasty in native coronary vessels. Circulation 1997; 96: 1454–1460

18. Fischman DL, Leon MB, Baim D et al. A randomized comparison of coronary stent placement and balloon angioplasty in the treatment of coronary artery disease. N Engl J Med 1994; 331: 1496–1501

19. Serruys PW, deJaegere P, Kiemeneij F et al. A comparison of balloon expandable stent implantation with balloon angioplasty in patients with coronary artery disease. N Engl J Med 1994; 331: 489–495

20. Colombo A, Hall P, Nakamura S et al. Intracoronary stenting without anticoagulation accomplished with intravascular ultrasound guidance. Circulation 1995; 91: 1676–1688

21. Schömig A, Neuman FJ, Kastrati A et al. A randomized comparison of antiplatelet and anticoagulant therapy after the placement of coronary artery stents. N Engl J Med 1996; 334: 1084–1089

22. Abdelmeguid AE, Whitlow PL. Coronary atherectomy: directional, rotational, and extraction catheters. In: White CJ, Ramee SR (eds) Interventional cardiology: new techniques and strategies for diagnosis and treatment. New York: Marcel Dekker, 1995: 175–200

23. Baim DS, Kuntz RE. Directional coronary atherectomy: how much lumen enlargement is optimal? Am J Cardiol 1993; 72: 65E–70E

24. Ellis SG, De Cesare NB, Pinkerton CA et al. Relation of stenosis morphology and clinical presentation to the procedural results of directional coronary atherectomy. Circulation 1991; 84: 644–653

25. Hinohara T, Rowe MH, Robertson GC et al. Effect of lesion characteristics on outcome of directional coro-

nary atherectomy. *J Am Coll Cardiol* 1991; 17: 1112–1120

26. Fishman RF, Kuntz RE, Carrozza JP *et al.* Long-term results of directional coronary atherectomy: predictors of restenosis. *J Am Coll Cardiol* 1992; 20: 1101–1110 .

27. Topol EJ, Leya F, Pinkerton CA *et al.* A comparison of directional atherectomy with coronary angioplasty in patients with coronary artery disease. *N Engl J Med* 1993; 329: 221–227

28. Stertzer SH, Rosenblum J, Shaw RE *et al.* Coronary rotational ablation: initial experience in 302 procedures. *J Am Coll Cardiol* 1993; 21: 287–295

29. Buchbinder M, Warth D, Zacca N *et al.* Multicenter registry of percutaneous coronary rotational ablation using the rotablator (Abstr). *Circulation* 1991; 84: 11–82

30. Cowley MJ, Warth D, Whitlow PL *et al.* Factors influencing outcome with coronary rotational ablation: multicenter results (abstract). *J Am Coll Cardiol* 1993; 21: 31A

31. Bertrand ME, Lablanche JM, Leroy F *et al.* Percutaneous transluminal coronary rotary ablation with Rotablator (European experience). *Am J Cardiol* 1992; 69: 470–474

32. Whitlow PL, Buchbinder M, Kent K *et al.* Coronary rotational atherectomy: angiographic risk factors and their relation to success/complication (Abstr). *J Am Coll Cardiol* 1992; 19: 334A

33. Popma JJ, Satler LF, Pichard AD *et al.* A quantitative analysis of factors affecting late angiographic outcome after rotational coronary atherectomy (Abstr). *J Am Coll Cardiol* 1993; 21: 31A

34. Reifart N, Vandormael M, Krajcar M *et al.* Randomized comparison of angioplasty of complex coronary lesions at a single center. Excimer laser, rotational atherectomy, and balloon angioplasty comparison (ERBAC) study. *Circulation* 1997; 96: 91–98

35. Abdelmeguid AE, Ellis SG, Whitlow PL *et al.* Discordant results of extraction atherectomy in old and young saphenous vein grafts: the NACI experience (Abstr). *J Am Coll Cardiol* 1993; 21: 442A

36. Litvack F, Eigler N, Margolis J *et al.* Percutaneous excimer laser coronary angioplasty: result in the first consecutive 3,000 patients. *J Am Coll Cardiol* 1994; 23: 323–329

37. Bittl JA, Ryan TJ, Keaney JF *et al.* Coronary artery perforation during excimer laser coronary angioplasty. *J Am Coll Cardiol* 1993; 21: 1158–1165

38. Ryan TJ, Faxon DP, Gunnar RM *et al.* Guidelines for percutaneous transluminal coronary angioplasty: a report of the American College of Cardiology / American Heart Association Task Force on Assessment of Diagnostic and Therapeutic Cardiovascular Procedures (Subcommittee on Percutaneous Transluminal Coronary Angioplasty). *J Am Coll Cardiol* 1988; 12: 529–545

CHAPTER 11

Diet, fat and cancer of the prostate

M. J. Hill

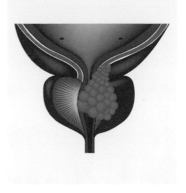

Introduction

Prostate cancer is one of the commonest cancers in Western societies. In a study by Levi *et al.* [1] it was ranked second in terms of male cancer mortality in three of the 26 European countries, third in four and fourth in all others except Bulgaria (where it was fifth) (Table 11.1). Compared with other cancer mortality, it is ranked lower than only lung and large bowel cancers. In terms of incidence, it is the commonest site for male cancer in Iceland, and second only to lung cancer in all Scandinavian countries, Germany, the Netherlands and many UK regions [1]. The lifetime risk of prostate cancer in men equals that of breast cancer in women in many countries. However, it is by far the least studied of the common cancers in either sex.

There are many reasons for this. One is that the incidence is very much higher than the mortality; traditionally, men are said to die with prostate cancer rather than of it. It is a cancer of old age, so that by the time epidemiologists develop a personal interest in it their research careers are coming to an end. In contrast, breast cancer can occur at a relatively early age when relatives working in cancer research are still young and active. In addition, there has been little public interest in prostate cancer until recently. Finally, data on the incidence of the cancer are very unreliable since, in many cases, the disease is diagnosed only at autopsy and the causes of relatively few deaths are confirmed in that way. Consequently, the European countries with the highest incidence and mortality rates for prostatic cancer are in Scandinavia (where until recently the autopsy rate was very high) and Switzerland (Table 11.2).

With the general increase in longevity seen throughout the Western world, the problem of prostate cancer is increasing. The precancerous condition, benign prostatic hyperplasia (BPH), is widely prevalent in older men in all parts of the world: 50% of men have the disease symptomatically by the age of 60, and 90% by the age of 85 [2]. Similarly, the progression to occult prostate cancer is widely prevalent in all countries, being detected in 30% of men over 50 years of age [2] and in a greater percentage in men over 70 years. However, there is no way of knowing which of these occult cases will become symptomatic and which will not. In Japan and other Asian countries, the disease usually stays at an early and asymptomatic stage and is diagnosed only at post-mortem examination, even though Japanese have a longer life expectancy than Europeans. In contrast, in Western populations, the severity of the disease increases with time and the mortality increases sharply with age (Table 11.3). Thus, as life expectancy increases, the magnitude of the problem will increase sharply.

Uncertainties regarding the management of prostate cancer and BPH also add to the problem [3]. Radical prostatectomy is advocated by some as soon as cancer is detected in biopsies; others advo-

Table 11.1. *Ranking of prostate cancer by mortality rate among 26 European countries*

Ranking	Countries
Second	Norway, Sweden, Switzerland
Third	Belgium, Denmark, Finland, Spain
Fourth	Austria, Czechoslovakia, England/Wales, France, Greece, Holland, Hungary, Ireland, Italy, Luxembourg, N. Ireland, Poland, Portugal, Romania, Scotland, East Germany, West Germany, Yugoslavia
Fifth	Bulgaria

Table 11.2. *Mortality from prostate cancer per 100 000 per annum in 23 European countries 1983–1987*

Country	Mortality	Country	Mortality
1. Switzerland	21.7	13. Ireland	15.4
2. Norway	20.8	14. UK	13.7
3. Sweden	18.9	15. Czechoslovakia	12.8
4. Iceland	18.5	16. Spain	12.7
5. Denmark	17.8	17. Portugal	12.5
6. Belgium	17.5	18. Italy	11.6
7. Holland	17.0	19. Poland	9.2
8. Finland	16.9	20. Greece	7.9
9. France	16.5	21. Bulgaria	7.4
10. Germany	16.3	22. Romania	6.8
11. Hungary	15.6	23. USSR	5.8
12. Austria	15.6		

Table 11.3. *Variation in mortality rates per 1000 per annum with age for prostate cancer in US white men**

Age (years)	Cancer mortality		
	Prostate	Breast	Cervix
0–4	0.07	0.05	0.02
5–9	0.02	0.01	0.00
10–14	0.02	0.01	0.00
15–19	0.04	0.03	0.02
20–24	0.03	0.21	0.28
25–29	0.03	1.53	1.47
30–34	0.03	5.72	3.96
35–39	0.07	13.55	7.46
40–44	0.26	27.12	11.78
45–49	0.92	43.34	15.51
50–54	3.65	58.47	18.28
55–59	11.09	69.25	19.92
60–64	29.91	78.65	21.87
65–69	66.82	87.29	23.32
70–74	134.15	103.41	25.68
75–84	285.16	132.77	29.36
85+	465.24	183.54	29.88

*Data for two other high profile cancer sites — breast and cervix — are added for comparison.

cate a 'watch and wait' policy on the grounds that many cancers do not progress rapidly to metastatic disease, and because of the often severe consequences of the surgery (e.g. erectile dysfunction, urinary incontinence). Under these circumstances it would seem to be prudent to make the study of prostate cancer prevention a major research priority.

Histopathology and precancerous lesions

This subject is dealt with in Chapter 9, but some consideration needs to be given to it here. Carcinogenesis, in general, is a multistage process with different aetiological agents acting at the different stages. The epidemiology of the overall process is a summation of the epidemiology of each of the stages, but the effect of an individual factor may be specific to a particular stage. Thus, in colorectal cancer, where the histopathological sequence is from normal mucosa to small adenoma with mild dysplasia, to adenoma growth, increasing severity of epithelial dysplasia and carcinoma, smoking is an important causal factor in the first stage of adenoma formation. However, it is not implicated in the progression from small adenoma to carcinoma. In studies of the overall process of colorectal carcinogenesis, smoking appears to be unimportant, even though more detailed study shows it to be important at the essential first stage.

There is a well-defined precursor lesion in prostate carcinogenesis — BPH — within which dysplasia can develop and progress through the stages of increasing severity until the lesion contains early focal carcinomas. At this stage the carcinoma is still asymptomatic (although the BPH is likely to be causing problems!) and slowly progressive, and so is termed 'latent cancer' by many [4]. In some cases, it progresses more rapidly to become symptomatic and ultimately fatal. In such cases, a firm diagnosis is readily made and confirmed histologically, and so is described as 'clinical cancer'. There is a further subgroup, known as 'occult prostate cancers' [4], where the disease metastasizes, and is diagnosed from those metastases, whereas the primary cancer remains undetectable.

A feature of the epidemiology of the disease is that, although the incidence of early prostatic carcinoma is relatively uniform geographically, the incidence of symptomatic disease is not. Using standard epidemiological techniques, therefore, the factors that cause asymptomatic disease to become symptomatic and to progress to metastatic disease can be studied. This is less difficult than trying to study the earlier stages of development of BPH and its progression to early carcinoma.

Diet and cancer of the prostate

In the study of the role of diet and nutrition in the causation of cancer, the tools available are (a) human epidemiology, (b) animal models, (c) in vitro and tissue culture studies, and (d) dietary intervention studies. All of these have their strengths and weaknesses, and these have been discussed elsewhere at length [5]. Suffice it to say at this point that the animal and in vitro model studies can give information only on the mechanisms of an already established relationship; they cannot provide any information on whether such a relationship between a dietary component and cancer risk exists for humans. In consequence, the two tools that are left are human epidemiology (as a guide to the relationships between nutrients, foods, food patterns and cancer risk) and intervention studies (to assess whether the relationships are causal or coincidental).

Epidemiological studies can be classified into (a) population, (b) case–control and (c) prospective studies. Again, each of these has its strengths and weaknesses. The early epidemiological studies of prostate cancer were well reviewed by Wynder et al. [6] and by Franks [4]; the relationship with diet has recently been updated by Pienta and Esper [7].

In population studies, (usually termed 'ecological', though they rarely study ecology), the diet patterns in a wide range of populations are correlated with the incidence of or mortality from the disease. This allows populations with a wide range of cancer risk and of dietary patterns to be compared. Armstrong and Doll [8] studied 32 countries from all continents and showed that there was a strong correlation between intake of total fat, meat and sugar and mortality from cancer of the prostate (Table 11.4). No such correlation was found with the incidence of the disease, but this was not surprising in view of the unreliability of incidence data. In earlier studies, Lea [9] and Howell [10] noted the same correlation with dietary fat. Since all population studies have to rely on essentially the same data, it is not surprising that such studies have continued to be unanimous in showing a correlation with total fat, animal fat, meat and sugar intake and with similar regressions (Table 11.4).

The main criticism of population studies is that the populations differ not only in their dietary patterns but also in many other respects, including climate, air and water pollution, geographical factors, personal hygiene and religious habits. This can be controlled for in case–control studies, where the controls are matched to the cases for many of these factors. The problem then is that, when these other factors are controlled for, the differences in diet patterns are

Table 11.4. *Correlation coefficients (r) between prostate cancer mortality and diet in 32 countries* and 41 countries†*

Diet factor	r	
	Armstrong and Doll (1975)*	Howell (1974)†
Total fat	0.74	0.73
Fats and oils	0.70	
Milk	0.66	0.70
Total protein	0.50	
Animal protein	0.67	
Meat	0.60	0.74
Cattle meat		0.75
Sugar	0.63	0.67
Eggs		0.50
Cereals	−0.60	
Pulses	−0.59	
Total energy intake	0.61	

*(Data from ref. 8)
†(Data from ref. 10)

often small, and the diets of uniformly exposed persons (one of whom was unlucky to develop the disease) are compared. In addition, when people are ill they tend to dislike their food and their diet can change subtly as a result of chronic symptoms. The diet must then be determined according to a time before symptoms took their effect, necessitating the use of diet recall, which is notoriously unreliable. This means that the results obtained are often very dependent on the choice of controlling factors. In consequence, case–control studies tend to give inconsistent results; it is not surprising, therefore, that whereas some case–control studies [11–13] give results that agree with those from the population studies, many others do not. For example, no relation between fat or meat intake and prostate cancer risk was found by Kaul *et al.* [14], Ohno *et al.* [15], Severson *et al.* [16], or Hsing *et al.* [17].

The prospective, or cohort study, involves the study of the current diet in a large cohort of healthy people. The cohort is then followed to see which members develop the cancer of interest.

These cases can subsequently be matched for age and location of residence to give a 'nested' case–control study with the diet determined prospectively. Thus, it has all the advantages of the case–control approach while avoiding many of the worst disadvantages. The major disadvantages of cohort studies are (a) the size of the cohort needed to yield a sufficient number of cases (cancer being a relatively rare disease), and (b) the length of time of follow-up needed to give sufficient numbers of cases. To study a large cohort over many years is costly in terms of money, time and expertise. A common way to get a quicker result is to have a large cohort and a very short follow-up. For example, in the Health Professionals Study of 51 529 men aged 40–75 years, diet was determined by a food-frequency questionnaire in 1986 with follow-ups in 1988 and 1990. By 1 January 1990, 126 new cases of advanced prostate cancer had been diagnosed. Of the nutrients studied, total fat was the most strongly correlated [relative risk (RR) in the highest intake quintile compared with the lowest = 1.79]. Within this food group, animal fat intake was significantly correlated (RR = 1.63), but the vegetable fat intake was not. With respect to specific foods, red meat carried the highest risk (RR = 2.64), whereas dairy fat carried no excess risk. It was concluded that decreasing red meat intake would reduce the risk of symptomatic prostate cancer.

As the follow-up in this study was so short, it might provide information about the role of diet in only the very last stages of the disease, leaving many questions unanswered. It is known that latent prostate cancer is widely prevalent and that the majority of such cancers remain latent. If a diet rich in red meat causes such cancers to progress more rapidly to symptomatic disease, then a decrease in red meat intake should be instantly accompanied by a decrease in cancer risk. However, if a long-term diet rich in red meat gives rise to a subgroup of apparently latent cancers that nevertheless progress rapidly to the symptomatic stage, then dietary change would affect risk much more slowly. The US diet has been rich in red meat for decades and, if the effects are on early disease stage, then the benefits of reducing meat intake might take a long time to emerge.

The Nutrition Society [18] has conducted a review of the literature on diet and cancer. For prostate cancer, they reviewed nine cohort studies (excluding Giovannucci *et al.* [19]); none showed meat or fat to be a risk factor and no general conclusions could be drawn from the findings. They also reviewed 12 case–control studies. Again, no general conclusions could be drawn, as some found a relationship with fat, meat, fruit or vegetables whereas others found no such relationship. The overall picture was of total confusion.

The role of other dietary factors

In recent years, interest has moved away from causal towards protective factors in the diet. A high intake of fruit and vegetables is associated with a decreased risk of cancer at a number of sites (Table 11.5) [20,21]. Block et al. reviewed 14 case–control studies of diet and prostate cancer and found that weight showed no relation between fruit and vegetable intake and cancer; four showed protection, while two showed a positive correlation [20]. In the huge North Italian study, the results were more positive, with an inverse dose–response relationship seen with both fruit and vegetable intake [21]. A strong role exists for male hormones in prostate carcinogenesis and plant products are a rich source of phyto-oestrogens — products that have an oestrogen-like action in the body. This may afford an explanation for the protective effect of fruit and vegetables in prostate cancer.

It is highly unlikely that antioxidant vitamins are responsible for the protective effect. Graham et al. observed an increase in prostate cancer risk with increased intake of vitamin C and of retinoids [11]. In the Alpha Tocopherol Beta Carotene (ATBC) Cancer Prevention Study, the group receiving supplements of beta carotene had an increased mortality from prostate cancer, whereas those receiving supplements of tocopherol (largely derived from fruit and vegetables) had a 33% decreased risk [22].

Regarding micronutrients in the diet, vitamin D deficiency has been postulated to be a risk factor for prostate cancer [23]. A large prospective study of long-term dietary supplementation with selenium showed a massive decrease in prostate cancers in those receiving the supplement [24]. This latter result is very exciting and should be replicated because of its potential public health implications.

Conclusions

Prostate cancer is one of the major causes of cancer death in Western males and the incidence and mortality is likely to continue to increase sharply as the population ages. In consequence, it is surprising how relatively little attention it receives compared with breast, cervical and ovarian cancer. In part, this is due to the reluctance of men (compared with women) to seek medical help, but this is a circular argument. The public is sceptical of the probable success of current treatment of prostate problems. Men would seek medical help for prostate problems with more enthusiasm if they felt that medicine could offer them anything other than the prospect of erectile dysfunction and incontinence with little apparent benefit. Those in the cancer-prevention field need to make men aware that their problems are not forgotten and that work is in progress.

It must be acknowledged, however, that the research on diet and prostate cancer is not showing clear results (Table 11.6). No doubt, at some stage, a large intervention study of the effect of

Table 11.5. *Correlation between fruit and vegetable intake and mortality from prostate cancer*

Study	Observation
Block et al. (1992) [20]	Reviewed 14 studies: four showed protection, two showed promotion and eight showed no effect
Negri et al. (1994) [21]	The North Italian study showed protection by both fruit and vegetables with a dose–response effect
Hirayama (1990) [25]	Very weak protective effect seen in those consuming green-yellow vegetables daily compared with less than daily consumption
Giovannucci et al. (1993) [19]	No protection by fruit and vegetables
ATBC Prevention Study (1996) [22]	Protection by alpha tocopherol

Table 11.6. *Summary of some epidemiological studies of diet and prostate cancer risk*

Study	Observation
Population studies	
Armstrong and Doll (1975) [8]	Strong correlation with total fat and meat, and protection by cereals
Howell (1974) [10]	Correlation with fat, meat, milk and sugar
Rose *et al.* (1986) [26]	Correlation with animal but not vegetable fat
Case–control studies	
Graham *et al.* (1983) [11]	Risk factors are animal fat, vitamin C and retinoids
Kolonel *et al.* (1983) [27]	Animal fat is a risk factor only for men over 75 years
Mettlin *et al.* (1989) [28]	Total fat is a risk factor
Mills *et al.* (1989) [29]	Total fat is a risk factor
Talamini *et al.* (1986) [13]	Meat and overweight risk factors
Heshmat *et al.* (1986) [12]	Total fat is a risk factor
Severson *et al.* (1989) [16]	No correlation with fat or meat
Kaul *et al.* (1987) [14]	No correlation with fat or meat
Ohno *et al.* (1988) [15]	No correlation with fat or meat in Japanese
Hsing *et al.* (1990) [17]	No correlation with fat or meat in American Lutherans
Prospective studies	
Hirayama (1990) [25]	Lower risk with high intake of green-yellow vegetables
Giovannucci *et al.* (1993) [19]	Increased risk with meat and animal fat but not with vegetable fat

decreased meat intake will be undertaken in the USA. Of more interest in the European context (where the meat intake levels are very much lower than US levels) is the possible use of selenium supplements. In the study by Clark *et al.*, the selenium was in the form of yeast selenomethionine (produced by feeding the selenium to yeasts) [24]. In this form, high intakes were well tolerated. At a recent symposium on micronutrients and human cancer in Aarhus, Denmark, the final consensus statement included a recommendation to the Danish Cancer Society that, in view of the relatively high mortality from prostate cancer in Scandinavia, they should support a study of such supplements in Denmark. If such a trial is undertaken, the results will be awaited with much interest.

References

1. Levi F, Maisonneuve P, Filiberti R *et al.* Cancer incidence and mortality in Europe. *Soz Praventivmed* 1989; 34(Suppl 2): 1–84
2. Griffiths S. Men's health. *Br Med J* 1996; 31(2): 69–70
3. Garnick MB. Prostate cancer; screening, diagnosis and management. *Ann Intern Med* 1993; 118: 804–818
4. Franks IM. Etiology, epidemiology and pathology of prostate cancer. *Cancer* 1973; 32: 1092–1095
5. Hill MJ. Diet and cancer; a review of the scientific evidence. *Eur J Cancer Prev* 1995; 5(Suppl 2): 3–42
6. Wynder EL, Mabuchi K, Whitmore WF. Epidemiology of cancer of the prostate. *Cancer* 1972; 28: 344–360
7. Pienta KJ, Esper PS. Is dietary fat a risk factor for prostate cancer? *J Natl Cancer Inst* 1993; 85: 1538–1540

8. Armstrong BK, Doll R. Environmental factors and the incidence and mortality from cancer in different countries with special reference to dietary practice. *Int J Cancer* 1975; 15: 617–631

9. Lea AJ. Dietary patterns associated with death rates from certain neoplasms in man. *Lancet* 1966; 2: 332–333

10. Howell MA. Factor analysis of international cancer mortality data and per capita food consumption. *Br J Cancer* 1975; 29: 328–336

11. Graham S, Haughey B, Marshall J *et al.* Diet in the epidemiology of cancer of the prostate gland. *J Natl Cancer Inst* 1983; 70: 687–692

12. Heshmat MY, Kaul L, Kovi J *et al.* Nutrition and prostate cancer; a case–control study. *Prostate* 1985; 6: 7–17

13. Talamini R, La Vecchia C, Decarli A *et al.* Nutrition, social factors and prostatic cancer in a North Italian population. *Br J Cancer* 1986; 53: 817–821

14. Kaul L, Heshmat MY, Kovi J *et al.* The role of diet in prostate cancer. *Nutr Cancer* 1987; 9: 123–128

15. Ohno Y, Yoshida O, Oishi K *et al.* Dietary beta carotene and cancer of the prostate: a case–control study in Kyoto, Japan. *Cancer Res* 1988; 48: 1331–1336

16. Severson RK, Nomura AMY, Grove JS, Stemmerman GN. A prospective study of demographics, diet and prostate cancer among men of Japanese ancestry in Hawaii. *Cancer Res* 1989; 49: 1857–1860

17. Hsing AW, McLaughlin JK, Schuman LM *et al.* Diet, tobacco use and fatal prostate cancer; results from the Lutheran Brotherhood cohort study. *Cancer Res* 1990; 50: 6836–6840

18. Nutrition Society. Diet and cancer. London: The Nutrition Society 1993: 4–167

19. Giovannucci E, Rimm E, Colditz GA *et al.* A prospective study of dietary fat and risk of prostate cancer. *J Natl Canc Inst* 1993; 83: 1571–1579

20. Block G, Patterson B, Subar A. Fruit, vegetables and cancer prevention. A review of the epidemiological evidence. *Nutr Cancer* 1992; 18: 1–29

21. Negri E, D'Avanzo B, Tavani A. The role of vegetables and fruit in cancer risk. In: Hill MJ, Giacosa A, Caygill CPJ (eds) Epidemiology of diet and cancer. Oxford: Ellis Horwood, 1994; 327–334

22. Alpha Tocopherol Beta Carotene Cancer Prevention Study. The effect of vitamin E and beta carotene on the incidence of lung cancer and other cancers in male smokers. *N Engl J Med* 1996; 330: 1029–1035

23. Schwartz GG, Hulka BS. Is vitamin D deficiency a risk factor for prostate cancer? *Anticancer Res* 1990; 10: 1307–1312

24. Clark LC, Combs GF, Turnbull BW *et al.* Effects of selenium supplementation for cancer prevention in patients with carcinoma of the skin. *JAMA* 1996; 276: 1957–1963

25. Hirayama T. Life-style and mortality. Basel: Karger, 1990

26. Rose, DP, Boyar AP, Wynder EL. International comparisons of mortality rates for cancer of the breast, ovary, prostate and colon and per capita food consumption. *Cancer* 1986; 58: 2663–2671

27. Kolonel LN, Nomura AMY, Hinds MW *et al.* Role of diet in cancer incidence in Hawaii. *Cancer Res* 1983; 43 (Suppl): 2397s–2402s

28. Mettlin C, Byers T, Natarajan N. Beta carotene and animal fats and their relationship to prostate cancer risk. *Cancer* 1989; 64: 605–612

29. Mills PK, Beeson L, Phillips RL, Fraser GE. Cohort study of the diet, lifestyle and prostate cancer in Adventist men. *Cancer* 1989; 64: 598–604

Male sexual dysfunction: diagnosis and treatment of erectile dysfunction

C. C. Carson

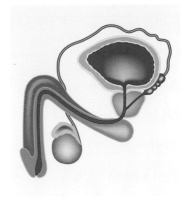

Introduction

Erectile dysfunction (ED), the preferred term to impotence, defines the inability to achieve and maintain an erection adequate for satisfactory sexual performance [1]. Epidemiological studies in both the USA and Europe have investigated the incidence and prevalence of ED in the male population. It has been estimated by the Massachusetts Male Aging Study that 5% of men over age 40, 10% of men in their 60s, and 20% of men in their 70s will have ED [2]. Patients over the age of 80 have a 30–50% prevalence of ED. Extrapolating these figures suggests that 20 million men in the USA may be suffering from ED; these numbers are clearly similar to those among European men. Until a decade ago, ED was suspected to be principally caused by psychological factors: in the 1970s, it was widely published that more than 90% of men with 'impotence' had a psychological basis for the condition. Pioneering studies in the past decade have elucidated the physiology of erectile function and the pathophysiology of ED, and have changed this concept. It is now clear that, in the majority of patients, ED has an organic aetiology.

Penile erectile function is a complex process requiring the combined neurological, endocrinological, psychological and vascular systems for satisfactory function. The aetiologies are, therefore, frequently overlapping and multifocal. In order to understand the causes and treatment for ED, it is important to review penile anatomy and the physiology of penile erection.

Anatomy of the penis

The penis is a specialized vascular organ composed of complex vascular tissue responsive to neurological impulses that create penile rigidity.

As discussed in chapter 2, it is composed of two paired corpora cavernosa and the corpus spongiosum, which contains the urethra, and is contiguous with the glans penis. The corpora cavernosa or penile erectile bodies are surrounded by a thick, fibrous sheath (tunica albuginea), which is relatively non-distensible, composed of elastic fibres and collagen which supports the rigidity of erectile function. The tunica albuginea is then surrounded by a second, gossamer, layer of fascia called Buck's fascia. Within these support structures there is a complex vascular sinusoidal network of spongy tissue which activates erection. Although the corpora cavernosa are generally considered separate, there is no clear septum between the two corpora in the distal portion of the penis and free vascular cross-communication is present. The corpora are composed primarily of sinusoids containing smooth muscle tissue and lined by endothelial cells. The corpus spongiosum is composed of similar spongy tissue but is surrounded by a less rigid, thinner tunica albuginea, resulting in less rigidity on activation.

The blood supply to the corpora cavernosa begins from the internal iliac arteries and travels to the internal pudendal arteries, which terminate in the arteries to the penis. These penile arteries include the dorsal artery to the penis above the tunica albuginea, the bulbo-urethral artery travelling within the corpus spongiosum lateral to the urethra and the central cavernosal arteries, which travel in the central portion of each of the paired corpora cavernosa and supply the blood for erection. A proximal perineal branch of the pudendal artery provides vascular supply to the perineal skin and scrotum. The dorsal artery of the penis is responsible for the blood supply of the penile skin and glans penis. The cavernosal arteries enter the corpora cavernosa at the hilum of each corpus and give rise to multiple helicine arteries which drain directly into the vascular lacunar spaces of the corpus cavernosum. Accessory pudendal arteries may also provide blood supply to the penis. These variable arteries may originate from the obturator artery, inferior pudendal artery, iliac trunk or inferior gluteal artery and frequently lie close to the prostate.

Venous drainage of the penis is important anatomically and functionally. The lacunar spaces or vascular sinusoids of the corpora cavernosa drain through subtunical veins beneath the tunica albuginea into the emissary veins by way of the deep dorsal vein of the penis. The deep dorsal vein ultimately culminates in the periprostatic venous plexus. The superficial dorsal vein, which lies above Buck's fascia, provides drainage primarily for the penile skin and culminates in the saphenous vein. The proximal penile shaft and proximal corpus cavernosum drains by way of veins exiting the crura of the corpora cavernosa and termed the crural veins, which join to form the internal pudendal vein. As with most venous systems, the venous drainage is variable and complex and has multiple intercommunications.

The nerve supply to the penis supplies sensation as well as corpus cavernosum vascular control. A pair of sympathetic nerves from S2–4 primarily control erectile function, while the sympathetic nerves from T11–L2 control detumescence and, ultimately, ejaculation. These autonomic nerve fibres form the pelvic plexus of nerves and enter the penis through the cavernous nerves, which course lateral and inferior to the prostate; these are the nerves that can be preserved during nerve-sparing radical prostatectomy. In addition to the autonomic nervous system, peripheral nerves form sensory and motor elements through a reflex arc in the sacral spinal cord.

Peripheral nerves containing sensory elements are also responsible for erectile function, especially maintenance of erection. Ultimate control of erectile function is through the central nervous system. Although the exact location of erectile stimulation in the central nervous system remains controversial, the median pre-optic area of the hypothalamus appears to be an integral part of psychogenic erectile stimulation.

Physiology of erection

Stimuli from the autonomic nervous system produce erections through a variety of neurotransmitters [3]. The most important neurotransmitter is nitric oxide (NO), which stimulates cyclic guanosine monophosphate (cGMP). Nitric oxide is formed from L-arginine by way of the enzyme NO synthase. The secondary neurotransmitter, cGMP, is ultimately responsible for smooth muscle relaxation in the corpus cavernosum, producing erection. cGMP is broken down in the corpus cavernosum by the enzyme phosphodiesterase (PDE) causing detumescence. The most active PDE in the corpus cavernosum is type 5. Further smooth muscle relaxation occurs via the cyclic adenosine monophosphate system, vasoactive intestinal protein and, ultimately, an intracellular calcium ion shift (Fig. 12a.1).

Once neurostimuli initiate the secretion of NO, the smooth muscle of the sinusoids of the corpora cavernosa begin to relax. Initial stimuli produce dilatation and relaxation of the central cavernosal artery and the helicine arterioles which supply blood to the lacunar spaces of the corpora cavernosa. Downstream relaxation and decrease in resistance of the lacunar spaces or sinusoids allow an increase in flow from these arteries into the sinusoids to produce a physical increase in pressure within the corpus cavernosum, increasing the pressure beneath the rigid tunica albuginea (Fig. 12a.2). The increase in pressure decreases venous outflow by compressing

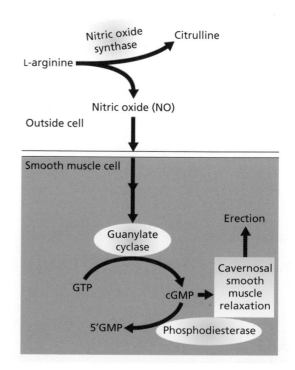

Figure 12a.1. *The erectile mechanism is mediated by neurotransmitters, of which nitric oxide is the most important.*

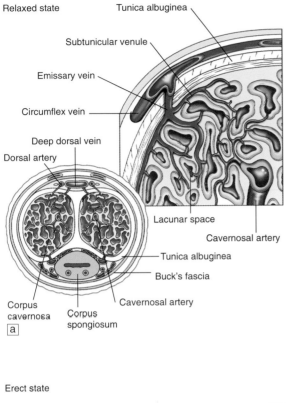

Relaxed state

Tunica albuginea

Subtunicular venule

Emissary vein

Circumflex vein

Deep dorsal vein

Dorsal artery

Lacunar space

Cavernosal artery

Tunica albuginea

Buck's fascia

Corpus cavernosa

Corpus spongiosum

Cavernosal artery

[a]

Erect state

Emissary vein

Circumflex vein

Lacunar space

Cavernosal artery

[b]

Figure 12a.2. *Erectile physiology: (a) cross-sectional anatomy of the penis in the flaccid state. Sinusoidal smooth muscle is contracted and blood flows from the internal pudendal arteries via the cavernosal arteries and the helicine arteries to the lacunar spaces and out through the open emissary veins; (b) during erection the smooth muscle of the sinusoids relaxes allowing blood to flow into the lacunar spaces. The resultant pressure compresses the emissary veins beneath the rigid tunica albuginea, reducing venous outflow.*

the subtunical venous channels against the tunica albuginea and producing a high-pressure rigid erection. Rigidity is enhanced by contraction of the perineal muscles, especially the bulbocavernosus and ischiocavernosus muscles. Once both psychological and physical stimuli have diminished, smooth muscle sympathetic tone increases, vasoconstriction occurs, NO is broken down by PDE type 5 and detumescence occurs.

Diagnosis of ED

History and physical examination

Sexual and general history are critical ingredients for diagnosis of ED and for planning appropriate therapeutic options for the patient. General history should include metabolic diseases, trauma, surgical procedures, smoking, current medications, recreational medication and alcohol use. The sexual history should differentiate between primary ED, in which the patient has had no previous erections, and secondary ED, where erection has been lost after previous normal sexual function. Associated ejaculatory dysfunction, diminished libido and changes in orgasm should also be investigated. Time of onset of ED is crucially important, as sudden onset is more common with psychogenic and post-surgical aetiologies, whereas gradual onset is more commonly associated with metabolic diseases, such as diabetes, thyroid disorders and hypercholesterolaemia. It is important to identify erectile function with other partners and during masturbation, as well as morning and nocturnal erections. The last successful intercourse should be queried, as well as interpersonal difficulty with partners, lifestyle changes, stress and possible depression. Psychogenic ED is a common aetiology produced by such psychological problems as performance anxiety characterized by fear of erectile failure, depression, obsessive compulsive disorder, psychiatric disorders, as well as interpersonal difficulties such as marital dysfunction. Problems with understanding sexual function as well as difficulty with sexual development may also produce psychogenic ED.

ED may be associated with medication use, requiring a careful history of both prescription and non-prescription medications (Table 12a.1). A careful medical history will also reveal any systemic diseases that may predispose to ED. These include a history of coronary artery disease with peripheral vascular disease, diabetes mellitus, renal failure, hypercholesterolaemia, neurological

Table 12a.1. *Medications associated with erectile dysfunction*

Psychotropic

- Benzodiazepines
- Amphetamines
- Barbiturates
- Opiates
- Tranquillizers
    - Phenothiazines
    - Butyrophenones
    - Thioxanthenes
- Antidepressants
    - MAO inhibitors
    - Tricyclics
    - Serotonin re-uptake inhibitors

Antihypertensives

- Diuretics (thiazides, spironolactone)
- Vasodilators
- Sympatholytics (methyldopa, reserpine)
- Beta blockers (propranolol, atenolol)
- Ganglion blockers (guanethidine)

Anticholinergics

- Atropine
- Diphenhydramine

Androgenic agents

- LHRH agonists
- Anti-androgens
- Oestrogen

Recreational agents

- Alcohol
- Marijuana
- Nicotine
- Cocaine

Others

- Clofibrate
- Cimetidine
- Digoxin
- Indomethacin

MAO, monoamine oxidase; LHRH, luteinizing-hormone-releasing hormone.

abnormalities including back surgery and trauma, thyroid disease, psychiatric diagnoses and alcohol and tobacco abuse. A surgical history may reveal surgical procedures associated with ED including radical pelvic surgery such as abdominal perineal resection, prostatectomy, cystectomy and pelvic trauma. Useful measurements of sexual dysfunction include sexual symptom scores or questionnaires as published by O'Leary and Rosen [4,5].

Physical examination is focused on the genitourinary system with special attention to the secondary sexual characteristics and genital development. The penis must be carefully examined to identify abnormalities, such as micropenis, Peyronie's disease or hypospadias. Testicular examination may reveal small, soft, atrophic testes or absent testes. Physical findings or unusual genetic syndromes such as Klinefelter's syndrome or Kallmann's syndrome can also be identified on careful physical examination. Peripheral pulses should be palpated to identify peripheral vascular disease and a focused neurological examination is necessary to identify decreased perineal, penile or suprapubic sensation. Elicitation of the bulbocavernosus reflex may also be helpful in identifying neurogenic abnormalities associated with ED. The prostate should also be carefully examined, since significant prostatitis may be associated with ED. Examination may also detect prostatic carcinoma or other abnormalities of the prostate.

Laboratory studies

Laboratory studies help to elucidate treatable causes of ED and any underlying, undiagnosed metabolic conditions. Urinalysis may identify glycosuria associated with undiagnosed diabetes mellitus or urinary infection. Serum studies should include serum testosterone, glucose, creatinine and a fasting lipid profile. If serum testosterone is low, free testosterone, luteinizing hormone (LH) and prolactin measurements may be required to differentiate pituitary from testicular abnormalities. In patients with significant renal failure and dialysis, a prolactin level is essential. Since hypogonadism and hyperprolactinaemia result in ED in only 1.7–35% of men with ED, these studies are frequently unfruitful [6]; they do, however, identify clearly treatable forms of ED.

Testosterone must be evaluated in the morning, since diurnal testosterone variation in normal physiological excretion results in the highest testosterone values between 0800 and 1000 hours; a late-afternoon testosterone may be abnormally low or borderline because of this diurnal variation. Primary or hypergonadotrophic hypogonadism is associated with an elevation in the pituitary hormones, LH and follicle-stimulating hormone. Most patients, however, have isolated decreases in serum testosterone associated with testicular testosterone deficiencies termed hypogonadotrophic. Patients with clear deficiencies in testosterone may benefit from testosterone replacement therapy.

Nocturnal penile tumescence monitoring

The association of nocturnal erections with rapid eye movement (REM) dream sleep has been well established. In 1970, Karacan reported the use of nocturnal penile tumescence monitoring to evaluate ED [7]. The RigiScan device used in these studies documents not only the presence or absence of erectile function but also its duration and rigidity; it can be used at home in the patient's own bedroom (Fig. 12a.3). The presence or absence of nocturnal erections may differentiate psychogenic, neurogenic and vasculogenic aetiologies and may be helpful in some patients with Peyronie's disease.

Pharmacological erection studies

Identifying a clear aetiology for ED is frequently difficult and the history, physical examination and laboratory studies may not clearly identify a cause for the patient's erectile problems. Additional specialized studies may be helpful in identifying patients for focused treatment.

Office injection of pharmacoactive agents to produce erections may be a helpful diagnostic procedure. The use of papaverine, phentolamine and prostaglandin E_1 (PGE_1) for both diagnosis and treatment has been quite common since the early 1980s. Virag and associates first identified the use of the vasoactive agent papaverine as a pharmacological screening procedure [8]. PGE_1 produces significant vasodilatation in the corpus cavernosum and, in normal patients, is associated with significant penile erection. A 20 µg dose of PGE_1 can be injected into a single corpus cavernosum to provide a full erection within 10–20 minutes and erectile maintenance for at least 15 minutes. A normal result following injection indicates normal vascular physiology, with adequate arterial flow and an intact veno-occlusive mechanism, and suggests a psychogenic, neurogenic or endocrine cause of the ED.

Unfortunately, however, abnormal findings are not specifically diagnostic of vascular disease [9]. Significant patient anxiety during the study

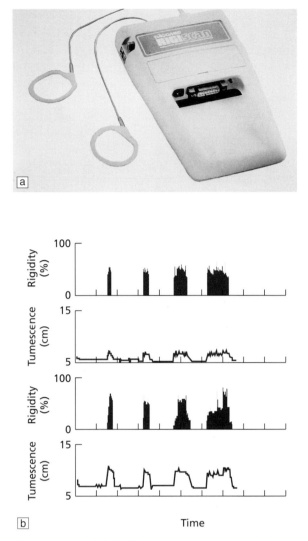

Figure 12a.3. (a) RigiScan home nocturnal penile tumescence monitor; (b) a normal RigiScan tracing with four erections of normal base and tip tumescence and rigidity.

can increase sympathetic tone in the corpus cavernosum, such that strong contraction of the corpus cavernosum smooth muscle tissue cannot be overcome by intracavernous injection [10]. Thus, despite repeat dosing, a negative study is not always diagnostic of arterial or venous abnormalities. In order to improve the response in such studies, vibratory stimulation, self-stimulation, or visual sexual stimulation after injection may be helpful. Similarly, second and third injections of vasoactive agents may be necessary to ensure maximum corpus cavernosum smooth muscle relaxation and accurate intracavernosal testing. A clearly abnormal study, however, suggests abnormal vascular physiology.

Further studies must be used to confirm these abnormalities. Duplex Doppler imaging provides information about the arterial inflow and can measure blood flow velocity in the cavernosal artery in both the contracted and relaxed state. Similarly, veno-occlusive abnormalities can be identified by pharmacocavernosometry and pharmacocavernosography [11]. Cavernosometry is performed by infusing normal saline into the corpus cavernosum to maintain an artificial erection while monitoring intracavernosal pressure. An inability to obtain or maintain pressure in the corpus cavernosum equal to or greater than the mean systolic blood pressure, with rapid drop in pressure and erection after infusion is stopped, is suggestive of a veno-occlusive abnormality. By following this infusion study with infusion of radiographic contrast media, the area and severity of venous leak can be documented radiographically. Accuracy depends on the adequacy of smooth muscle relaxation and it is frequently necessary to use two or three doses of vasoactive agent, with the caveat that priapism after the investigation must be treated aggressively.

Treatment of ED

In the past decade, a variety of new treatment alternatives have been introduced. Similarly, additional treatment options are being investigated throughout the world with new medications and devices based on recent knowledge of erectile physiology.

Psychogenic ED

Treatment of purely psychogenic ED continues to be frustrating and controversial. Masters and Johnson reported a 70% success rate in 1970 after 5 years of follow-up using behaviour-oriented therapy called sensate focus exercises [12]. Sensate focus emphasizes sensuality rather than sexual performance to promote self-discovery and interpersonal communication. It permits investigation of physical sexual stimulation without the pressure of sexual performance. The usual sensate focus treatment programme is designed to treat patients with significant performance anxiety and includes multiple sessions with significant partner co-operation. These programmes are difficult for single men and those patients with marital dysfunction.

In addition to performance anxiety, it is important to identify other relationship problems, lack of sexual performance, difficulty with intimacy and major or minor depression. Treatment of depression must be carefully designed, since many antidepressant medications result in ED, and serotonin re-uptake-inhibiting antidepressants often produce delayed ejaculation. Trazodone is an excellent agent for treatment of patients with depression and ED; however, patients must be warned of the possibility of priapism [13].

Endocrine treatment

Patients with early-onset diabetes mellitus, or diabetes mellitus associated with peripheral neuropathy, may benefit from regulation of their blood sugars. Although such regulation does not frequently result in restoration of erectile function, it may improve the erections of patients with partial ED. Patients with hypogonadism can be treated with a variety of preparations to restore erectile function. Patients with significant hyperprolactinaemia should be considered for bromocriptine treatment once satisfactory evaluation of the cause of their elevated prolactin has been completed. Patients with chronic renal failure and dialysis will usually respond poorly to testosterone replacement alone without management of high prolactin levels.

In patients with clear hypogonadal hypogonadism, testosterone replacement may be helpful. It is important to realize that increases in testosterone in the ageing male may result in changes in prostate size. Subsequently, prostate-specific antigen levels should be monitored on a regular basis; in addition, regular digital rectal examination should be performed to identify any changes in prostate size or consistency. Testosterone may be replaced using oral medications, intramuscular injection or transdermal delivery systems. Oral testosterone can be administered as multiple daily doses of a 17-alkyltestosterone, such as methyltestosterone or fluoxymesterone [14]. Because the oral androgen replacement is via metabolites of testosterone, the serum testosterone levels are not as effectively influenced. Similarly, hepatoxicity even at low doses of oral testosterone has been reported. Finally, the normal metabolites of testosterone, including oestradiol and dihydrotestosterone (DHT), are not increased by the use of oral medications. Intramuscular injections can be used for sustained-release testosterone replacement: injections at 2–4-week intervals result in the least physiological testosterone replacement with very high testosterone levels within 2–3 days of injection and subsequent declining testosterone levels to a nadir at approximately 14 days. Metabolites of testosterone are likewise not adequately restored with testosterone injection therapy. Transdermal delivery systems have been designed to improve the diurnal testosterone levels: use of these skin patches enables normal testosterone levels and normal daily variation to be reproduced pharmacologically. Transdermal delivery systems can be used on either the scrotum or overlying major muscle groups. Controlled transdermal delivery systems have been used effectively to provide therapy for female hormone replacement, smoking cessation, angina and analgesia. If men apply these transdermal testosterone patches in the evening prior to bedtime, a peak testosterone level will occur in the morning as normal; similarly, oestradiol and DHT levels will be restored. Multiple investigators have reported improvements in hypogonadal men whose testosterone levels are normalized, with subsequent increased energy, libido, sexual function and mood improvement. Side effects include local skin irritation and dermatitis, which can be treated with local application of corticosteroid ointment.

Oral pharmacological agents

A variety of oral agents have been used for the treatment of ED without convincing controlled clinical trials. The most commonly used of these agents is yohimbine, an indole alkaloid derived from the bark of the tree *Pausinystalia yohimba* [14]. This agent, which has been available for many years, causes alpha-2-adrenergic blockade, both peripherally and centrally. In a small controlled study of the effect of yohimbine on men with psychogenic ED, Morales and colleagues have demonstrated improvement in erectile function in 31%, compared with 5% of men taking placebo [14].

Trazodone, a commonly prescribed antidepressant, can also be used as a precoital tablet to enhance erectile activity. It stimulates serotonin (5HT) receptors in the midbrain erectile centre and has peripheral alpha-inhibitory activity; it can be given at a dose of 50–100 mg, 1–2 hours before coitus. Because priapism is a complication of this medication, patients must be warned of potential adverse events [13].

Newer oral agents designed with the understanding of the physiological mechanism of erectile function are now (or will soon be) available. These include sildenafil, apomorphine and oral phentolamine. Sildenafil (Viagra) is a PDE5 inhibitor that reduces the breakdown of cGMP in the corpus cavernosum, prolonging smooth muscle relaxation in erectile function. Clinical studies, both in-home and office-based, have demonstrated the effectiveness of sildenafil in treating ED of various aetiologies [15]. Sildenafil is administered 30–60 minutes before coitus and is statistically significantly better than placebo in providing erectile function. Apomorphine (Spontain) has been used in the laboratory to produce erections in laboratory animals for many years. It derives its function from central nervous system effects in the hypothalamus and is a serotonin stimulator. The sublingual preparation introduced by Heaton and colleagues has provided a tolerable administration technique for this agent [16]. Apomorphine is administered 30 minutes prior to coitus and has been shown to produce excellent erectile function in double-blind placebo-controlled studies, both in office and home settings. Side effects include nausea and vomiting, but are experienced by a small minority of patients and rarely affect patient compliance. Sublingual phentolamine has alpha-adrenergic-blocking activity, producing relaxation of the corpus cavernosum smooth muscle. Studies have demonstrated improved erectile function compared with placebo in a substantial number of patients.

Intracavernosal injection therapy

The use of pharmacoactive smooth muscle relaxation to treat ED has been in common practice since the early 1980s (Fig. 12a.4) [8]. At that time it was demonstrated that agents injected directly into the corpus cavernosum relaxed smooth muscle tissue by reducing adrenergic sympathetic tone, producing erectile function for a controlled period of time. A variety of agents have been used to produce erection, including papaverine, phentolamine and PGE_1. Currently, PGE_1 in the form of alprostadil is most often prescribed for this purpose. Injectable alprostadil (Caverject) is widely used in the USA and the UK and effectively produces erection by stimulating neurotransmitter secretion in the penis. It can be used alone or in combination with papaverine and phentolamine as 'trimix'. A multicentre study of 550 men demonstrated that 70% of patients achieved an erection satisfactory for coitus which lasted at least 30 minutes [17]. A total of 77% of sexual partners reported good or very good erection and 74% reported improvement in the marital relationship. Side effects include penile pain and prolonged erection or priapism.

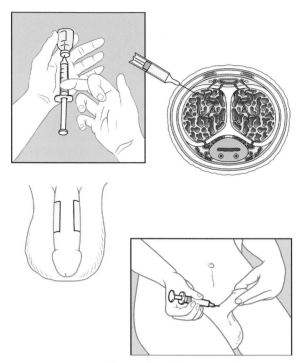

Figure 12a.4. *Technique for self-injection of vasoactive agents for erection.*

In order to avoid troublesome priapism, it is necessary to titrate the effective dose in an office setting. Doses usually range from 5 to 60 μg, depending on vascular function and the aetiology of ED.

Papaverine alone and in combination with phentolamine has been used since the early 1980s to produce erectile function clinically and diagnostically [11]. Papaverine is a direct smooth muscle relaxant which relaxes the trabecular smooth muscle of the corpus cavernosum and produces erections which may last for several minutes or several hours. Because of its very rapid and precipitous dose–response curve, risk of prolonged erections and priapism is greater than that with alprostadil, although the associated corpus cavernosum pain and discomfort is less with this agent. Combinations of papaverine with phentolamine result in a better erectile response than papaverine alone and enable a reduction in papaverine dose; duration of erection is also improved. Phentolamine is a short-acting, non-selective alpha-blocker producing vascular smooth muscle relaxation. Phentolamine is usually added to papaverine in a dose of 0.5–1 mg/ml.

Technique
Although there are few contraindications to the use of intracavernosal injection of vasoactive agents, relative contraindications include haematological abnormalities such as leukaemia, sickle-cell disease and significant coagulopathies. Patients with poor manual dexterity must depend on their partners for injection. Initial injection should be performed in the clinic setting with a medical professional demonstrating the technique and monitoring the response to the injected agent. Alprostadil is usually started at a dose of 1.25 μg in patients with normal vascular symptoms and 2.5 μg for older patients or those with vascular compromise. Papaverine and phentolamine combinations start with a mixture of 30 mg/ml papaverine with 0.5 or 1 mg/ml phentolamine; treatment is initiated with 0.5–1 ml of the mixture for neurogenic or psychogenic patients and 0.3–0.4 ml in patients with vascular compromise. The erection should be monitored for rigidity and duration and, if adequate, the dose trial can be continued. If inadequate, however, dose escalation can be performed in a home setting (with reliable patients) or by additional office visits if necessary.

Treatment failure or dropout occurs in approximately 80% of patients over the first 12 months of usage. Although this dropout rate can be reduced by careful follow-up and encouragement, many patients request therapeutic alternatives because of lack of spontaneity, discomfort from injection and inadequate erectile function. Systemic side effects of these agents are infrequent and occur in only 1% of patients: hypotension, dizziness and hepatotoxicity have been reported occasionally. The most difficult side effect, however, is that of prolonged erection or priapism. Patients must be carefully instructed that, if erections last more than 4 hours, they must seek immediate treatment for detumescence. Delayed treatment of a prolonged erection can result in priapism and ultimately corpus cavernosum fibrosis from ischaemia and loss of subsequent erectile function. Initial treatment is begun by aspiration of blood from the corpus cavernosum using a 14–19-gauge needle. Aspiration of 50–100 ml of blood will frequently decompress the corpus cavernosum and permit detumescence. If this fails to resolve the prolonged erection, injection of an alpha-agonist such as phenyl-ephrine should be initiated. This can be performed by single injection or by lavage of the corpus cavernosum through the previously inserted aspiration needle. Patients should be carefully monitored for cardiac abnormalities such as tachycardia and hypertension when administering alpha-agonists. This is especially important with agents such as metaraminol and adrenaline.

Intra-urethral delivery

Recently, intra-urethral delivery of PGE_1 has been introduced [18]. The agent in the form of a gel is administered through the medicated urethral system for erection (MUSE). MUSE is available in concentrations of 125, 250, 500 and 1000 μg PGE_1 and is self-administered. Supplementation can be performed using a constriction band at the base of the penis. Responses to MUSE administration have been variable and vary with the aetiology of ED. The use of this technique, however, eliminates the need for injection and is more comfortable and acceptable to many patients.

Vacuum constriction device

Vacuum constriction devices have been available since they were first patented in 1917 by Dr Otto Lederer. They have been medically prescribed since the 1980s. These devices aspirate blood into the penis through a vacuum tube placed around the penis, producing engorgement of the corpus cavernosum with trabecular smooth muscle relaxation. The blood is maintained within the corpus cavernosum by use of a constricting band placed at the base of the penis to maintain venous stasis and without decreased arterial inflow. Although these devices produce erectile function satisfactorily in as many as 80% of patients, they may be uncomfortable, obstruct ejaculation and produce other untoward side effects [19].

The vacuum chamber consists of a cylinder placed over the penis and closed at the opposite end (Fig. 12a.5). The closed end is attached to a vacuum pump and the constriction band is placed on the proximal portion of the open cylinder. The cylinder is then sealed to the skin at the base of the penis and the vacuum pump activated. Once an erection has been established, the constriction

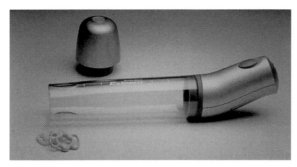

Figure 12a.5. *Vacuum erection device with constriction rings. (Reproduced with permission from Timm Medical Devices, Augusta, GA, USA.)*

ring is displaced from the proximal cylinder onto the base of the penis in order to maintain the erection. Usually erection can be maintained for up to 30 minutes before discomfort and oedema require removal of the constriction ring.

Patients should not use the vacuum constriction device if they have haematological abnormalities such as anticoagulant use, leukaemia, or sickle-cell disease. Complications of these devices include Peyronie's disease and plaque formation, decreased penile sensation and temperature, and postejaculatory discomfort.

Surgical treatment

Arterial revascularization may be indicated in patients with documented arterial abnormalities who are non-smokers and less than 40 years of age, and where penile Doppler ultrasound and arteriography demonstrates an isolated traumatically induced lesion resulting in decreased arterial inflow. Revascularization is performed using the inferior epigastric artery, which is dissected free from the underside of one or both rectus muscles and transferred to the base of the penis. Microscopic anastomosis is carried out between the inferior epigastric artery in an end-to-end or end-to-side fashion with the deep dorsal artery of the penis. This technique redirects blood from the inferior epigastric artery to the central cavernosal arteries and may be effective in as many as 65% of patients who are carefully selected [20].

As high blood flow rates produce erectile function in the corpora cavernosa, the integrity of the arterial supply is critical for normal erectile function. Patients with arterial lesions (usually acquired traumatically), in whom there is no significant atherosclerosis or atherosclerotic risk factors, may therefore be suitable for penile arterial revascularization or deep dorsal vein arterialization. Specific arteriographic visualization of the internal pudendal arteries and central cavernosal arteries is, however, essential to diagnose arterial compromise. Once diagnostic studies have demonstrated arterial abnormalities, arteriography following stimulation of the corpus cavernosum with vasoactive agents will document arterial abnormalities in the internal iliac vessels. Arterial revascularization should also be considered in lesions unlikely to respond to percutaneous transluminal angioplasty. Although this procedure usually has few complications, excessive arterial blood flow may result in priapism or glans penis hyperaemia, and the anastomosis may become occluded during the postoperative period. Patients are encouraged to avoid sexual activity for approximately 6 weeks after the operation. The alternative forms of surgical intervention must be discussed with all patients selected for arterial revascularization, including the possibility of penile prosthesis implantation.

Venous incompetence is more difficult to treat. Previously, venous ligation was carried out for patients with veno-occlusive abnormalities. The outcome of these surgical procedures, however, has been poor. Sustained surgical success has been identified in less than 40% of patients, with an additional 40% of patients responding to a combination of surgery and injectable agents [21]. Postoperative complications — including penile shortening, decreased penile sensation, recurrent venous incompetence and wound infection — as well as inadequate success rates have eliminated this surgical option for most patients. Preferred treatments are intracavernosal injection of pharmacological agents, vacuum constriction device or penile prosthesis implantation.

Penile prosthetic implants

Surgically implantable penile prostheses have been used for restoration of erectile function for more than 20 years [22]. Patient/partner satisfaction is usually quite high and is higher than other forms of treatment for ED. Many types of penile prosthesis are available, classified as either semi-rigid or inflatable; these implants provide satisfactory penile rigidity, normal sensation, erectile size and excellent patient/partner satisfaction [23]. Patients should be chosen for penile prosthesis implantation if simpler, less-invasive procedures are inadequate for producing erections or are not well tolerated by patient or partner. A careful discussion regarding the implantation, outcomes and complication of penile prosthesis should be held with patient and partner prior to surgery.

Semi-rigid rod prosthesis

The semi-rigid rod was the first penile prosthesis to be implanted widely for the treatment of ED. A variety of designs of semi-rigid rod prostheses are currently available, but all consist of two flexible rods or cylinders which can be varied in length by trimming or adding measured extensions at the proximal portion to fit the individual patient's measurements (Fig. 12a.6). These permanent devices are quite satisfactory for sexual activity, although the major caveat is the presence of an erect penis when not sexually active. Mechanical malfunction can occur, but the prin-

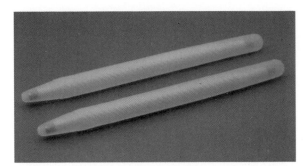

Figure 12a.6. AMS 600 *semi-rigid rod penile prosthesis*.

cipal complication is penile prosthesis infection.

Inflatable penile prostheses

Inflatable penile prostheses have been implanted widely since the mid-1970s. They are available as self-contained, two-piece and three-piece designs and consist of individual paired cylinders implanted in the penis with a proximal reservoir and distal activation pump. Because only a small amount of fluid is transferred during erection, these cylinders approximate semi-rigid rod prostheses in their inflated position. They are hydraulically hinged during deflation, providing improved positionability, but not complete flaccidity. Implantation is similar to that used for semi-rigid rod penile prostheses.

Two-piece penile prostheses contain completely inflatable cylinders and a scrotal pump/reservoir (Figs. 12a.7, 12a.8). The pump/reservoir provides a limited, but usually adequate, volume of fluid to be transferred for inflation and deflation of the prosthesis. The prosthesis provides better inflation and deflation than the self-contained inflatable penile prosthesis, but deflation and flaccidity are usually compromised because of the low volume of fluid transferred between pump and cylinders. Implantation of this device can be performed infrapubically or periscrotally in a fashion similar to that of three-piece inflatable penile prostheses.

Three-piece inflatable penile prostheses are the most complex, yet the most cosmetically and physiologically desirable prosthetic devices available (Figs. 12a.9, 12a.10). Two paired, hollow, inflatable cylinders are placed in the corpora cavernosa and connected to a small pump device, which is positioned in the most dependent portion of the scrotum lateral to the testicles. This device is used to inflate and deflate the cylinders and stimulate erection. The solution used to activate the device is stored in a reservoir, which is placed

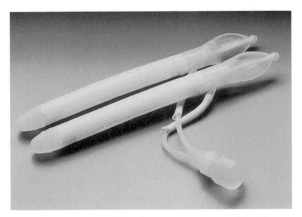

Figure 12a.7. *AMS Ambicore two-piece inflatable penile prosthesis.*

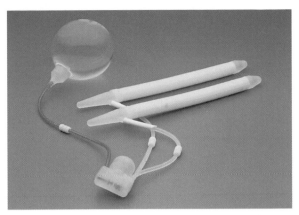

Figure 12a.10. *AMS 700 Ultrex inflatable penile prosthesis.*

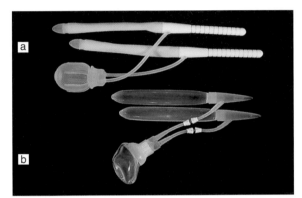

Figure 12a.8. *Two-piece inflatable penile prostheses: (a) Surgitek Uniflate 1000; (b) Mentor GFS.*

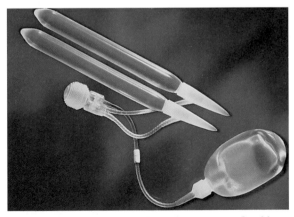

Figure 12a.9. *Mentor Alpha 1 three-piece inflatable penile prosthesis.*

beneath the rectus muscles of the abdomen and is neither visible nor palpable. Because of the significant volume of fluid provided by this reservoir, inflation and deflation are optimized. The erect state provides a larger girth and length, and more satisfactory erection, while deflation provides a completely flaccid and normal-appearing penis for concealment beneath clothing. Modification and redesign of these devices in the 1980s have improved patient satisfaction and lowered mechanical malfunction rates below 5% [24].

Postoperative care

Following surgical implantation of a penile prosthesis, patients are begun on antibiotics 1 hour prior to surgery and maintained on them for at least 72 hours afterwards. Following discharge patients are advised to use ice and analgesics for approximately 48 hours. Patients are asked to check the position of the pump for 4–6 weeks prior to activation of the prosthesis in order to maintain its dependent location and to ensure that the cylinders are maintained in a flaccid position during this healing stage. Postoperative complications have diminished markedly with design improvements. Inflatable penile prostheses, however, may be associated with more mechanical complications, including fluid leak, which occurs in approximately 5% of patients over a 3-year period. Because the fluid contained within the prosthesis is water or normal saline, leaks themselves do not produce significant morbidity but do result in prosthesis inactivation. Leaks usually occur in the cylinders or in the high-pressure portion of the device and require surgical exploration and replacement of malfunctioning portions.

The most difficult and disastrous complication of penile prostheses is infection, which occurs in 3–5% of patients. Higher infection rates can be expected in patients following prosthesis revision and in patients with autoimmune diseases or diabetes, or who are immunocompromised. Treatment requires prosthesis removal and usually subsequent healing prior to replacement. Other complications include penile prosthesis erosion, prolonged pain, reduced penile length and sensation; however, these are infrequent.

References

1. NIH Consensus Conference. Impotence. NIH Consensus Development Panel on Impotence. *JAMA* 1993; 270: 83–91

2. Feldman H, Goldstein I, Hatzichristou DG *et al*. Impotence and its medical and psychological correlate: results of the Massachusetts Male Aging Study. *J Urol* 1994; 150: 54–61

3. Carson CC. Pharmacologic treatment of erectile dysfunction. *Urol Int* 1995; 2: 7–9

4. O'Leary M, Fowler F, Lenderking W *et al*. A brief male sexual function inventory for urology. *Urology* 1995; 46: 697–705

5. Rosen R, Riley A, Wagner G *et al*. The Index of Erectile Dysfunction (IED): a multidimensional scale for assessment of ED. *J Urol* 1996; 155: 342A

6. Johnson AR, Jarow JP. Is routine endocrine testing of impotent men necessary? *J Urol* 1992; 147: 1542–1543

7. Karacan I. Clinical value of nocturnal penile erection in the prognosis and diagnosis of impotence. *Med Aspects Hum Sex* 1970; 4: 27–29

8. Varag, R, Frydman D, Legman M *et al*. Intracavernous injection of papaverine as a diagnostic and therapeutic method in erectile failure. *Angiology* 1984; 35: 79–84

9. Lerner SE, Melman A, Christ GJ. A review of erectile dysfunction: new insights and more questions. *J Urol* 1993; 149: 1246–1255

10. Borirakchanyavat S, Lue TF. Evaluation of impotence. *Urology* 1997; 7: 12–23

11. Kirby RF. Impotence: diagnosis and management of male erectile dysfunction. *Br Med J* 1994; 308: 957–961

12. Masters, WH, Johnson VE. Human sexual inadequacy. London: Churchill, 1970

13. Carson CC, Mino RD. Priapism associated with trazodone therapy. *J Urol* 1988; 139: 369–371

14. Morales A, Heaton JP. The medical treatment of impotence: an update. *World J Urol* 1990; 8: 80–83

15. Boolell N, Gepi-Attee S, Gingell JC, Allen MJ. Sildenafil, a novel effective oral therapy for male erectile dysfunction. *Br J Urol* 1996; 78: 257–261

16. Heaton JPW, Morales A, Johnstone B *et al*. Recovery of erectile function by the oral administration of apomorphine. *Urology* 1995; 45: 200–206

17. Linet OI, Ogring FG. Efficacy and safety of intracavernosal alprostadil in men with erectile dysfunction. *N Engl J Med* 1996; 334: 873–877

18. Padma-Nathan H, Hellstrom WJ, Kaiser FE. Treatment of men with erectile dysfunction with transurethral alprostadil. Medicated Urethral System for Erection (MUSE) Study Group. *N Engl J Med* 1997; 336: 1–7

19. Bosshardt RJ, Farwerk R, Sikora R *et al*. Objective measurement of the effectiveness, therapeutic success and dynamic mechanisms of the vacuum device. *Br J Urol* 1995; 75: 786–791

20. Goldstein I. Arterial revascularization procedures. *Semin Urol* 1996; 4: 252–258

21. Kerfoot WW, Carson CC, Donaldson JT, Kliewer MA. Investigation of vascular changes following penile vein ligation. *J Urol* 1994; 153: 884–887

22. Carson CC. Current status of penile prosthesis surgery. *Probl Urol* 1993; 7: 289–297

23. Steege JF, Stout AL, Carson CC. Patient/partner satisfaction. *Arch Sex Behav* 1986; 15: 393–399

24. Woodworth BE, Carson CC, Webster GD. Inflatable penile prosthesis: effect of device modification on functional longevity. *Urology* 1991; 38: 533–536

Male sexual dysfunction: the male menopause

W. D. Dunsmuir

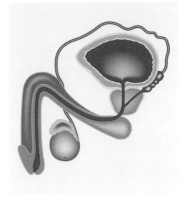

Introduction

The concept of a male menopause has been debated for many years. Many clinicians and patients have identified symptoms during the mid-life period that are comparable to those described by women whose reproductive life is drawing to a close. For women, much of the experience is concomitant with the endocrine changes that occur with ovulatory failure: these include fatigue, depression, irritability, hot flushes and reduced libido, as well as the cessation of menses. For many women, some of these symptoms can be ameliorated by hormone replacement therapy (HRT), which also provides many long-term benefits such as reductions in osteoporotic bone disease, in cardiovascular morbidity and in dementia.

As many middle-aged men frequently describe a similar constellation of symptoms, it would seem reasonable to suppose that their experience — or the male menopause — may also have an endocrine basis. However, as the menopause is a normal physiological process in ageing, it should not be regarded as a disease.

Definition, size of the problem and male:female ratio

Estimating the size of the problem is confounded by the concept of definition. For women, the menopause can only be accurately defined retrospectively as the time when the last menses occurred. The perimenopausal period — or climacteric — includes several years preceding last menses when menstrual irregularity begins and endocrine fluctuations can be measured. Longitudinal studies have suggested that the perimenopause begins on average at 47.5 years of age and the duration of the transition to last menses is about 4 years [1]. However, there is

much cross-cultural and socio-demographic variation in the perception of the menopause. For example, many African and Asian cultures simply accept the menopause as being a state of nature [2–5]. This frequently differs in Western societies where the transition period is often regarded as a disease state for which help can be sought. One population-based survey in Scotland found that 22% of women experiencing the transition perceived their symptoms to be a problem [4]. However, the proportion of these women who actually seek help is much smaller, and this too varies between countries. An Oxfordshire (UK)-based survey found that only 4.4% of women in the age range 40–69 consulted their general practitioners for advice regarding climacteric symptoms and less than half of those accepted HRT [5]. In countries such as Canada, the USA, Australia and Holland, a higher proportion of climacteric women receive HRT (9–12%) – at least for a limited period [6,7]. However, in all of these studies, comparisons are difficult because the breadth of definition varies. Indeed, a brief survey of the recent history of menopausal studies has seen the pendulum swing both back and forth; the original broad definition and rating scale proposed by Kupperman in 1953 [8] was gradually reduced by most investigators to the two symptoms of vasomotor flushing and genital atrophy. This was largely to facilitate the logistics of study, but also because these are the only two symptoms that are consistently remedied by HRT (see below). More recently, a new international Menopause Rating Scale (MRS) has been re-introduced with weighted scores that include sexual dysfunction (such as loss of libido) and bladder function, in addition to the core symptoms of genital atrophy and hot flushing [9].

To quantify the problem in men is even more difficult. No international rating scales have been proposed. Furthermore, there is no finite event, symptom or measurement by which the male menopause can be identified. Those who support the concept of a male menopause usually do so in terms of nebulous symptom complexes. These are often correlated with other equally ill-defined biochemical parameters, such as 'hypogonadism', again alluding to an endocrine cause. Furthermore, much of the lay public equate the male menopause with erectile failure. Using this symptom as a surrogate measure for the more ethereal menopause would quite simply be wrong. However, if the more holistic view of disease is considered, then the reported 52% incidence of erectile dysfunction in men aged 45–55 years, as described in the Massachusetts Male Aging Study [10], might conceal additional problems that could conceivably be menopausal in nature. In support of this notion are other population studies that have found that at least 40% of middle-aged men report some kind of sexual dysfunction [11]. However, there are inconsistencies, and other comparable studies have estimated the problems of sexual function to be considerably less. For example, in a cross-sectional survey of men aged 40–49 years, although 25% of these men expressed worry about their sexual function, only 10% reported a deterioration in performance compared with a year previously [12]. Furthermore, only about 1% of men described extreme sexual dissatisfaction, erectile dysfunction or loss of libido [12].

Direct comparisons of male and female climacteric symptoms are difficult to evaluate for many other reasons. First, there are gender differences in the way that individuals respond to ill-health. Vulnerability is a characteristic largely concealed by men — they regard it as a threat to their masculinity. Second, society has not evolved the infrastructure for men of mid-life to share their fears and failings with their contemporaries or their doctors. Furthermore, one must also assume that cultural variations in perception exist equally for men as for women. A male:female menopausal incidence ratio cannot be quoted and biological equivalence should not be assumed.

Aetiology: evidence for an endocrine-based menopause

Changes in circulating testosterone concentrations

The evidence that the male menopause has an endocrine basis comparable to the female experience is drawn from studies that have documented changes in male serum hormone concentrations with age. Many studies have reported that circulating testosterone (T) decreases with age [13]. Most of these reports are from cross-sectional studies and therefore have several limitations. First, it is known that both illness and stress will reduce circulating T [14]; as such, cross-sectional studies may be confounded by the effects of age-related illness [15]. Second, there is huge interindividual variation: many healthy elderly men have T concentrations markedly greater than young men [13]. Third, cross-sectional studies may also be confounded by age-related nyctihemeral variations. For instance, it has been well demonstrated that although there is no decrease in the frequency of pulsed daily T secretions, the pulsed amplitude is often reduced in older men [16]. For this reason, it may be difficult to demonstrate an age difference in the late afternoon. Furthermore, few data describe differences in the patterns of daily T secretion, which may be of greater biological importance. Certainly, it has been reported that sensitivity to pulsed gonadotrophins is reduced in older men and this may reduce the nyctihemeral peaks of T secretion [17].

Despite these limitations, two large cross-sectional studies that have tried to correct for body mass and age-related disease have concluded that there *is* a real decline in T with age [18,19]. Estimates of a 1% reduction per year between the age of 40 and 70 years have been described [18]; others have calculated that mean T values at 75 years are about two-thirds of those at age 25 [20]. However, definitive answers to the question of T decline with age will be provided only by longitudinal studies. Few have been performed, but one small study, the New Mexico Aging Process Study [21], has followed the sequential endocrine changes in elderly men (61–87 years) for up to a 14-year period. In this group, a general decline in T was reported, the average rate of decrease being 110 ng/dl for every decade. In other words, there is a marginal decrease that may not be apparent if corrected for body mass index. Furthermore, the importance of this study should not be overestimated as it is reporting on changes in elderly rather than middle-aged men.

What then, is the significance of these possible slight decreases in measurable T? Clearly, such reductions are not of the same magnitude as those of oestradiol seen in women. However, many critics feel that these reports misrepresent the more fundamental 'bioavailability' of T to the man of mid-life years. As circulating T is bound to sex-hormone-binding globulin (SHBG), only a small fraction is available to the target tissues. Hepatic production of SHBG increases with age and it has been suggested that the biologically active T available for the target tissues is reduced in ageing men [22]. Indeed, when the 'free testosterone index' (FTI) is calculated, then it is apparent that there may be a more marked reduction in biologically available T in some men [23].

The concept of an FTI is widely held by many endocrinologists. However, one should be cautious before assuming that it really is of any true clinical significance for the man in his mid-life years. First, the physiological regulation of T is under the control of a negative endocrine loop. As such, decreases of biologically 'available' T should be reflected by a concomitant rise in serum gonadotrophic luteinizing hormone (LH). This is rarely the case and a true diagnosis of 'hypogonadism' should include raised LH in the definition. Indeed, the one longitudinal study that has addressed this question found that, even in elderly men, only 10% demonstrated an elevation in LH concentration; furthermore, this was not necessarily sustained [21]. Second, the assumption that SHBG is an inert molecule that 'sequesters' T is probably also inaccurate and several authorities are challenging the functional model as described above [24]. Indeed, SHBG is a biologically active molecule with its own unique plasma membrane receptor. It has the facility to bring T to the target tissue and enhance the nuclear steroidal effect, even in the absence of the steroidal hormone itself [25]. Alone, or in combination with its 'jockey' molecule (i.e. T), SHBG can promote the growth of both androgen-dependent prostate cells [26] and germ cells in vitro [27]. The T-binding capacity of SHBG also displays a circadian variation and therefore the FTI can vary even within a 24-hour period [28]. SHBG exists in different molecular forms and its function alters, depending on the sialic acid content [29]; the regulation of these different forms is not understood but concentrations of SHBG are profoundly altered by many other factors, such as lipoglucose metabolism [30] and exercise [31]. It has even been suggested that SHBG functions as a buffer in response to circadian and exercise-induced fluctuations in T [28]. Clearly, understanding of the FTI and the true biological relationship of T and SHBG is in its infancy.

Peripheral androgen receptor (AR) status

Understanding of androgen action becomes even further obscured on consideration of the relationship of circulating T concentrations to the target tissue response. In other words, how well do measurements of serum T reflect the events occurring at the AR? The androgen-mediated responses relating to male behaviour and to sexual and erectile function are extraordinarily complex. To gain an understanding of the complexity, some of the mechanisms of AR action must be considered. However, it should be realized that most of the molecular studies described below are based on animal models and caution is necessary when interpreting extrapolations to the human.

The AR is an intracellular protein that mediates the biological actions of T and 5-alpha-dihydrotestosterone (DHT). This receptor modulates the expression of genes and gene networks in a cell- and tissue-specific manner and is found in both males and females. However, there are many differences in the AR response between the two sexes (sexual dimorphism). ARs are also ubiquitous, found in many tissues outside the genitourinary tract: these include cells in arteries, skin, sweat glands, hair follicles, cardiac and skeletal muscle, bladder, skin, liver, kidney and gastrointestinal tract.

In general, T will undergo a differential metabolism: it will be either reduced at the 5-alpha position to DHT or aromatized to oestrogenic compounds. DHT has no oestrogenic activity. In animal studies, both androgen and oestrogen receptors are often co-localized. This is particularly noted in areas of the brain associated with sexual behaviour — notably the medial preoptic nucleus, amygdala, septum, anterior hypothalamus and hippocampus [32]. Clearly, the target effect will depend not only on the steroids supplied but also on the enzyme systems that are present locally within the tissues.

The effects of AR stimulation are also known to be age dependent. One obvious example is the upregulation of AR that occurs in many tissue and organ systems at puberty. This phenomenon can be illustrated in the erectile (cavernosal) tissue of the penis. In the rat, human and most other mammalian species, there is a dense population of ARs in infancy. At the onset of puberty there is a marked increase in 5-alpha-reductase activity. However, in the fully developed adult phallus, AR expression and 5-alpha-reductase activity is barely discernible [33]. This suggests that during the 'pubescent' years, AR-mediated activity in the penis relates to organogenesis. The cessation of phallic growth seems to be determined by the switching-off of the AR gene and does not correlate with the concentration of any circulating androgen [34]. In the mature phallus, excess stimulation of the AR will not initiate further growth. However, in the adult penis, the low level of AR expression would appear to mediate alternative functions: these include the maintenance of cavernosal smooth muscle contractility [35] and nitric oxide-mediated penile erection [36]. Furthermore, for this 'adult' function, the active androgen appears to be DHT rather than T [37].

Finally, the regulation of AR can be altered in many other situation-specific ways. Castration of the rat can upregulate AR in the brain while simultaneously downregulating expression in the prostate [38]. Very rapid changes in AR expression can be determined by measuring AR mRNA in response to specific stimuli. Examples in the rat include copulation [39] and even the presence of the female scent [40]. In this respect, AR activation is being induced by neurohumoral systems, seemingly independent of circulating androgen [41]. This almost certainly has direct corollaries in the human: for instance, most adult human males who have suffered bilateral castration for testicular cancer receive depot T replacement therapy; this naturally declines throughout the 3-week treatment interval. Recent studies have shown that no aspect of sexual function is related to the absolute circulating T concentrations: indeed, both visually stimulated erections and nocturnal penile tumescence are maintained throughout the treatment cycle, irrespective of the fact that there is a sixfold variation in T concentration [42]. Clearly, from both the animal and human clinical studies reported, there is plenty of evidence to suggest that circulating T measurements are a poor reflection of AR status. In view of the complexities of the biological systems involved, the true significance of an individual's serum T concentration is far from clear. As such, the diagnostic use of the term 'hypogonadism' is probably not of any great value for the vast majority of men.

Changes in the androgenic adrenal steroid hormones

In recent years, attention has turned to other androgenic steroid hormones that may be contributory to the male menopause symptom complex. Dehydroepiandrosterone (DHEA) and the sulphonated hepatic metabolite (DHEAS) are present in much greater concentrations than T. It has been reported that these molecules start to decline from the age of about 20 years so that, by 60 years of age, the measurable values have fallen to about one-third of the young adult concentra-

tion [43]. This reduction is much more marked than the changes in T, but is still not analogous to the precipitous drop in oestradiol seen following the female climacteric. The role of the androgenic adrenal steroids in the male menopausal symptom complex remains to be explored.

Investigations

Possibly as a consequence of popular press publications, many men have recently been encouraged to request investigations for their mid-life symptoms. However, does the identification of a single, low, early morning T measurement help to identify 'menopausal' patients in whom HRT may be beneficial? There are some clinicians who believe that it does, but there are few data on the peer-reviewed database to either support or refute such a hypothesis. Certainly, on the basis of a population screen, one would expect 2.5% of men to have a serum T concentration reported as 'below normal'. This is simply because most laboratories will report the 'normal' range as being all values that fall within 1.96 standard deviations of a log-normal distribution. Whether the group of 'tail-enders' have any symptoms relevant to the menopausal symptom complex is not known. However, if the reported studies of endocrine testing in erectile dysfunction clinics are used as a surrogate marker for the menopause, the useful diagnostic yield is again found to be low. Two large studies have reported the yield of significant endocrinopathies in impotent men to be 1.7 and 2.1%, respectively [44,45]. In these two studies, an initial screen of serum T was complemented by further investigations (prolactin and gonadotrophins) only if a serum T concentration below 220 ng/dl was found. A similar study, which has used a higher cutoff for defining a 'low' T (< 300 ng/dl), reported a 12.1% significant endocrinopathy rate for a similar group of men [46]. Clearly, the incidence of abnormal endocrine profiles in such men is low. Furthermore, in each of these studies the authors have commented on the high cost of these investigations. Despite this, many clinicians believe that reassuring men that their 'hormone levels' are normal has an important psychological benefit, and an NIH conference (1993) firmly recommended the measurement of T in the evaluation of men with erectile dysfunction [47]. However, the rationale for using any endocrine screen should be based on whether such tests help to identify a group of men who will benefit from HRT.

Treatment administration

HRT can be administered in several different ways. These different modes of androgen delivery are summarized below, followed by a description of the efficacy of supplementation.

Oral administration

Oral T is rapidly inactivated by the liver; however, 17-alpha-alkylation of the steroid molecule reduces hepatic inactivation to make oral therapy practical (stanozolol, nandrolone, dianabol). Long-term use is still limited by the risk of hepatotoxicity. Furthermore, as both the parent compound and the metabolites remain in the 17-alpha-alkylated form, it is difficult to monitor therapy by measuring serum T concentrations. Indeed, therapeutic doses will actually suppress endogenous gonadotrophin and testosterone secretions. These are the oral androgenic steroids widely used by athletes for potential anabolic benefit.

Mesterolone (Pro-Viron; 1-methyltestosterone) and testosterone undecanoate (Restandol, Andriol; a 17-beta-carboxylic acid ester) are oral preparations largely used in clinical practice. They do not appear to have significant hepatotoxic effects but adsorption is erratic and unpredictable. Despite these shortcomings, these two preparations still account for between 26 and 75% of the total androgen market in the Western World. New oral androgen delivery systems include sublingual preparations and slowly degradable microcapsules.

Depot preparations

Esterification of the T molecule at the 17-beta position allows for a slowly hydrolysable form that can be given as a depot injection. The two preparations that have been most extensively studied are testosterone cyprionate and testosterone enanthate (Primoteston). These need to be given every 2–3 weeks. However, the most commonly prescribed depot preparations are combinations of several esters, such as Sustanon. Treatment with ester preparations can be monitored by measuring serum T concentrations. However, the shortcomings of this form of administration relate to the pharmacokinetic hills and troughs. Chronic administration may have detrimental cardiovascular effects due to the increased oestrogen and haematocrit (see below). Finally, the oily injections can be painful and need to be repeated every several weeks.

Transdermal patches

Transdermal patches have recently been introduced into clinical practice and provide a delivery system whereby T can be delivered in a dose-dependent manner relative to the size of the patch. Peak T concentrations are achieved after 8 hours. There are two distinct advantages of this mode of administration: first, the diurnal pattern of T secretion can be more closely mimicked; second, the application to certain parts of the skin — such as the back and the scrotum — allows for a substantial proportion of the T to be converted to DHT, owing to the high 5-alpha-reductase activity in these skin areas. It would appear that DHT is the more active androgen in peripheral genitourinary tissues. Furthermore, it has also been suggested that DHT may be the most potent circulating androgen driving male sexual behaviour [48]. In addition, high circulating concentrations of DHT tend to suppress T and therefore the aromatizable substrate. Thus, serum oestrogens may also show a decline and this may have benefits in both reducing cardiovascular risks and in protecting against the development of prostatic hypertrophy. Finally, the main problem with these patches seems to be contact dermatitis and patch adherence. The reported incidence of skin problems has ranged between 12 and 32%, and the scrotal region appears to be the preferable site of application [49].

Treatment efficacy

Short-term benefits

In men, the clinical effectiveness of androgen supplementation with respect to improvements in mood, energy, flushing and libido is largely anecdotal. The first publications to describe such improvements are both over 50 years old. In the first publication, a series of case reports are described in men, all of whom had some physical cause for testicular hypofunction or non-function [50]. In the second, patients were selected on the basis of reduced measurable T with concomitant elevation of urinary gonadotrophins [51]. In other words, patients were truly hypogonadal. Since that time, publications on the treatment of male menopausal symptoms have largely been sporadic, mainly case reports and largely outside the context of clinical trials. Likewise, most of these reports have suggested that, if treatment is to be effective, then selection of patients should be dictated by a measurable reduction in FTI. Contemporary trials in men who are both eugonadal and hypogonadal are in the recruitment process and, at the time of writing, no clear statements on efficacy can be made.

However, using potency as a surrogate indicator for the potential efficacy of HRT, the many clinical trials that have been repeated over the last 30 years can be summarized. For men who are profoundly hypogonadal (such as those who have undergone castration or pan-pituitary failure), T replacement therapy will promote a marked improvement in erectile and ejaculatory frequency including spontaneous and nocturnal penile erections [52]. However, in eugonadal and the mildly hypogonadal normal gonadotrophic (MHNG) group of men (i.e. low T with no elevation of LH), the results of HRT are disappointing: a profound subjective response is seen in only a very few patients. For the MHNG group, although positive subjective responses have been reported to occur in about 9% of men given oral supplementation [53], similar studies have failed to show any real measurable improvements in erectile function — although increases in libido were reported by about one-third of such men [54]. Other studies have suggested that, of the MHNG group, it is only those with minimal erectile dysfunction that improve with treatment [55].

When intramuscular depot T esters are given, the results — although slightly more encouraging — are similar. For eugonadal men there may be some enhanced rigidity of nocturnal penile tumescence (NPT) [56] and increases in genital sensation (sensual response) [57]. In general, however, no real improvements in subjective erections are achieved [57]. For the MHNG group, one study has reported improvements in libido in 70% of men, and increases in erectile function sufficient to restore vaginal penetration in 50% [58]. This particular study is also of interest in that a substantial proportion of men in the placebo group also reported significant improvements. Furthermore, measurable differences in serum T concentrations were not apparent between the placebo and treatment crossovers. This later finding supports the previous discussion, which questioned the value of measuring serum T in otherwise apparently normally androgenized males.

In summary, other than in profoundly hypogonadal men (with raised gonadotrophins), the results of HRT are variable and often disappointing. For MHNG men, HRT may improve libido,

and if erectile dysfunction is minimal, then responses to supplementation are occasionally achieved. However, reliable studies for men with menopausal symptoms are lacking. Furthermore, although the results of most studies are not encouraging, it should be remembered that individual polymorphisms to androgen response undoubtedly occur and dramatic idiosyncratic improvements may be seen in an (as of yet) unidentifiable group of men. Finally, substantial trials using the new transdermal androgen delivery systems have not yet been reported.

Long-term benefits

The long-term benefits of HRT in men are not yet known. Although osteoporotic bone disease does not present the same magnitude of clinical problems for male as for female subjects, T therapy improves bone mineral density in hypogonadal men as measured by quantitative computed tomography [59]. In eugonadal men, T supplementation may result in an increase in lean body mass and possibly a decline in bone resorption as assessed by urinary hydroxyproline excretion [60]. The mechanisms of T action on bone metabolism are not clear; however, it has been proposed that reduced T results in a decrease in peripheral aromatization to oestrogen — oestrogen having an osteotrophic action. Alternatively, reduced T causes a decrease in calcitonin secretion, the latter being a potent inhibitor of bone resorption. T supplementation has also been reported to increase hand-grip strength [61] and may reduce visceral body fat [62].

Safety issues and guidelines for shared care

In practice, 70–90% of all androgens prescribed for erectile failure and climacteric symptoms are given without any prior investigations. This suggests that most clinicians are happy to treat patients empirically, despite the overwhelming evidence that T therapy is unrewarding, particularly in eugonadal men. This empirical approach to treatment is, of course, perfectly reasonable, as long as long-term treatments can be shown to be safe. Unfortunately, the controversy surrounding HRT in men not only is poorly studied but also is confounded by conflicting indirect evidence.

Many aspects of the safety of HRT relate to the mode of administration. It has already been mentioned that the oral 17-alpha-alkylated agents are hepatotoxic. Furthermore, many of these same agents have also been shown markedly to reduce serum concentrations of high-density lipoprotein (HDL) and increase low-density lipoprotein (LDL) [63]; this may increase the risk of cardiovascular morbidity. Indeed, as it is these agents that are largely used by athletes for the potential anabolic–androgenic effects, it is not surprising that fatalities from myocardial infarction and stroke have been reported in athletes consuming these drugs.

With regard to the injectable esters, the effects of HRT on fat metabolism are conflicting: some studies have reported favourable changes in serum cholesterol, HDL and LDL lipoprotein profiles [60], whereas others have found the opposite [64]. The transdermal patches do not appear significantly to affect cholesterol and lipoprotein homoeostasis [65].

T replacement may also result in weight gain due to an increase in lean body mass and fluid retention. Furthermore, several studies have also reported an increase in haematocrit in patients treated with injectable esters [60]. In addition, it is known that oestrogens can increase cardiovascular mortality in men (a paradox, in that they seem to be cardio protective in women), and excess aromatization of injectable esters has been shown to increase serum oestradiol concentrations [66]. Taken together, the possible detrimental effects that depot T supplementation may have on oestrogen status, haematocrit and lipoprotein/cholesterol homoeostasis could result in an increased risk of cardiovascular disease. This link has not been shown, although it remains a concern.

The excess aromatization of T to oestradiol can have several other effects. First, bothersome gynaecomastia can occur as a result of this peripheral conversion. Second, increased intraprostatic oestrogen is thought to be important in the pathogenesis of benign prostatic hyperplasia (BPH) [67]. Indeed, the combination of excess T and oestradiol may promote the development of BPH and several studies have documented an increase in prostatic volume with T therapy [62]. However, it has also been suggested that the application of T patches can actually result in a decrease in prostate volume due to the preferential transdermal conversion of T to DHT — rather than oestrogen [68]. Despite these claims, more extensive recent investigations have refuted these findings and reported fairly marked increases in prostate size with transdermal T therapy [69]. It should also be noted that this increase in prostate volume was maximal by 3 months of treatment and did not

continue to increase with prolonged administration.

Perhaps the greatest safety concern relates to prostate cancer. It is well known that microscopic foci of prostate cancer are found in the prostates of at least one-third of men over the age of 50 [70]. It is also well known that T will promote prostate cancer growth both in animal tumour models and in vitro [71]. Furthermore, there have been reports of prostate cancer developing in athletes taking high doses of androgenic–anabolic steroids [72]. It has also been suggested that the higher incidence of prostate cancer in Black males may relate to higher serum T concentrations [73]. Another study in elderly men found that T administration resulted in an increase in prostate-specific antigen (PSA) concentration in most men; furthermore, this increase was sustained in 30% of men despite treatment withdrawal [68]. However, no link between HRT and prostate cancer has been shown. It should also be appreciated that the World Health Organization considers that the long-term high-dose administration of T for male contraceptive regimens is safe [74]. To date, the safety issues are not resolved and multicentre controlled clinical trials for both the safety and efficacy of the newer transdermal delivery systems are currently under way at the Johns Hopkins University (Baltimore, USA), the University of Utah (USA) and the Karolinska Hospital in Stockholm (Sweden). Until these issues have been resolved, it would seem sensible for all patients who start on HRT to have an estimation of PSA and a digital rectal examination (DRE) prior to beginning treatment. If either of these give abnormal results, then an appropriate search for prostate cancer should begin. Patients should be warned of the potential risks and uncertainties and encouraged to undergo routine 6-monthly health checks. In view of the uncertainties with respect to cardiovascular morbidity, these checks should include assessments of PSA, haematocrit, and HDL- and LDL-cholesterol, in addition to a DRE.

Future directions and the application of evidence-based medicine

It will be clear from the foregoing discussion that there are many problems in defining the male menopause and identifying the patients who may benefit from HRT. The efficacy and safety issues are still being questioned, and the problems in conducting and executing clinical trials are legion. The fundamental problem remains one of definition: even for those clinicians working in the field of the female climacteric, the methodological shortcomings have always related to this limitation. The finite event for women (the cessation of menses) can be defined only retrospectively: until this point, the start (or existence) of 'the transition' can be alluded to. This is at odds with a basic axiom of scientific methodology: if there is no objective way of detecting when a phenomenon is either present or absent, then it cannot be quantified. An interesting analogy would be to try to relate sexual promiscuity in adolescent boys to a 'teenage' variable based upon the time since the voice broke.

Traditionally, those who have tried to help men with mid-life symptoms have defined the menopause in terms of reduced FTI [23]. However, the vast majority of men who have fatigue, depression, irritability, hot flushes, impotence and loss of libido have normal endocrine profiles. This then, might be to deny treatment to many men who would benefit from it if their individual condition truly had an endocrine basis. Indeed, such men may escape identification on the basis of a normal FTI.

For all these reasons, the prospect of designing adequate prospective randomized trials is unlikely. Further studies are required to define the molecular basis of the mid-life changes that are truly caused by endocrine aberrations. For instance, as seems likely in women, it may well be that symptoms relate to rapid fluctuations in hormone concentrations rather than to gradual deficiency states. To this end, the day-to-day nyctihemeral variations in hormone concentrations need to be studied in symptomatic and non-symptomatic men. If more specific endocrine changes can be elucidated, then men can be more satisfactorily categorized for clinical trials. Indeed, it is highly likely that individual idiosyncratic responses to T replacement therapy do occur, but these 'positive' responders may have been lost in large trials (or may be 'lost' in large future trials).

New systems for androgen application are now available and it may well be that previous clinical impressions of T efficacy and safety are no longer applicable. The new transdermal delivery systems have pharmacokinetics that approximate more closely the normal male physiology. For this reason alone, all the same questions need to be re-addressed. Indeed, the potential long-term benefits (such as retention of body strength and muscle mass) and the safety implications will become apparent only many years from now. Finally, the future of male HRT may not depend on the delivery of steroidal hormones. Indeed, it has been predicted that the future of HRT in women may ultimately be more successfully delivered through the development of selective oestrogen receptor modulators (SERMs). Two such agents — draloxifene and raloxifene — have been evaluated in double-blind, placebo-controlled, short-term phase II clinical trials. Favourable results in terms of bone metabolism were found without any proliferative endometrial effects. In addition, reductions in serum cholesterol were also reported — an effect not seen with conventional HRT. The development of similar selective androgen-receptor modulators (SARMs) can be envisaged. These might be expected to provide the favourable aspects of tissue-specific androgenic stimulation without the other, broader consequences of the steroidal androgens.

In summary, this is an exciting era in understanding the biology of the ageing male. New androgen delivery systems are creating opportunities to treat some men effectively, but it is not yet known who these men are. It is important that the previous concepts of male physiology are modified and that a definition should be sought of the conditions that will respond to the evolving androgen delivery systems available. The onus is on each of the clinicians involved in this field to avoid the demand to treat individuals empirically. Trials should be conceived and conducted so that the answers to the questions that have baffled practitioners over the last 50 years are not equally elusive in the next millennium. Only when such trials have been conducted will it be possible accurately to quantify the efficacy of HRT and to assess the real risks, and risks/benefits, to the prostate and cardiovascular system, respectively.

References

1. McKinlay SM, Brambilla DJ, Posner JG. The normal menopause transition. *Maturitas* 1992; 14: 103–105
2. Boulet MJ, Oddens BJ, Lehert P *et al.* Climacteric and menopause in seven South-East Asian countries. *Maturitas* 1994; 19: 157–176
3. Holmes-Rovner M, Padonu G, Kroll J *et al.* African-American women's attitudes and expectations of menopause. *Am J Prev Med* 1996; 12: 420–423
4. Porter M, Penney GC, Russell D *et al.* A population based survey of women's experience of the menopause. *Br J Obstet Gynaecol* 1996; 103: 1025–1028

5. Barlow DH, Brockie JA, Rees CM. Study of General Practice consultations and menopausal problems. Oxford General Practitioners Menopause Study Group. *Br Med J* 1991; 302: 274–276

6. Blumberg G, Kaplan B, Rabinerson D *et al.* Women's attitudes towards menopause and hormone replacement therapy. *Int J Gynaecol Obstet* 1996; 54: 271–277

7. Harby K. Menopause: disease state or state of nature? Implications for molecular medicine. *Mol Med Today* 1996; 2: 414–417

8. Utian WH. Pieter Van Keep Memorial Lecture. Menopause — a modern perspective from a controversial history. *Maturitas* 1997; 26: 73–82

9. Hauser GA, Huber IC, Keller PJ *et al.* Evaluation of climacteric symptoms (menopause rating scale). *Zentralbl Gynakol* 1994; 116: 16–23

10. Feldman HA, Goldstein I, Hatzichristou DG *et al.* Impotence and its medical and psychosocial correlates: results of the Massachusetts Male Aging Study. *J Urol* 1994; 151: 54–61

11. Solstad K, Hertoft P. Frequency of sexual problems and sexual dysfunction in middle-aged Danish men. *Arch Sex Behav* 1993; 22: 51–58

12. Panser LA, Rhodes T, Girman CJ *et al.* Sexual function of men ages 40 to 79 years: the Olmsted County Study of Urinary Symptoms and Health Status Among Men. *J Am Geriatr Soc* 1995; 43: 1107–1111

13. Purifoy FE, Koopmans LH, Mayes DM. Age differences in serum androgen levels in normal adult males. *Hum Biol* 1981; 53: 499–511

14. Woolf PD, Hamill RW, McDonald JV *et al.* Transient hypogonadotrophic hypogonadism caused by critical illness. *J Clin Endocrinol Metab* 1985; 60: 444–450

15. Harman SM, Tsitouras PD. Reproductive hormones in ageing men. Measurement of sex steroids basal luteinizing hormone and Leydig cell response to human chorionic gonadotrophin. *J Clin Endocrinol Metab* 1980; 51: 35–40

16. Tenover JS, Bremner WJ. The effects of normal aging on the response of the pituitary–gonadal axis to chronic clomiphene administration in men. *J Androl* 1991; 12: 258–263

17. Greenstein A, Chen J, Perez ED, Mulligan T. Characteristics of men interested in evaluation of erectile dysfunction. *Int J Impot Res* 1994; 6: 199–204

18. Gray A, Feldman HA, McKinlay JB, Longcope C. Age, disease, and changing sex hormone levels in middle-aged men: results of the Massachusetts Male Aging Study. *J Clin Endocrinol Metab* 1991; 73: 1016–1025

19. Simon D, Preziosi P, Barrett-Connor E *et al.* The influence of aging on plasma sex hormones in men: the Telecom Study. *Am J Epidemiol* 1992; 135: 783–791

20. Vermeulen A. Clinical review 24: androgens in the aging male. *J Clin Endocrinol Metab* 1991; 73: 221–224

21. Morley JE, Kaiser FE, Perry HM III *et al.* Longitudinal changes in testosterone, luteinizing hormone, and follicle-stimulating hormone in healthy older men. *Metabolism* 1997; 46: 410–413

22. Nahoul K, Roger M. Age-related decline of plasma bio-available testosterone in adult men. *J Steroid Biochem* 1990; 35: 293–299

23. Carruthers M. Male menopause — fact or fiction? *Br J Sex Health* 1995: 17–19

24. von Schoultz B, Carlstrom K. On the regulation of sex-hormone-binding globulin — a challenge of an old dogma and outlines of an alternative mechanism. *J Steroid Biochem* 1989; 32: 327–334

25. Nakhla AM, Romas NA, Rosner W. Estradiol activates the prostate androgen receptor and prostate-specific antigen secretion through the intermediacy of sex hormone-binding globulin. *J Biol Chem* 1997; 272: 6838–6841

26. Nakhla AM, Khan MS, Rosner W. Biologically active steroids activate receptor-bound human sex hormone-binding globulin to cause LNCaP cells to accumulate adenosine $3',5'$-monophosphate. *J Clin Endocrinol Metab* 1990; 71: 398–404

27. Gerard A, Bedjou R, Clerc A *et al.* Growth response of adult germ cells to rat androgen-binding protein and human sex hormone-binding globulin. *Horm Res* 1996; 45: 218–221

28. Yie SM, Wang R, Zhu YX *et al.* Circadian variations of serum sex hormone binding globulin binding capacity in normal adult men and women. *J Steroid Biochem* 1990; 36: 111–115

29. Fonseca ME, Mason M, Ochoa R *et al.* Changes in molecular forms of sex hormone binding globulin during menstrual cycle and menopause. *Ginecol Obstet Mex* 1996; 64: 508–516

30. Reed MJ, Cheng RW, Simmonds M *et al.* Dietary lipids: an additional regulator of plasma levels of sex hormone binding globulin. *J Clin Endocrinol Metab* 1987; 64: 1083–1085

31. Zmuda JM, Thompson PD, Winters SJ. Exercise increases serum testosterone and sex hormone-binding globulin levels in older men. *Metabolism* 1996; 45: 935–939

32. Clancy AN, Bonsall RW, Michael RP. Immuno-histochemical labelling of androgen receptors in the brain of rat and monkey. *Life Sci* 1992; 50: 409–417

33. Godec CJ, Bates H, Labrosse K. Testosterone receptors in corpora cavernosa of penis. *Urology* 1985; 26: 237–239

34. Berger FG, Watson G. Androgen-regulated gene expression. *Ann Rev Physiol* 1989; 51: 51–65

35. Baba K. Effects of testosterone on smooth muscle in the isolated rabbit corpus cavernosum penis. *Nippon Hinyokika Gakkai Zasshi* 1993; 84: 1783–1790

36. Baba K, Yajima M, Carrier S *et al.* Effect of testosterone on the number of NADPH diaphorase-staining nerve fibres in the rat corpus cavernosum and dorsal nerve. *J Urol* 1995; 153: 506A

37. Lugg JA, Rajfer J, Gonzalez-Cadavid NF. Dihydrotestosterone is the active androgen in the maintenance of nitric oxide-mediated penile erection in the rat. *Endocrinology* 1995; 136: 1495–1501

38. Burgess LH, Handa RJ. Hormonal regulation of androgen receptor mRNA in the brain and anterior

pituitary gland of the male rat. *Brain Res Mol Brain Res* 1993; 19: 31–38

39. Wood RI, Newman SW. Mating activates androgen receptor-containing neurons in chemosensory pathways of the male Syrian hamster brain. *Brain Res* 1993; 614: 65–77

40. Hermkes A, Probst B. Neural androgen receptors and scent marking of male gerbils: modulation by females. *Physiol Behav* 1992; 51: 1179–1182

41. Osada T, Hirata S, Hirai M *et al.* Detection and levels of androgen receptor messenger ribonucleic acid in the rat brain by means of reverse transcription-polymerase chain reaction. *Endocr* 1993; 40: 439–446

42. van Basten JP, van Driel MF, Jonker-Pool G *et al.* Sexual functioning in testosterone-supplemented patients treated for bilateral testicular cancer. *Br J Urol* 1997; 79: 461–467

43. Orentreich N, Brind JL, Vogelman JH *et al.* Longitudinal measurements of plasma dehydro-epiandrosterone sulphate in normal men. *J Clin Endocrinol Metab* 1992; 75: 1002–1004

44. Maatman TJ, Montague DK. Routine endocrine screening in impotence. *Urology* 1986; 27: 499–502

45. Johnson AR, Jarow JP. Is routine endocrine testing of impotent men necessary? *J Urol* 1992; 147: 1542–1543

46. Nickel CJ, Morales A, Condra M *et al.* Endocrine dysfunction in impotence: Incidence, significance and cost effective screening. *J Urol* 1984; 132: 40–43

47. NIH Consensus Development Panel on Impotence. Impotence. *JAMA* 1993; 270: 83–90

48. Mantzoros CS, Georgiadis EI, Trichopoulos D. Contribution of dihydrotestosterone to male sexual behaviour. *Br Med J* 1995; 310: 1289–1291

49. Jordan WP, Jr. Allergy and topical irritation associated with transdermal testosterone administration: a comparison of scrotal and nonscrotal transdermal systems. *Am J Contact Dermatol* 1997; 8: 108–113

50. Werner AA. The male climacteric: additional observations of thirty-seven patients. *J Urol* 1943; 49: 872–882

51. Heller CG, Myers GB. The male climacteric, its symptomatology, diagnosis and treatment. *JAMA* 1944; 126: 472–477

52. Burris AS, Banks SM, Carter CS *et al.* A long-term, prospective study of the physiologic and behavioral effects of hormone replacement in untreated hypogonadal men. *J Androl* 1992; 13: 297–304

53. Morales A, Johnston B, Heaton JW, Clark A. Oral androgens in the treatment of hypogonadal impotent men. *J Urol* 1994; 152: 1115–1118

54. Morales A, Johnston B, Heaton JP, Lundie M. Testosterone supplementation for hypogonadal impotence: assessment of biochemical measures and therapeutic outcomes. *J Urol* 1997; 157: 849–854

55. Carani C, Zini D, Baldini A *et al.* Effects of androgen treatment in impotent men with normal and low levels of free testosterone. *Arch Sex Behav* 1990; 19: 223–234

56. Carani C, Scuteri A, Marrama P, Bancroft J. The effects of testosterone administration and visual erot-ic stimuli on nocturnal penile tumescence in normal men. *Horm Behav* 1990; 24: 435–441

57. Davidson JM, Kwan M, Greenleaf WJ. Hormonal replacement and sexuality in men. *Clin Endocrinol Metab* 1982; 11: 599–623

58. Nankin HR, Lin T, Osterman J. Chronic testosterone cyprionate therapy in men with secondary impotence. *Fertil Steril* 1986; 46: 300–307

59. Behre HM, Kliesch S, Leifke E *et al.* Long-term effect of testosterone therapy on bone mineral density in hypogonadal men. *J Clin Endocrinol Metab* 1997; 82: 2386–2390

60. Tenover JS. Effects of testosterone supplementation in the aging male. *J Clin Endocrinol Metab* 1992; 75: 1092–1098

61. Morley JE, Perry HM III, Kaiser FE *et al.* Effects of testosterone replacement therapy in old hypogonadal males: a preliminary study. *J Am Geriatr Soc* 1993; 41: 149–152

62. Marin P, Holmang S, Jonsson L *et al.* The effects of testosterone treatment on body composition and metabolism in middle-aged obese men. *Int J Obes Rel Metab Disord* 1992; 16: 991–997

63. Thompson PD, Cullinane EM, Sady SP *et al.* Contrasting effects of testosterone and stanozolol on serum lipoprotein levels. *JAMA* 1989; 261: 1165–1168

64. Berglund L, Carlstrom K, Stege R *et al.* Hormonal regulation of serum lipoprotein A levels: effects of parenteral administration of estrogen or testosterone in males. *J Clin Endocrinol Metab* 1996; 81: 2633–2637

65. McClure RD, Oses R, Ernest ML. Hypogonadal impotence treated by transdermal testosterone. *Urology* 1991; 37: 224–228

66. Bagatell CJ, Heiman JR, Matsumoto AM *et al.* Metabolic and behavioral effects of high-dose, exogenous testosterone in healthy men. *J Clin Endocrinol Metab* 1994; 79: 561–567

67. Geller J. Overview of benign prostatic hypertrophy. *Urology* 1989; 34: 57–63

68. de Lignières B. Transdermal dihydrotestosterone treatment of 'andropause'. *Ann Med* 1993; 25: 235–241

69. Meikle AW, Arver S, Dobs AS *et al.* Prostate size in hypogonadal men treated with a nonscrotal permeation-enhanced testosterone transdermal system. *Urology* 1997; 49: 191–196

70. Franks LM. Latent carcinoma of the prostate. *J Pathol Bacteriol* 1954; 68: 603–616

71. Noble RL. Androgen use by athletes: a possible cancer risk. *Can Med Assoc J* 1984; 130: 549–550

72. Roberts JT, Essenhigh DM. Adenocarcinoma of prostate in 40-year-old body builder. *Lancet* 1995; 2: 742

73. Ross R, Bernstein L, Judd H *et al.* Serum testosterone levels in healthy young black and white men. *J Natl Cancer Inst* 1986; 76: 45–48

74. Word Health Organization Task Force on Methods for the Regulation of Male Fertility. Contraceptive efficacy of testosterone-induced azoöspermia in normal men. *Lancet* 1990; 336: 955–959

CHAPTER 13

Infertility in men

L. S. Ross

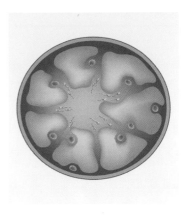

Introduction

Infertility is the inability of a couple either to achieve pregnancy or to carry a pregnancy to live birth. In the USA, it is estimated that 10% of married couples have primary infertility (are unable to conceive a first pregnancy) and 10–15% experience secondary infertility (have one child but cannot conceive a second time). Over one billion dollars per year are spent in the USA on treatment of infertility. The expenditures worldwide are not known but are clearly increasing each year, making this a major health issue.

Traditionally, women have sought fertility services when unable to become pregnant, and the focus of medical evaluation has been directed toward 'female factors'. With more interest and study of the problem it has become clear that 'male factors' are an equally important cause of infertility: in approximately 40% of infertile couples, a female factor only is found; in 30%, a male factor alone is identified, and in 30%, both male and female factors occur. Because more than one-half of all infertility involves the male, it is critical that physicians and patients have an understanding of the causes of male factor infertility; only through treatment of the 'couple' will the best results be achieved.

'Clinical infertility' has been defined as the inability of a couple of prime reproductive age (16–30 years) to conceive after 12 months of unprotected intercourse. Because many couples delay marriage and family building to a later age, evaluations are initiated after 3–6 months of failure if either partner is over 30 years of age.

Male reproductive physiology

The pituitary and testis interact to stimulate the development and maturation of the male reproductive cell, the spermatozoon. These two organs begin to differentiate at 3 months of embryonic life and are fully developed anatomically at birth; they do not begin to function until puberty. Spermatogenesis in the male and ovarian regulation in the female are similar in that the hypothalamus, stimulated by a variety of neurotransmitters, produces gonadotrophin-releasing hormone (GnRH) [1]. GnRH stimulates release of follicle-stimulating hormone (FSH) and luteinizing hormone (LH), both of which have direct effects on the testis and ovary. A schematic view of these interactions in the male is shown in Figure 13.1.

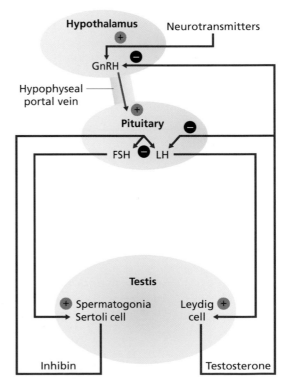

Figure 13.1. *Spermatogenesis: diagram showing hormonal regulation. FSH, follicle-stimulating hormone; GnRH, gonadotrophin-releasing hormone; LH, luteinizing hormone; +, stimulation; −, suppression.*

FSH acts directly on the Sertoli cell, which communicates with germ cell paracrine factors, resulting in active regulation of germ-cell development. The Sertoli cell releases inhibin and other factors that regulate the release of FSH. LH stimulates the testis interstitial cell (Leydig cell) to produce testosterone, which is then converted to its most biologically active form, dihydrotestosterone (DHT), by the action of the enzyme 5-alpha-reductase. DHT acts both in the testis tubule to further spermatozoon maturation and in the epididymis to stimulate motility.

In the testis tubules, spermatogonia (primordial diploid cells) differentiate into mature haploid sperm in an orderly process [2,3]. This cellular differentiation is controlled by specific genes. Although the hormonal regulation of spermatogenesis is well understood, the nature of genetic control is at a much earlier stage of study.

Mature spermatozoa travel from the testicular tubular lumen through the rete testis to the epididymis and vas deferens, and then to the ejaculatory ducts which exit in the urethra. Here the spermatozoa mix with secretions from the seminal vesicles and prostate; the fluid is ejaculated as semen. Ejaculation is a complex phenomenon of co-ordinated peristalsis of the epididymis, vas deferens, seminal vesicle and ejaculatory duct. This wave of activity is accompanied by rhythmic contraction of the bulbocavernosus and perineal muscles and closure of the bladder neck, resulting in propulsion of the semen from the urethra.

On ejaculation, semen coagulates and spermatozoa are trapped in the thick mucoid secretion. The semen liquefies in 30–60 minutes and the spermatozoa are released [4,5]. In the vagina, spermatozoa will swim through the cervical os into the uterine cavity and ultimately enter the fallopian tubes. It is there that spermatozoa encounter the ovum and fertilization takes place.

Because of the complex developmental and delivery mechanisms necessary to bring a single spermatozoa and ovum together for conception, it is not difficult to understand the number of problems that can develop in the male alone to prevent pregnancy.

Clinical evaluation of the infertile male

Given the shared processes that lead to conception, it is clear that any workup for infertility must be a simultaneous evaluation of both partners. For the male, this should consist of a thorough urological medical history, with emphasis on factors that can affect reproduction. Table 13.1 outlines many childhood and adult diseases and surgical procedures that could affect spermatozoon production or transport. Table 13.2 lists medications, industrial agents, non-surgical medical therapies and 'recreational' drugs that may act as gonadotoxins. Patients should also be questioned about sexual function, frequency of intercourse and use of lubricants, some of which are spermicidal.

Table 13.1. *Adult and childhood factors affecting fertility*

Adult surgery

Herniorrhaphy

Orchiectomy (testis cancer, torsion)

Pelvic, inguinal or scrotal surgery

Retroperitoneal surgery

Transurethral resection of prostate

Y–V plasty of bladder

Genetic factors

Androgen receptor deficiency

Cystic fibrosis

Kallman's syndrome

Childhood diseases

Delayed puberty

Herniorrhaphy

Testicular torsion

Testicular trauma

Undescended testis, orchiopexy

Y–V plasty of bladder

Infections

Mumps orchitis

Sexually transmitted diseases

Tuberculosis

Viral, febrile

Table 13.2. *Gonadotoxins*

Alcohol

Androgenic steroids

Cannabis

Cocaine

Chemicals (pesticides)

Chemotherapeutics

Cimetidine

Nicotine

Nitrofurantoin

Radiation

Sulfasalazine

Thermal exposure

The physical examination should emphasize the male reproductive tract, while ensuring complete evaluation of other systems that may play a part (e.g. endocrine system). General body habitus should be noted, with attention to overall development of secondary sex characteristics, hair distribution and morphometrics. Examination of the genitalia should assess the descent of both testes into the scrotum and include a measurement of testis size (normal volume ≥ 30 ml; long axis > 3 cm) and consistency (firm, full). Careful palpation should confirm the presence of the vas deferens and a complete epididymis bilaterally. The epididymis should be non-tender with no swelling or masses. The penis should be examined for hypospadias or any abnormality that might affect deposition of spermatozoa in the vagina.

Scrotal varicoceles have been recognized as a significant cause of infertility since Tulloch's first description in 1955 [6]. The varicocele can be diagnosed only with the patient in the upright position and is felt as a dilatation of the internal spermatic veins. This 'bag of worms' abnormality is often accentuated as the patient performs a Valsalva manoeuvre. Confirmation can be obtained with a portable office Doppler or with colour duplex ultrasound screening, provided that the patient is tested in the upright position. Varicoceles occur in 15% of the male population, but are found in 35–50% of infertile men [7]. They occur most commonly on the left side

(80–90%) but occasionally on the right or bilaterally (10–20%) [8].

Finally, the prostate should be evaluated by digital rectal examination to rule out benign or malignant enlargement or prostatitis. Any palpable enlargement of the seminal vesicle that may suggest ejaculatory duct obstruction should be noted.

Laboratory testing for infertility

Semen analysis

Men are much easier to evaluate for infertility than women, owing to the external location of the reproductive organs. In addition, the male gametes can be retrieved and subjected to complete analysis. The standard semen analysis is the primary laboratory test in evaluation of male infertility. As semen can vary considerably, even in fertile men, at least two samples a minimum of 4 weeks apart should be collected. The standard semen analysis includes measurement of volume, density (spermatozoa/ml), total motility (percentage of cells), percentage progressive motility, morphology (percentage of normal forms), viscosity and pH [9]. Sperm agglutination and the presence of white blood cells (WBCs) will also be recorded. The finding of WBCs must be confirmed with special stains, such as CD 45 monoclonal antibody, as many infertile men slough immature round spermatozoon forms in the semen [10]. Mistaking these cells for WBCs leads to an erroneous diagnosis of infection or 'prostatitis' and, as a consequence, to unnecessary and ineffective treatment of the patient and often the spouse.

Testing for fructose, a sugar produced by the seminal vesicle, is performed when no spermatozoa are present in the semen (azoöspermia). Absence of fructose may mean obstruction of the ejaculatory ducts or absence of the seminal vesicle, which may or may not be accompanied by absence of the vasa deferentia. Semen volumes less than 1 ml are also suggestive of obstructed ejaculatory ducts. The World Health Organization range of values for normal semen analysis is given in Table 13.3.

Sperm function studies

Although the standard semen analysis is a good screen for assessing male fertility, it does not always detect a male factor. In some couples where initial male and female evaluations are negative and clinical infertility persists, more sophisticated semen testing may be revealing. The sperm penetration assay tests the ability of

Table 13.3. *World Health Organization criteria for normal semen analysis (on at least two occasions)*

Semen parameter	Value
Volume	1.5–5.0 ml
Density	> 20 x 10^6/ml
Motility	> 60%
Forward progression	> 2 (scale 1–4)
Morphology	> 60% normal forms
Leucocytes	< 1 x 10^6/ml
Agglutination	None
Hyperviscosity	Drop-like, or thread not > 2 cm

the human spermatozoon to enter a zona-free mammalian egg (usually golden hamster) and begin the fertilization reaction. This study was developed in 1976 by Yanagimachi and coworkers while studying laboratory techniques for human in vitro fertilization [11]. They demonstrated that trypsin digestion of the zona pellucida of mammalian eggs allowed cross-species fertilization. They also discovered that the rate of penetration of such eggs by human spermatozoa correlated quite well with pregnancy rates, leading to the use of this study in some centres as a measure of sperm fertilizing capacity and as a predictor of success of in vitro fertilization procedures. Some controversy over the accuracy and predictive value of this test exists, owing to the lack of standardized technique and result reporting. In the author's laboratory, the test is run against a control (normal donor semen), giving a comparative measure of the patient's potential fertilizing capacity.

Another test of sperm function is the hemizona assay, in which the ability of spermatozoa to bind to human zona pellucida is assessed [12]. These studies are labour intensive and thus very expensive compared with a standard semen analysis. They are not a replacement but are used as an adjunct or arbiter when appropriate. The hypoosmotic swelling test (HOS test) [13] evaluates the integrity of the sperm cell membranes, and acrosin assays (triple stain, antibody, biochemical assay) measure completeness and activity of the acrosome, which is involved in sperm–egg interaction [10,14].

Antisperm antibodies

The role of antisperm antibodies in infertility remains controversial [15]. Circulating and seminal plasma serum antisperm antibodies have been measured in both men and women, and early attempts to link their presence to infertility were not convincing [16]. Some studies have shown that the distribution of these free circulating antibodies is similar in fertile and infertile populations. More recent evidence suggests that fertility may be compromised in men with antibodies directed at the spermatozoa. These antibodies are detected with the immunobead test, in which antihuman immunoglobulin antigen (IgA, IgG, IgM) is bound to polyacrylamide spheres that attach to antibodies on the sperm cell surface [17]. It is believed that these sperm-surface antibodies may affect motility (tail bound) or inhibit egg penetration (head bound).

Sperm cervical mucus penetration tests

The ability of spermatozoa to migrate through and penetrate cervical mucus correlates with fertilizing potential, both in vivo and in vitro [18]. Utilization of the partner's cervical mucus (Kremer test) is unreliable and impossible to standardize [19]. Several commercial tests using bovine cervical mucus are available and more accurate (Penetrak, Serono and True-Trax, Humagen) [20].

Hormonal screening

Owing to hormonal regulation and stimulation of spermatogenesis, defects in hormonal production can influence fertility. Although obvious hormonal diseases — such as Kallman's syndrome, hyper/hypothyroidism and Klinefelter's syndrome — are detected by history and physical examination, screening of pituitary gonadotrophins (FSH, LH) and testosterone may detect mild forms of pituitary and testicular dysfunction that can influence the semen and fertility.

Hyperprolactinaemia can cause oligospermia by affecting the uptake and binding of testosterone; it may also result in erectile dysfunction. Subclinical adrenal hydroxylase deficiency can result in mild oligo-asthenospermia and can be detected with serum dehydroepiandrosterone and testosterone measurement [21]. In patients with azoöspermia or severe oligospermia (counts ≤ 3 × 10^6 spermatozoa/ml), elevations of FSH greater than or equivalent to twice the upper limit of normal indicate testis failure and usually preclude further testing and treatment.

Other diagnostic tests

Diagnostic ultrasound

Ultrasound is a safe and effective modality allowing imaging of organs and assessment of blood flow. Small, portable directional Doppler units are useful in the office setting to detect or confirm the presence of varicoceles [22]. Colour duplex Doppler ultrasonography can provide even more accurate confirmation of varicoceles, as well as identification of the number of venous tributaries, their size and the direction of venous flow. Transrectal ultrasound (TRUS) has become the standard for imaging the prostate and guiding biopsy for detection of prostate cancer. As this technology can image the seminal vesicles, ampulla of the vas deferens and the ejaculatory ducts, it can be used to diagnose ejaculatory duct obstruction [23,24].

Testis biopsy

In the past, testis biopsy was frequently used to diagnose many fertility disorders. With modern hormonal screening studies and non-invasive imaging such as TRUS, testis biopsy and operative vasography have a much more limited role. Today, biopsy is reserved for patients with normal serum FSH, azoöspermia, normal-size testes, palpable vas deferens and epididymis, and fructose-positive normal-volume semen. Here, biopsy allows differentiation between patients with microtubular obstructive disease who are candidates for microsurgical reconstruction and patients with disorders of spermatozoa development. Vasography, if indicated, should not be performed at the time of testis biopsy, but should be reserved for the definitive microsurgical exploration and repair. Independent vasography at the time of biopsy does not add useful information and may result in unnecessary obstruction at the site of vasography.

Treatment
Varicocele

Treatment of varicoceles should be limited to men with clinical infertility and abnormal semen parameters. In this setting, treatment can yield semen improvement rates of 50–70% and pregnancy rates of 35–60%. Treatment options include open surgical ligation under local, regional or general anaesthesia (with or without optical magnification for identification of venous tributaries and other cord structures), laparoscopic vein ligation, or transvenous embolization.

Infections

Infections involving the testis (orchitis), epididymis (epididymitis), prostate (prostatitis) and bladder/urethra (cystitis/urethritis) can affect spermatozoon production and/or function and motility. It has been shown that exotoxins from *Escherichia coli* can significantly alter sperm motility [25]. Positive culture tests should prompt the use of appropriate antibiotics. Some drugs are to be avoided because of detrimental effects on spermatogenesis: principal among these are the nitrofurantoins.

Hormonal causes

Significant thyroid dysfunction, hypogonadotrophic hypogonadism (Kallman's syndrome), or pre-pubertal adrenogenital syndrome should be treated early in order to preserve fertility. Occasionally, adult patients are seen with Kallman's syndrome; if these are treated with replacement therapy (chorionic and menotrophins) before the age of 30, they may recover spermatogenesis. Some andrologists believe that subclinical forms of hypogonadotrophic hypogonadism and adrenal hydroxylase deficiency exist and that appropriate therapy with exogenous pituitary hormone and suppression with prednisone or dexamethasone, respectively, can enhance impaired fertility in these men.

Retrograde ejaculation

In retrograde ejaculation, the ejaculate flows retrogradely into the bladder because of incomplete closure of the bladder neck. Such lack of closure can result from bladder neck injury following surgery (open or transurethral resection of the bladder neck/prostate neck, diabetes mellitus (neurovascular damage), sympathetic nerve injury during retroperitoneal or pelvic surgery, or congenital displacement of the ejaculatory ducts at the bladder neck. The diagnosis is made when large numbers of sperm are found in the postejaculatory urine of azoöspermic and severely oligospermic patients with low semen volume. Men with diabetes or sympathetic nerve injury may respond to oral pseudoephedrine or similar sympathomimetic agents, which will promote forward ejaculation by increasing bladder neck tone [26,27]. Those with traumatic bladder neck injury usually require postejaculation catheterization and sperm recovery for artificial insemination [28].

Anejaculation

Some patients with retroperitoneal or pelvic nerve injury, or with spinal cord injury, suffer from anejaculation. The sensation of ejaculation may occur, owing to contraction of the bulbocavernosus muscles during sexual stimulation, but there is no forward ejaculation and no spermatozoa are found in postejaculatory urine. The lack of ejaculation results from inability of the muscles of the vas deferens, seminal vesicles and prostatic ducts to contract and propel spermatozoa and seminal fluid into the urethra. Options for treatment include vibratory stimulation of the glans penis, electro-ejaculation using rectal probes and surgical extraction of sperm from the vas deferens, epididymis or testis. Semen and spermatozoa obtained by these techniques are used for artificial reproductive techniques [29].

Ejaculatory duct obstruction

Obstruction of the ejaculatory ducts may be the result of infection (prostatitis, urethritis, seminal vesiculitis), injury to the ducts (traumatic, iatrogenic), or congenital anomaly (müllerian duct cyst). Classically, these patients have low-volume (0.5–1.0 ml), fructose-negative, azoöspermic semen. As late as the mid-1980s, only about 40 cases had been reported in the literature and results of therapy were usually dismal [30]. Diagnosis involved cystoscopy with attempted catheterization of the ejaculatory ducts and/or surgical vasography. With the introduction of diagnostic TRUS, the diagnosis can be made non-invasively. In addition, some investigators feel that there is a significant pool of infertile men with fructose-positive low-volume semen and severe oligo-asthenospermia who have partial ejaculatory duct obstruction diagnosed on TRUS by finding enlarged seminal vesicles and dilated ejaculatory ducts. Many of these patients respond to transurethral resection of the ducts with increase in semen volume and improvement in semen parameters [31].

Microtubular obstructive disease

Men with obstruction of the vas deferens or epididymis account for 8–10% of azoöspermic patients. Vasal obstruction is most typically iatrogenic (vasectomy, vasal injury during herniorrhaphy, or pelvic or scrotal surgery), but may be congenital (partial atresia). Epididymal occlusion may also be iatrogenic, but is more frequently the result of infection (epididymitis) or a congenital problem in which the vas deferens and epididymis fail to unite during embryonic development.

Patients with microtubular obstruction present with normal-volume, fructose-positive azoöspermia and have normal-size testes and normal serum FSH and testosterone. Modern microsurgical techniques allow correction of these problems with reasonably high success rates. Vasovasostomy patency rates as high as 90% and vaso-epididymostomy rates of 70% can be achieved [32]. Unfortunately, long-standing dilatation of the epididymis with entrapped spermatozoa often leads to epididymal damage, which affects sperm quality.

Congenital absence of the vas deferens

A very few men with azoöspermia have bilateral congenital absence of the vasa (CAV), which may or may not be associated with absence of the seminal vesicle. Thus, the presence or absence of semen fructose is not a reliable diagnostic clue. Because the vasa are easily palpable, the diagnosis can be made by failing to feel the structure in an azoöspermic male. These patients can reproduce by having surgical extraction of sperm from the epididymis or testis for in vitro fertilization [33]. CAV may be associated with the gene defect (CFTR) that causes cystic fibrosis, and all CAV patients should be screened prior to attempting conception. Unilateral CAV also occurs, but is not usually associated with infertility.

Non-obstructive azoöspermia

The majority of azoöspermic patients have pretesticular or primary testicular disorders. The primary conditions include spermatogenic arrest, in which the testis tubules contain both spermatogonia (precursor sperm stem cells) and Sertoli cells (sustentacular cells); however, the spermatogonia do not go through full development and maturation to adult diploid sperm, and in the Sertoli cell-only syndrome, no spermatogonia are identified in the tubules. Spermatogenic arrest is thought to be due to defects in the genetic regulation of sperm maturation; the cause of Sertoli cell-only syndrome is unknown. There is no therapy to restore spermatogenesis in either condition. Recent studies have shown that, in both conditions, generous testis biopsies may occasionally yield tiny pockets of mature spermatozoa. Advances in assisted reproductive techniques allow such small numbers of spermatozoa to be cryopreserved for egg fertilization.

Idiopathic oligospermia

Even with an extensive workup, in as many as 20% of men, abnormal semen analyses and infertility will not have an identifiable aetiology.

Attempts to treat these patients have focused on empirical therapies with varying degrees of success. The use of thyroid hormone or testosterone in the absence of specific endocrinopathy is to be condemned. 'Testosterone rebound', as reported in older literature, not only fails to yield clinically significant results but also has been noted to produce prolonged azoöspermia in some men. The most commonly used empirical therapy is based on the notion that hypergonadotrophic stimulation of eugonadotrophic men may stimulate increased spermatozoon production. Thus, oral administration of clomiphene citrate and intramuscular injection of human chorionic and menotrophins have been reported to stimulate spermatogenesis in idiopathic infertile men. Unfortunately, there are few controlled data to support these findings. Other drugs, including tamoxifen, kallikrein and pentoxifylline, have been used in non-controlled studies with variable results [34]. Finally, a wide variety of 'over-the-counter' remedies — including vitamins, herbs and tonics — have been recommended, but no data are available on their efficacy.

Assisted reproductive techniques (ART)

Intra-uterine insemination

Insemination of a partner's sperm into the uterine cavity during timed or stimulated ovulatory cycles is an integral part of the treatment for men with ejaculatory failure and retrograde ejaculation. The semen obtained by vibratory stimulation or electro-ejaculation in the former and that recovered from the bladder in the latter is generally treated by separation of the sperm cells from seminal plasma and/or urine and resuspension in a sterile laboratory medium prior to insemination (sperm wash). This technique may also be useful in men with low-volume semen.

In vitro fertilization (IVF)

There are a number of techniques for the combination of human eggs and spermatozoa outside the female, with re-implantation of zygotes or embryos. Traditionally, these techniques were developed to treat couples in whom the female partner had obstructed or absent fallopian tubes, preventing transport of the sperm to the egg for natural conception. The indications for this technique have been broadened to include it as an option for male factor infertility where low sperm numbers or lack of motility preclude natural fertilization. Even this method has had poor results when sperm concentrations are below 1×10^6 to 5×10^6 progressively motile spermatozoa per ejaculate [35].

Intracytoplasmic sperm injection (ICSI)

Variations of IVF have been developed in cases of low sperm count or poor sperm motility. Artificial disruption of the zona pellucida (zona drilling) and subzonal injection of spermatozoon have been tried with success. Most notable has been the development of intracytoplasmic sperm injection (ICSI) where a single spermatozoon is placed directly into the egg cytoplasm with a micropipette [36]. Thus only a single spermatozoon, motile or immotile, is needed to yield an embryo capable of producing a viable pregnancy. This technique offers the possibility of conception to men with severe oligo-asthenospermia. In other conditions, such as CAV and unreconstructable vasal or epididymal lesions, small numbers of spermatozoa surgically extracted from the epididymis or directly from the testis can be used fresh or cryopreserved for ICSI [33]. Furthermore, patients with conditions thought to be untreatable are sometimes candidates for this therapy. In some patients with germ cell aplasia (Sertoli cell-only syndrome) or spermatogenic arrest, generous biopsies may yield a few mature spermatozoa sufficient for ICSI. ICSI and IVF have been suggested by some as the treatment of choice for most male-factor infertility. However, it is much more cost-effective to treat most primary male problems in a way that allows for natural conception, the method favoured by most couples.

Conclusions

Infertility is a problem affecting a significant proportion of couples of childbearing age. It is clear that male factors play a part in over 50% of couples. Recent advances in the diagnosis and treatment of men with fertility problems make it imperative for physicians treating clinical infertility to evaluate the male partner thoroughly. Because the majority of male factors can be treated, the success rate for any couple attempting conception will depend on management of both the female and male partner.

Acknowledgements

The author wishes to thank Dr Craig Niederberger for reviewing the manuscript,

Karen Lewak for her editorial suggestions and Carolyn Seydel for preparing the chapter.

References

1. Belchez PE, Plant TM, Nakai Y et al. Hypophyseal response to continuous and intermittent delivery of hypothalamic gonadotropin-releasing hormone. *Science* 1978; 202: 631–633

2. Clermont Y. The cycle of the seminiferous epithelium in man. *Am J Anat* 1963; 112: 35–45

3. Schulze C. Morphological characteristics of the spermatogonial stem cells in man. *Cell Tissue Res* 1979; 198: 191–199

4. Huggins C, Neal W. Coagulation and liquefaction of semen: proteolytic enzymes and citrate in prostate fluid. *J Exp Med* 1942; 76: 527–541

5. Bunge RG. Some observations on the male ejaculate. *Fertil Steril* 1970; 21: 639–644

6. Tulloch WS. Varicocele in subfertility: results of treatment. *Br Med J* 1955; 2: 356

7. Lipshultz LI, Greenberg SH. Varicocele and male subfertility. In: Sciarra JJ (ed) Gynecology and obstetrics, Vol. 66. Hagerstown: Harper and Row, 1987: 1

8. Saypol DC. Varicocele. *J Androl* 1981; 2: 61–71

9. Amelar RD, Dubin L, Schoenfeld C. Semen analysis. *Urology* 1973; 2: 605–611

10. WHO laboratory manual: The examination of human semen and sperm–cervical mucous interactions, 3rd ed. Cambridge: Cambridge University Press, 1992

11. Yanagimachi R, Yanagimachi H, Rogers BJ. The use of zona-free animal ova as a test system for the assessment of the fertilizing capacity of human spermatozoa. *Biol Reprod* 1976; 15: 471–476

12. Oehringer S. Diagnostic significance of sperm–zona pellucida interaction. *Reprod Med Rev* 1992; 1: 57

13. Jeyendran RS, VanderVen HH, Perez-Pelaez M et al. Development of an assay to assess functional integrity of the human sperm membrane and its relationship to other semen characteristics. *J Reprod Fertil* 1984; 70: 219–228

14. Kennedy WP, Kaminski JM, VanderVen HH et al. A simple clinical assay to evaluate the acrosin activity of human spermatozoa. *J Androl* 1989; 10: 221–231

15. Haas GG. Antibody-mediated causes of male infertility. *Urol Clin North Am* 1987; 14: 539–550

16. Coombs RRA, Rümke P, Edwards RG. Immunoglobulin classes reactive with spermatozoa in the serum and seminal plasma of vasectomized and infertile men. In: Bratanov K (ed) Second International Symposium on Immunology of Reproduction. Bulgaria: Bulgarian Academy of Sciences Press, 1972

17. Clarke GN, Elliott PJ, Smaila C. Detection of sperm antibodies in semen using the immunobead test: a survey of 813 consecutive patients. *Am J Reprod Immunol* 1985; 7: 118–123

18. Alexander NJ. Evaluation of male infertility with an in vitro cervical mucus penetration test. *Fertil Steril* 1981; 36: 201–208

19. Kremer J. A simple penetration test. *Int J Androl* 1965; 10: 209

20. Niederberger CS, Lamb DJ, Glinz M et al. Tests of sperm function for evaluation of the male: Penetrak and True-Trax. *Fertil Steril* 1993; 60: 319–323

21. Ross L. Routine hormonal screening of infertile men: is it worthwhile? *J Urol* 1981; 126: 756–758

22. Ross L. Diagnosis and treatment of infertile men: a clinical perspective. *J Urol* 1983; 130: 847–854

23. Belker AM, Steinbock GS. Transrectal prostate ultrasonography as a diagnostic and therapeutic aid for ejaculatory duct obstruction. *J Urol* 1990; 144: 356–358

24. Jarow JP. Transrectal ultrasonography of infertile men *Fertil Steril* 1993; 60: 1035–1039

25. Teague NS, Boyarsky S, Glenn JF. Interference of human spermatozoa motility by *Escherichia coli*. *Fertil Steril* 1971; 22: 281–285

26. Kedia K, Markland C. The effect of pharmacological agents on ejaculation. *J Urol* 1975; 114: 569–573

27. Gilja I, Parazajder J, Radej M et al. Retrograde ejaculation and loss of emission: possibilities of conservative treatment. *Eur Urol* 1994; 25: 226–228

28. Urry RL, Middleton RG, McGavin S. A simple and effective technique for increasing pregnancy rates in couples with retrograde ejaculation. *Fertil Steril* 1986; 46: 1124–1127

29. Shaban SF, Seaman EK, Lipshultz LI. Treatment of abnormalities of ejaculation. In: Lipshultz LI, Howards SS (eds) Infertility in the male. St Louis: Mosby Year Book, 1997: 423–438

30. Ross LS. Ejaculatory duct obstruction. In: Garcia CR, Mastroianni L, Amelar RD, Dubin L (eds) Current therapy of infertility — 3. Philadelphia: Decker, 1988; 225–228

31. Meacham RB, Hellerstein DK, Lipshultz LI. Evaluation and treatment of ejaculatory duct obstruction in the infertile male. *Fertil Steril* 1993; 59: 393–397

32. Belker AM, Thomas AJ Jr, Fuchs EF et al. Results of 1469 microsurgical vasectomy reversals by the vasovasostomy study group. *J Urol* 1991; 145: 505–511

33. Ross LS, Yuan J, Dolgina R et al. Routine testicular sperm extraction (TESE) during microsurgical vasal and epididymal reconstruction is safe and effective. *J Urol* 1997; 157: 168

34. Jarow JP. Non-surgical treatment of male infertility: empiric therapy. In: Lipshultz LI, Howards SS (eds) Infertility in the male. Philadelphia: Mosby Year Book, 1997: 410–422

35. Redgment CJ, Yang D, Tsirigotis M et al. Experience with assisted fertilization in severe male factor infertility and unexplained foiled fertilization in vitro. *Hum Reprod* 1994; 9: 680–683

36. Palermo GD, Joris M, Devroey P, Van Steirteghem AC. Pregnancies after intracytoplasmic injection of a single spermatozoon into an oocyte. *Lancet* 1992; 4: 17–18

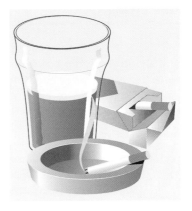

CHAPTER 14

Men as risk takers

S. Griffiths

Introduction

The stereotypes of little boys and girls focus around the notion that they are different, not only biologically but also in their behaviour. Parents do not usually choose a present for their son from the glittering range of Barbie or Cindy dolls, and if they choose a doll it will be more like Action Man (Fig. 14.1), with his guns and ropes and equipment which allows him to carry out daring feats and rescue bids. This stereotyping does, inevitably, over-simplify the differences between boys and girls. Many parents would immediately tell you of their positive efforts to encourage a less-biased approach to the upbring-

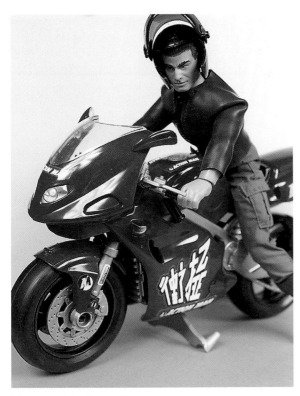

Figure 14.1. *Action Man.*

ing of their children, and will cite the footballs given to their daughters and the educational toys given to their sons. But stereotyping reflects the cultural expectation on boys as they grow up — the expectation that they will be risk takers. Men are expected to be tough, independent and strong. This expectation is reflected in the way they treat their health, with a strong focus on fitness and the body as a machine. It is also reflected in the way that they behave — driving faster, smoking more, drinking to excess and being more violent.

That men take greater risks with their health than women is evident from the statistics. In the UK, men die at a younger age than women; on average, 5 years sooner. They are three and a half times more likely to die from coronary heart disease under the age of 65, they have a suicide rate at least double that of women; they are more likely to smoke, drink and be overweight; and they are more likely to contract human immunodeficiency virus (HIV)/autoimmune disease (AIDS). These statistics reflect higher levels of risk taking, which is also indicated by men's use of health care: they are less likely to turn up for their 'well man' checks than are women, but are more likely to be more severely ill by the time that they get to their doctor. This chapter does not seek to explain such behaviours; instead it focuses on what is known and what might be done to improve the health of men of all ages.

The size of the problem

In his annual report of 1992, the Chief Medical Officer of England described the different health profiles for men and women, highlighting the fact that, although the male birth rate is higher — with 106 male births for every 100 female births — men have a consistently higher mortality [1]. Foetal mortality is higher among males, and the 20% higher pattern of infant mortality is reflected in all ages thereafter. In 1991, an 18-year-old man had an 80% chance of survival to 65 years of age compared with the 88% expectation of a woman of the same age.

This is not a new finding and is one that is common across the developed world. Comparing mortality as a ratio between men and women shows that excess deaths tend to occur in young male adults and can be attributed to accidents, suicide and AIDS. The smaller peak at around 65 is due to higher death rates from coronary heart disease and lung cancer [2]; in 1992, 70% of all male deaths were as a result of circulatory diseases and cancer. Causes of male deaths vary, as would be expected, with age. Road accident-related deaths are highest amongst men aged 15–34, accounting for one-fifth of the deaths in this age group.

However, this picture is not as simple as aggregated statistics would suggest. As one would suspect, men are not a homogeneous group. Recent work shows that there is a social class gradient for mortality in men and that this gradient is increasing [3]. Compared with social class I, social class V men have almost three times the rate of mortality and social classes IIIM and IV have nearly double the mortality. Put another way, young men aged 20–24 in social class V at death experience the same mortality rates as do men 20 years older, in social class I. The social class differentials for stroke, lung cancer, accidents and suicides are even greater. In addition, the differentials between social class I and social class V have widened since the 1970s, despite the overall downward trend. In simple terms, men who are better off are getting healthier at a faster rate than those who are less well off.

Looking in more detail at causes of death for men aged 20–64, 33% of deaths were from neoplasms (cancers), almost 40% from diseases of the circulatory system and 12% from external causes of injury and poisoning. Lung cancer is the most common cancer, and deaths account for 29% of all cancer deaths, with a class gradient that reflects higher rates amongst the less affluent. The same gradient, that of greater mortality in social class V, is seen for circulatory diseases — heart disease and stroke. For these diseases, social class V mortality is twice that of the whole of England and Wales, and three times that of social class I. Mortality from accidents and suicides is four times greater in social class V than in social class I. This is particularly reflected in motor vehicle accidents, which are three times more common in social class V. Men

who are unemployed are more than twice as likely to commit suicide; men who are single, widowed or divorced are three times as likely. Men with AIDS, men in prison and abusers of drugs and alcohol are also more likely to commit suicide. Statistics that do not fit with this trend include a higher death rate from skin cancer in social class I and a greater number of deaths from HIV infection in social classes II and IIIN.

Reasons for this growing differential are not well understood, but less-affluent men are under increased social stress from economic insecurity, lack of secure employment and changing social expectations. Boys are doing less well in school than girls. This is backed up by recent government reports suggesting the need for an increase in male primary school teachers as 'role models' for boys. There seems little way out of the poverty trap for many, so taking risks is both a means of expression and a symptom of alienation.

Mortality statistics are of use as indicators of health, but it is not only death rates that reflect differences between the health of men and women. Available data show that for most illnesses, men are less likely than women to consult their general practitioners, yet their hospital admission rates for diseases such as coronary heart disease and stroke are higher. Men are more likely to wait until their symptoms are more severe before seeking help. They are also less likely to attend health checks or dental checks than are women. Studies of long-term sickness show that there are no significant differences in the number of men and women who report chronic or long-standing illness. However, men in lower socio-economic groups are more likely to define their health as fair or poor than either women in comparable groups or men in higher socio-economic groups.

Aetiology

It is not just the illnesses experienced by men that differ from those of women, it is health behaviour as well. When the Men's Forum published its *Men's Health Review* [4], media coverage included headlines referring to the popular television programme *Men Behaving Badly*, an image which perhaps sums up the stereotypical beer-drinking, fun-loving, risk-taking lifestyle which young men aspire to. The review stresses that it is the interaction of biological, social and behavioural factors that needs to be addressed if men's health is to be improved. Specific risk-taking activities that affect men's health are detailed below.

The statistics quoted above highlight the damage that risk-taking behaviour causes to health. Some of those that require closer analysis are discussed below.

Smoking

The commonest causes of death are heart disease and lung cancer. Both are related to smoking tobacco, and men have traditionally smoked more than women. Trends are changing, however: in 1972, the death rate due to heart disease and lung cancer in men was five times that in women; in 1992, it was only double. This is a clear demonstration of the impact that changing lifestyles has on both women and men. Although more men smoke, more will have tried and succeeded in giving up. Until Richard Doll's study of smoking in doctors, which linked tobacco with lung cancer, male doctors had high rates of smoking; now it is rare to find male doctors who smoke. However, the number of young women who smoke continues to rise, and this change in behaviour is storing up future health problems.

It can also be argued that the statistics are symptomatic of the blurring of gender roles that is occurring. In his recent book, *The Future of Men*, Dave Hill highlights the theme that the future is female [5]. His summary that:

'. . . As girls do better and better at school, boys trail behind; as women secure more and better jobs, men become more intimate with the schedules of daytime TV; while men kill themselves with increasing frequency, women lead lives that are not only longer, but also sweeter.'

is an obvious parody, but rings true. Such sentiments reflect that, in the last decade, most Western societies have restructured their economies. There are more part-time jobs and fewer manual jobs. The employment market is more responsive to portfolio careers than to jobs for life, and it is argued that women cope with this ambivalence better than do men.

Not only do women increasingly expect to go out to work, they are expected to do so; hence, the current social policy initiatives in the UK, such as after-school support for single parents. This alters the stereotypical image of men as breadwinners and women as housewives caring for children. Some of this reflects the necessities created by the increasing breakdown of families, but much is a reflection of the wishes of women to be equal. This change in stereotypical roles

has blurred the boundaries of what it is to be male or female. It is no longer acceptable to assume that domestic labour is the domain of women. Much is being written about the phenomenon of the new man — a caring, sharing individual, eschewing the socially prescribed male role to share domestic duties. But how far are roles really changing? There are a variety of reactions to the pressure to change man's traditional role. One is to re-emphasize macho behaviour, possibly as a response to the threat that the breaking down of traditional barriers creates for many men, be they at a personal or a social level. The result of this is reflected in the differing patterns of morbidity and mortality associated with risk-taking behaviour.

Road traffic accidents

One of the areas of risk taking that kills disproportionately more young men than women is road traffic accidents (Fig. 14.2). In 1992, three-quarters of deaths from accidental injuries were to men between the ages of 15 and 64, and 46% of accidental deaths in men were due to motor vehicle accidents. Young men are also more likely to have accidents when driving than are young women. Risk-taking behaviour — combined with lack of experience, alcohol and, to a lesser extent, drugs — are significant factors in accident causation in this group.

Mental health

There is a body of literature about the relationship between masculinity and mental health, which is not described here. Statistics show that men are less likely to suffer from depression or anxiety than women, but are as likely to be diagnosed schizophrenic. The diagnosis is more likely to be made at a younger age in men, peaking at

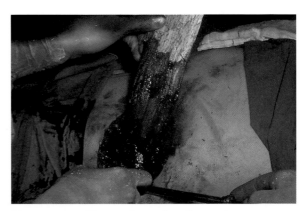

Figure 14.2. *Victim of a road traffic accident.*

between 15 and 24 years. Particular groups of men (e.g. the homeless) are more likely to be severely mentally ill. More than 10 times as many men as women are to be found among those who live in hostels for the homeless and 30–50% of them suffer from severe mental illness. Young Afro-Caribbean men are more likely to suffer from severe mental illness and to be admitted to secure wards. Commenting on these and other statistics, Chan suggests that improvement in the health of men from ethnic minorities will depend on the reduction of stress generated by unemployment, poor housing and other forms of racism, as reflected in the suicide statistics, particularly for young men [6].

Suicide

Suicide is associated not only with previously diagnosed mental illness but also with a variety of social factors. Hawton emphasizes that we need to consider suicide as a spectrum from vague thoughts about suicide through more serious thoughts, a suicidal act either with little or no suicidal intent or considerable intent, to completed suicide [7]. For every one teenage suicide there are 100 attempts. It has been suggested that, at some time, 10–20% of teenagers entertain quite serious suicidal ideas. This is particularly worrying, since between 1980 amd 1990 the suicide rate in 15–84-year-old males increased by 85%, particularly among 20–24-year-olds. The following contributory factors have been suggested:

- Rising rates of unemployment;
- Increasing alcohol and drug abuse;
- Increasing rates of family breakdown;
- Increasing availability of dangerous methods;
- HIV/AIDS.

Not only have male suicides increased, but more young men are attempting suicide. The most common problems of young suicide attempters are difficulties in interpersonal relationships with partners or relatives, unemployment and employment difficulties and substance abuse. The behaviour is often repeated and there is a significant risk of successful suicide among older male teenagers.

Substance abuse

Substance abuse (Fig. 14.3) is more common in men than in women and, in the UK, nearly 90% of boys have drunk alcohol by the time that they are 13. Of 13–17-year-olds, 25% get into arguments and fights after drinking alcohol and 1000

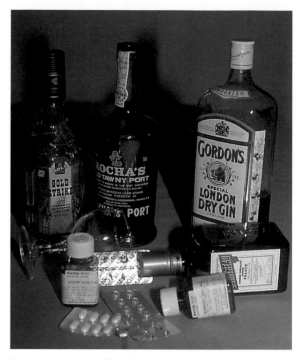

Figure 14.3. *Drink and drugs: substances open to abuse.*

children under 15 years of age are admitted to hospital each year with acute alcohol poisoning [8]. Alcohol is a contributory cause of road traffic accidents and is correlated with the incidence of crime. About one-fifth of convicted prisoners, the vast majority of them male, have an alcohol- or drug-related problem. Alcohol is implicated as a factor in 60% of homicides, 75% of stabbings, 70% of beatings, 40% of domestic violence incidents and 20% of child abuse, most of which are committed by men. Prisoners are four times as likely as their peer group to describe themselves as drinking 'quite a lot' or as drinking 'heavily'. A study by Gunn found that 8.6% of sentenced prisoners had a primary diagnosis of alcohol dependence or abuse [9], and Maden found that 15.4% of remand prisoners were alcohol dependent [10].

Drug misuse is also associated with crime, and three-quarters of opioid addicts notified to the Home Office are men. Of registered drug misusers, 75% have a criminal record, usually related to their use of drugs. In 1988, half the drug offenders in the UK were aged 21–29 years, with 88% being men.

HIV/AIDS

Another example of a disease that affects more men than women in the UK is AIDS. The majority of men in the UK who become infected are homosexuals, although the proportion of such cases is continuing to fall; in contrast, the proportion of cases in which infection is acquired through intercourse between women and men is rising.

A worrying aspect of health behaviour of young men is the finding that, despite knowing the risks of infection, many fail to practise safe sex by using condoms. One study of users of sexually transmitted disease clinics found that one-third of male attenders never used condoms in the first 3 months of a new relationship and over 50% of them failed to use them after 3 months. There is continuing evidence of unsafe sex among young gay men, who are now the main focus for health promotion efforts in the UK.

Further evidence of risk taking in sexual activity by men is found in studies of men who travel abroad. Another study from a clinic of genitourinary medicine indicated that about one-third of patients admitted to having intercourse abroad with a new partner and only 42% consistently used condoms. Although this is a small study, the results must be a cause for concern.

Heart disease

Coronary heart disease is a major killer, killing more men than women. It is closely related to individual lifestyle factors, such as smoking, as well as to social and environmental influences. The challenge to reduce deaths for those under 65 years of age remains a key target for the UK Government.

Male-specific diseases

The risks that men take by ignoring their health can contribute to greater morbidity and mortality from male-specific diseases, such as those of the prostate and the testes. Prostate cancer is extremely common and yet a *Reader's Digest* study found that only half of the men interviewed knew that the prostate gland affects only men and only one in 10 could locate the gland on a diagram of the male body — something more women could do [11]. Body awareness underlies the efforts being made to encourage young men to examine their testes for lumps, particularly since testicular cancer, if diagnosed early, has a good prognosis.

Addressing the issues

Men are more reluctant to go to their doctor for a variety of reasons, ranging from reluctance to have a medical examination to issues such as being too busy and fear of wasting a doctor's time. A study involving Scottish men found that they trusted their doctors but usually went to their families first for advice, were reluctant to attend for 'well person' checks, and were unlikely to go to their doctors for emotional problems [12]. The idea of 'well man' clinics was attractive, but attendance was low. The picture from this survey is fairly typical of other surveys and poses the problem of how to persuade men to be more health conscious and to take a more positive attitude to healthy living and less risk-taking.

Solutions to this challenge lie at several levels — individual, educational and community. For individual men, there is a need to provide both the information and the opportunity to improve knowledge and understanding of health-related risks and what can be done to make sure that opportunities for prevention are taken up. This needs to occur across the age spectrum, starting in schools. There is a growing understanding among those providing personal and social education for schoolchildren that, rather than merely providing knowledge, other approaches are needed. Particular emphasis is being placed on developing self-esteem — promoting feelings of self-worth and ability to cope with peer pressure. Initiatives to help older men to understand more about their health and what they need to do to keep healthy are increasingly building on approaches that recognize men's interests. Examples include Health Works in Dorset, where focus groups identified that men were generally reluctant to face health problems, but they did regret loss of fitness and were concerned with their appearance. They also recognized that a good way of reaching men is through the workplace [13]. Workplace teams of men who are overweight compete to lose weight by lifestyle changes, such as diet and exercise.

Links to sport are also a way of engaging men in health-related activities. An example of this comes from Coventry health promotion, who initiated a health promotion programme for men, endorsed by the city's football team, which was based on local competition and sports-related prizes. Such approaches, aimed at reaching men in their normal settings (e.g. at work and watching sport), are an attempt to raise awareness among men of the risks they take in ignoring their health.

Although outreach to individuals is important, men will be happy with their new image only if it is the one reflected to them in the media. Ian Wylie has argued that male icons are often those associated with tragic death from lifestyles associated with 'sex, drugs and rock and roll': Coleridge, Shelley and Beethoven in the 19th century; Jim Morrison, Rock Hudson, Kurt Cobain and James Dean in the 20th [14]. He argues that much of the targeted advertising about health fails to understand the world-view of the target audience — the glamour of tragedy and risk taking — thus failing to have an impact on risky behaviour. In the same vein, the Health Education Authority has recently called for less cigarette smoking on screen, since smoking is often glamorized within film.

Statistics show, however, that men hearing the health messages are less likely to be those at greatest risk, who (even if they hear them) may well not be motivated to act. To address the growing gap in health inequalities, more needs to be done about the fundamental causes of ill-health (i.e. the social environment in which we live). The links between poverty and ill-health are clear. The links between drugs, crime, violence, imprisonment and unemployment and the ill-health of men highlight the need not only to educate young men nor merely to concentrate on lifestyle changes for the motivated: the root cause of much of the inequalities within men's health lies with their lack of employment and resources to live in a way that will result in better health.

Recognition that there is a shift away from manual tasks towards more technological and computerized means of production has led to national initiatives to give new skills to men who might have earned their living from manual labour. Improving men's health requires composite effort from those constructing the social and economic environment in which we live, as well as individual factors and influences. The risks men take in their lifestyles, coupled with the risky social environment in which they live, need to be addressed if their health is to be improved.

References

1. On the state of the public health. London: HMSO, 1992: 79–107
2. On the state of the public health. London: HMSO, 1992: 81
3. Drever F, Whitehead M. Health inequalities. Series D S No. 15. London: HMSO, 1997
4. Men's health review. London: RCN, 1996
5. Hill D. The future of men. Weidenfeld and Nicholson, 1997
6. Chan M. Ethnicity and men's health. Report of conference: Men's Health Matters, July 1995. The Medicine Group
7. Hawton K. By their own hand. Br Med J 1992; 304: 1000
8. Macfarlane A. The user: drug use by young people. Oxford: Oxford University Press, 1996: 27–29
9. Gunn J. Personality disorders and forensic psychiatry. Criminal Behaviour and Mental Health 1992; 2: 202–211
10. Maden A, Taylor C, Brooke D, Gunn J. Mental disorders in remand prisoners. London: Institute of Psychiatry, 1996
11. Court C. Survey reveals men's ignorance about health. Br Med J 1995; 310: 759
12. Taylor H (compiler and analyser), Riddoch L. (ed). Scotsman; 23 May, 1996
13. Baker P. Men only: is there a role for the well man clinic? Healthlines (HEA); December 1996: 17–18
14. Wylie I, Strong T. Communicate more effectively with men. Report of conference: Men's Health Matters. London: The Medicine Group, 1995

CHAPTER 15

Sexually transmitted diseases and men

J. F. Jovanovich

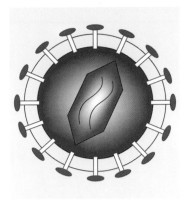

'There are, however, other human diseases that pass directly from host to host with no intermediary carrier and with minimal delay.' [1]

Introduction

A number of diseases that have caused major health concerns and plagues throughout history have been shown to require vectors for their transmission. Other diseases, such as tuberculosis, are not transmitted in this way, but are acquired directly from host to host. Sexually transmitted diseases (STDs) are included in this category. Although no vector is required for their transmission, the direct spread of an STD from one host to another necessitates an act of sexual intimacy.

Transmission of disease through sexual intimacy includes such pathogens as *Treponema pallidum*, *Neisseria gonorrhoeae* and *Chlamydia trachomatis*, which primarily infect the genitalia and genital regions. There are also other organisms that are not thought of as being sexually transmitted because this may not be the usual manner of their spread. These pathogens, however, may reside, pass through, or accidentally enter the pharynx, rectum, anus, and other mucosal areas involved in sexual intimacy. Because of this association they are capable of being transmitted by sexual activity. Such pathogens include, among others, the hepatitis A virus (HAV), the hepatitis B virus (HBV) and *Giardia lamblia*. Thus, the list of STDs and their causative organisms is substantially increased (Table 15.1).

The incidence and prevalence of STDs continue to increase. According to the World Health Organization, the estimated annual incidence of curable STDs — such as syphilis, gonorrhoea, chlamydia and trichomoniasis — is 33.3 million cases worldwide. The number of initial physician office visits for herpes simplex virus

Table 15.1. *Possible aetiologies of sexually transmitted diseases*

Bacteria

> *Treponema pallidum*
> *Neisseria gonorrhoeae*
> *Chlamydia trachomatis*
> *Mycoplasma hominis*
> *Ureaplasma urealyticum*
> *Haemophilus ducreyi*
> *Calymmatobacterium granulomatis*
> *Shigella* species
> *Campylobacter* species

Protozoa

> *Giardia lamblia*
> *Entamoeba histolytica*
> *Trichomonas vaginalis*
> *Isospora belli*
> *Cryptosporidia* species
> *Microsporidia* species

Viruses

> Herpes simplex
> Cytomegalovirus
> Epstein–Barr virus
> Papillomavirus
> Poxvirus
> Hepatitis A
> Hepatitis B
> Hepatitis C
> Human immunodeficiency virus

Ectoparasites

> *Phthirus pubis*
> *Sarcoptes scabiei*

(HSV) and human papillomavirus (HPV) infections has risen continually since 1966 (Figs. 15.1 and 15.2). Since the late 1970s the prevalence of

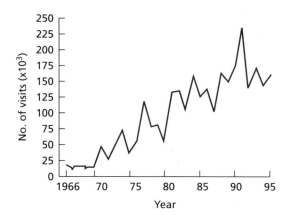

Figure 15.1. *Initial visits to physicians' offices for genital herpes simplex virus infections in the USA, 1966–1995 [43].*

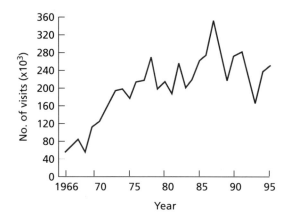

Figure 15.2. *Initial visits to physicians' offices for human papillomavirus (genital warts) in the USA, 1966–1995 [43].*

HSV-2 infections has increased by 30% [2]. Unfortunately, patients previously diagnosed with the human immunodeficiency virus (HIV) also return with other STDs [3] suggesting unprotected sexual activity that allows acquisition of an STD and transmission of HIV. This information implies an unfortunate failure of prevention and educational efforts.

STDs are a major health problem. Nothing has brought this more to light than the AIDS epidemic, which has been a significant cause of morbidity and mortality worldwide. Prevention of infection has been the only means available to stop the epidemic because there is still no cure and no vaccine to prevent HIV transmission. That the presence of other STDs may actually aid in the transmission of the HIV agent is of prime importance to all concerned.

STDs other than AIDS are also associated with significant morbidity and mortality. Infertility and reproductive complications may be seen. Malignancies may be the result of these infections, such as those seen with HPV [4]. Some of these infections may have a prolonged course, such as the chronic and persistent forms of hepatitis seen with HBV that eventually lead to cirrhosis. Others, such as HSV are 'recurrent' and the cause of physical and emotional discomfort to the patient.

Millions of dollars are spent annually on treating these STDs. One problem arising is that of drug resistance to some of the agents commonly prescribed to treat these infections. This trend is also being identified with newer agents such as the fluoroquinolones [5–7]. Antimicrobial resistance is not a new concern but is highlighted by the resistance problems seen in other areas of infectious diseases.

Gay health issues

Men who have sex with other men (MSM) are at an increased risk for STDs. This includes men who identify themselves as gay and men who may not, but who still engage in sex with other men for whatever reason. The rates of infection seen for most STDs are disproportionately higher in these men than in their strictly heterosexual counterparts.

In addition to these higher rates of the 'traditional' STDs such as syphilis, gonorrhoea and chlamydia, these men also experience other sexually encountered infections such as those caused by enteric bacteria, parasites and viruses. This fact has suggested that many 'tropical medicine' patients seen by parasitologists in the late 1970s have actually been gay men presenting with STDs such as amoebiasis and giardia [8]. Many of these infections present clinically, whereas others are asymptomatic and remain undetected. Unfortunately, the latter are more likely to be unknowingly transmitted.

Non-infectious problems such as trauma to the anus or rectum and allergies to lubricants are also encountered. These traumatic problems are the result of sexual practices and can produce mucosal tears, fissures, and inflammation [9]. Bleeding, rectal pain, burning and mucopurulent discharge may be the presenting symptoms and are similar to those encountered with STDs.

All gay men do not have the same risk for STDs. The sexual behaviour, not the sexual orientation, of this population accounts for the high incidence of STDs. A number of criteria are important in determining risk of exposure [10]. An increased number of sexual partners, anonymous partners, and the nature of specific practices such as anal intercourse and oral–anal contact may account for some of these differences. Some of these practices also occur in the heterosexual population but their role in the transmission of pathogens is less appreciated [11]. Sexual practices in the lesbian population differ and account for a lower incidence of STDs, including HIV [12]: often there are fewer sexual partners, and woman-to-woman contact is a less efficient means for transfer of infection.

The male anatomy itself constitutes a risk factor for transmission of infection. The penis and urethra can be exposed to infection when inserted into body cavities such as the mouth, rectum or vagina. Conversely, an infection of the urethra can be transported deep into these cavities by the penis and the force of ejaculation [13,14].

Many STDs seen in MSM occur in the rectum. This may be attributed to the moist, warm environment of the perirectal area. Rectal mucosal tearing that can occur with sexual activity allows efficient entry for pathogens into tissues and the bloodstream. This mechanism explains the high and 'unsafe' level of risk for infection associated with anal intercourse.

Psychosocial, cultural and political factors relate to the increased incidence of STDs in the gay population. Medical services may be under-utilized because these men feel uncomfortable seeking attention when it requires open admission of their sexual preference. The medical services that are offered may be incomplete because of the attitude, lack of understanding and, perhaps, prejudice by health care providers. In 1996 the Council on Scientific Affairs of the American Medical Association updated earlier recommendations on the *Health Care Needs of Gay Men and Lesbians in the United States* in an attempt to understand and deal with these issues [15].

Obtaining a history

An inquiry of sexual orientation and sexual practices is vital to any evaluation of a patient for STDs [16]. Patients may not readily volunteer information in any medical situation, whether the problem be cardiac, pulmonary or sexual. The only way to obtain specific information is by asking specific questions. One study [17] found that, although physicians asked new patients about their history of STDs, less than half regularly asked about sexual preference and less than one-third asked about oral or anal sexual practices or the number of sexual partners.

In obtaining such information it is important that the physician's questions be completely understood. Too often, patients will give a negative reply, simply because they do not understand what is being asked. Medical terminology that may be unfamiliar to the patient should be avoided. It may be necessary to use phrases and colloquial terminology with which the patient is more familiar. In some cases anatomical terms and sexual activities may need to be discussed in 'street terms' to facilitate communication.

The physician needs to feel comfortable in eliciting a sexually related history [18]. An honest, open and non-judgemental communication needs to be established. Different interviewing techniques and styles are available to aid the physician in achieving effective communication (Table 15.2). It

Table 15.2. *Interviewing techniques*

Open-ended questioning	Can you tell me about your sexual behaviour?
Open-ended questioning with explanatory preface	It's important to know the type of sexual activity you engage in so that I can evaluate you thoroughly... Can you tell me?
Direct formal questioning (*may limit communication*)	Do you engage in homosexual activity?
Indirect formal questioning	Do you have sex with other men?
Closed-ended questioning (*discourages communication*)	I assume that you don't engage in homosexual activity?
Judgemental questioning (*undesirable; unjustified*)	You're not homosexual are you?

is necessary to remember that it is not only *what you ask*, but *how you ask it*.

Symptoms experienced by the patient are usually brought to attention immediately. Frequently, these symptoms, such as urethral discharge, appear to be obviously related to an STD; at other times, however, symptoms such as rectal pain may not seem to be sexually related and further questioning may be in order. It is important to remember that a patient with one STD is likely to have one or more concomitant STDs. All the body sites involved in sexual contact need to be determined and this will involve obtaining information about sexual practices.

Information should be obtained about any past history of STDs. A related review of symptoms is also required. Inquiry should be made about sexual partners and their number. It should not be assumed that sexual partners are necessarily of the opposite sex. A time-frame of sexual exposure is also important, since the time of exposure can help to rule out some infections and indicate others as a possibility.

The examination

The physical examination will be directed by the patient's symptoms and by the review of the patient's history and sexual behaviour. A systematic approach will assist in providing a thorough evaluation. Table 15.3 provides an overview of the different body regions, with attention given to possible physical findings and aetiologies.

The patient's general appearance should be noted, together with any type of skin rash or disseminated lesions. The head and neck should be inspected with particular attention to the mouth and pharynx. Evidence of lymphadenopathy should be sought. The cardiovascular and respiratory systems should be carefully examined and the abdomen should be evaluated for any evidence of hepatosplenomegaly. Attention should also be directed to the joints and extremities for any evidence of arthritis that may be associated with STDs.

In examining patients for STDs, most of the attention becomes focused on the genital region since this is the site of most problems. In examining the penis and scrotum, any external lesions should be detected. In uncircumcised males the foreskin should be retracted. Attention should be directed to the urethral meatus. The urethra may be 'stripped' or the patient may be requested to 'milk' the urethra for any evidence of discharge.

Patients should not void for an hour prior to the time of the examination because the force of urinating may remove any discharge that is present. Any evidence of inguinal adenopathy should be determined.

The perianal region and anus are examined externally, and digital rectal examination may be necessary. Attention may need to be directed to the prostate. Anoscopy should be considered in patients with anorectal symptoms or a history that suggests infection of this area.

Appropriate specimens for smears, culture and pathology should be obtained during the examination and blood samples should be sent for serological studies. In some instances, stool samples may need to be obtained for ova and parasite examination.

STD syndromes

STDs can present clinically in many ways. Patients often present with a particular complaint, such as 'I have this ulcer' or 'I've been having drainage'. At times, the presentation may not initially lead the clinician to think of an STD, such as when the patient complains of diarrhoea or of being tired and having a rash. However, further history taking and examination should point the clinician in the direction of the correct diagnosis and treatment. The patient's presenting complaint directs attention to a differential diagnosis of the specific presenting problem or syndrome. The following sections specifically detail common syndromes, clinical presentation, diagnosis and treatment. It is important to remember that one or any combination of these syndromes can occur at any one time.

Genital ulcer syndrome

Genital ulcerations are seen in syphilis, chancroid and lymphogranuloma venereum (LGV). The genital lesions of HSV-1 or HSV-2 present as vesicular eruptions if seen early (Fig. 15.3), but can present as ulcerations after these initial vesicles have ruptured (Fig. 15.4). Granuloma guinale, also known as donovanosis, is caused by *Calymmatobacterium granulomatis* and may present as an ulceration. It is also important to be aware that genital ulcer disease increases the risk of HIV transmission.

Syphilis is caused by infection with *T. pallidum* and chancroid by infection with *Haemophilus ducreyi*. LGV is secondary to infec-

Table 15.3. *Physical examination findings associated with sexually transmitted diseases and their aetiologies*

Region	Finding	Possible aetiologies
General appearance	Fever; weight loss	HIV disease
	Jaundice	HAV, HBV, HCV, EBV, CMV
Cutaneous areas	Ulcers	Primary syphilis, chancroid, HSV-1, HSV-2, VZV, LGV
	Papules	Condylomata acuminata, molluscum contagiosum, Kaposi's sarcoma, disseminated *Neisseria gonorrhoeae*
	Maculopapular rash	Secondary syphilis
Eyes	Conjunctivitis	*Neisseria gonorrhoeae*
Mouth	Vesicles/ulcers	HSV-1, HSV-2, HIV
Pharynx	Exudative pharyngitis	HIV, EBV, CMV, *Neisseria gonorrhoeae*, chlamydial pharyngitis
	White plaques	Thrush, hairy leukoplakia (EBV)
Lymph nodes	Generalized adenopathy	Secondary syphilis, HIV, EBV, CMV, HBV
Abdomen	Hepatomegaly	HAV, HBV, HCV, EBV, CMV
Genitalia	Ulcers	Primary syphilis, chancroid, LGV, granuloma inguinale, HSV-1, HSV-2, trauma
	Urethral discharge	*Neisseria gonorrhoeae*, agents of non-gonococcal urethritis
	Papules	Condylomata acuminata, molluscum contagiosum
	Erythematous rashes	Fungal infections, fixed drug eruptions, contact dermatitis
Perianal region	Ulcers	Primary syphilis, HSV, LGV, traumatic fissures
	Proctitis, proctocolitis and enteritis	*Neisseria gonorrhoeae*, LGV, chlamydia, syphilis, HSV, amoebic proctitis, trauma
	Papules	Condylomata acuminata, condylomata lata
	Dermatitis	Fungal infections
Extremities	Arthritis	Disseminated *N. gonorrhoeae*

HIV disease, human immunodeficiency virus disease; HAV, hepatitis A virus; HBV, hepatitis B virus; HCV, hepatitis C virus; EBV, Epstein–Barr virus; CMV, cytomegalovirus; HSV-1, herpes simplex virus 1; HSV-2, herpes simplex virus 2; VZV, varicella zoster virus; LGV, lymphogranuloma venereum.

tion with the LGV serovars (L_1, L_2 and L_3) of *Chlamydia trachomatis*. Other *C. trachomatis* serovars are seen with urethritis and are discussed later in this chapter. Patients with primary syphilis or chancroid are more likely to have an ulcer present. Although an ulcer may be seen in the early stage of LGV, it usually goes unnoticed. The most common clinical presentation of LGV occurs in the second stage, where tender inguinal adenopathy is the major finding.

Trauma that occurs as a result of sexual activity (Fig. 15.5) and drug allergies (Figs. 15.6 and 15.7)

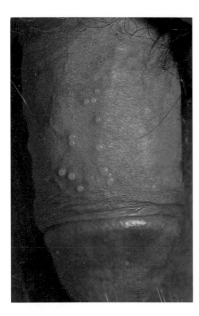

Figure 15.3. Herpes simplex *virus, vesicular stage*. (*Reproduced from ref. 44 with permission*.)

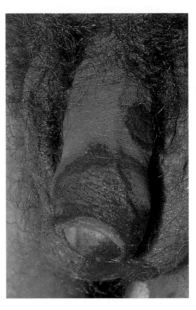

Figure 15.6. *Fixed drug eruption*. (*Reproduced from ref. 47 with permission*.)

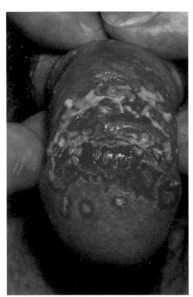

Figure 15.4. *Ulcerous* herpes simplex *virus*. (*Reproduced from ref. 45 with permission*.)

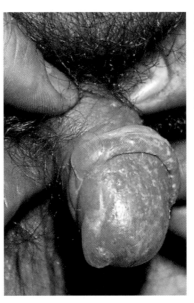

Figure 15.7. *Bullous drug eruption*. (*Reproduced from ref. 48 with permission*.)

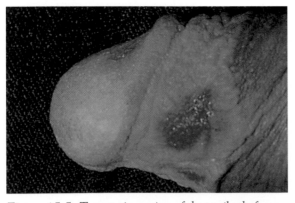

Figure 15.5. *Traumatic erosion of the penile shaft secondary to oral sex. (Reproduced from ref. 46 with permission of Glaxo Wellcome Inc.)*

can also present as ulcerations. Further facts obtained in the history are useful in elucidating this finding. A history of antibiotic usage could suggest a fixed drug eruption that has become ulcerated through scratching. The use of lubricants can suggest an allergy that can present similarly.

The time of onset of the lesion(s) may be helpful in arriving at the diagnosis (Table 15.4). A historical point that can aid in the diagnosis is whether the lesions are recurrent, as is seen with HSV. Another important clue to the diagnosis is whether the lesion is painful: classically, the chancre of syphilis is painless unless infected; however, the lesions of chancroid and the ulcera-

Table 15.4. *Incubation periods associated with genital ulcer diseases*

Infection	Incubation period (days)
Syphilis	3–90 (average 21)
Chancroid	5–7
LGV	3–30
HSV	2–7
Donovanosis	8–80

LGV, lymphogranuloma venereum; HSV, *herpes simplex virus.*

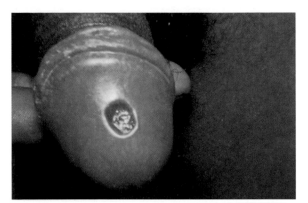

Figure 15.8. *Chancre of primary syphilis, penis. (Reproduced from ref. 49 courtesy of US Department of Health, Education and Welfare.)*

tions seen with HSV are associated with pain and discomfort.

Physical findings on examination are also important. The characteristics of the ulceration are helpful diagnostically. For example, the number of ulcers may favour one diagnosis over another: the chancre of syphilis tends to be single, but can be multiple, especially in patients with HIV; the lesions of chancroid usually are multiple; those seen with HSV-1 and HSV-2 tend to occur 'in a crop'.

It is also important to pay particular attention to the appearance of the ulcer: in the chancre seen with primary syphilis, the lesion is 'punched out' with a clean base and raised borders and is indurated to palpation (Fig. 15.8); the lesion of chancroid is irregular and 'ragged' with a necrotic base and is not indurated (Fig. 15.9); in granuloma inguinale the bases of the lesions are beefy red and friable (Fig. 15.10).

It is noteworthy that these ulcerations are also seen on other body parts: the chancre of primary syphilis may be seen on the lips, tongue and tonsillar areas (Fig. 15.11); whereas chancroid is not commonly seen on other body areas; although 75% of HSV-2 infections are below the waist, HSV-2 can also occur as gingivostomatitis (Fig. 15.12) and can further spread to other body parts by auto-inoculation (Fig. 15.13); HSV-1 can present in the same manner.

Another important body site where ulcers are frequently encountered is the perianal region and rectum, following anal intercourse. The chancre of syphilis is usually asymptomatic when located in the anorectal area (Fig. 15.14). Symptoms, when present, are usually mild and may lead to a non-infectious diagnosis such as haemorrhoids.

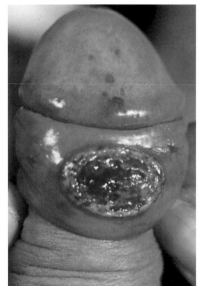

Figure 15.9. *Chancroid. Tender, eroded nodule with marked surrounding erythema and oedema. (Reproduced from ref. 50 with permission.)*

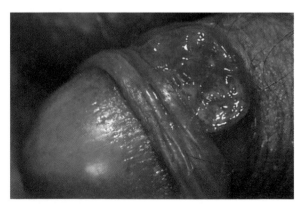

Figure 15.10. *Donovanosis. A button-like papule with central ulceration, a beefy-red base, and a sharply demarcated margin. (Reproduced from ref. 51 with permission.)*

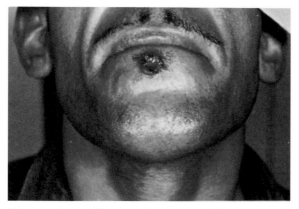

Figure 15.11. *Chancre of primary syphilis, lower lip. (Reproduced from ref. 52 courtesy of US Department of Health, Education and Welfare.)*

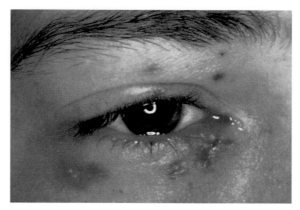

Figure 15.13. Herpes simplex *virus infection of the eye. (Reproduced from ref. 53 with permission of Glaxo Wellcome Inc.)*

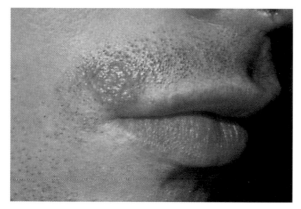

Figure 15.12. *Orofacial* herpes simplex *virus infection, often HSV-2, reflecting sexual practices. (Reproduced from ref. 53 with permission of Glaxo Wellcome Inc.)*

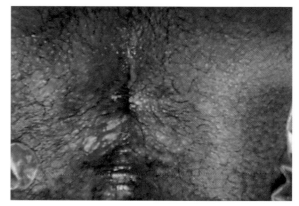

Figure 15.14. *Perianal chancre of primary syphilis. (Reproduced from ref. 52 courtesy of US Department of Health, Education and Welfare.)*

Painful herpetic lesions may also be seen in the perianal region. At times these lesions may also be asymptomatic. Painful lesions of chancroid can be confused clinically with those of HSV infection. LGV usually presents as proctocolitis and asymptomatic lesions of granuloma inguinale can also be seen following anal intercourse.

The presence of adenopathy may also be helpful diagnostically: painless, firm regional adenopathy can be seen with the primary chancre of syphilis; tender regional adenopathy is seen with chancroid and HSV infections. The adenopathy associated with LGV is usually tender and unilateral; the lymph nodes become enlarged and are almond shaped; the 'groove' sign occurs where the inguinal ligament makes a linear depression between the enlarged inguinal and femoral lymph nodes (Fig. 15.15).

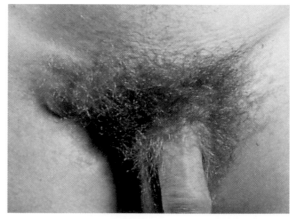

Figure 15.15. *The 'groove sign' of lymphogranuloma venereum: marked, tender lymphadenopathy occurring in the femoral and inguinal lymph nodes separated by a groove made by Poupart's ligament. (Reproduced from ref. 54 with permission.)*

Confirmatory diagnosis of the ulceration is based on some type of laboratory confirmation. This can include looking for the responsible organism on Gram staining or phase microscopy, culture, and serological testing. However, laboratory testing may not confirm or provide a diagnosis in up to 25% of cases. In such cases, the clinician must rely on clinical grounds for making the diagnosis.

The diagnosis of syphilis can be accomplished by dark-field examination of suspicious lesions or serological testing. Serous transudate from a moist lesion is examined for the typical corkscrew spiralling motion of *T. pallidum* organisms. This type of microscopy is not always available and most clinicians rely on serological testing.

The two types of serological tests available to aid in the diagnosis of syphilis are non-treponemal tests (NTTs) and treponemal tests (TTs). Each of these detects a different antibody that is produced in response to infection with *T. pallidum* [19,20].

NTTs include the Venereal Disease Research Laboratory test (VDRL) and the rapid plasma reagin test (RPR). NTTs detect *non-specific* antibodies made against a lipoidal antigen produced when *T. pallidum* interacts with host tissue. NTTs are carried out in serial dilution, correlate with disease activity and are the preferred means to monitor patients with syphilis [21].

The TTs used in clinical practice are the fluorescent antibody absorbed test (FTA-ABS) and the *T. pallidum* haemagglutination assay (TPHA). These tests, which detect *specific* treponemal antibody, are technically more difficult and costly to perform; hence, their value as screening methods is limited.

NTTs and TTs are used in tandem in the diagnosis of syphilis [22]: basically, the NTT is used to screen for the infection and the TT is used for confirmation. The reactivity of either of these tests is based, in part, on the stage of syphilis encountered and other technical factors. In some instances, this makes the serological diagnosis of syphilis challenging.

Not all instances of a positive test, however, indicate an infection with *T. pallidum*: other conditions can give rise to a positive NTT or TT. False-positive NTTs can be seen *acutely* in situations where there is a strong immunological stimulus, such as immunization or acute infections and during pregnancy. False-positive NTTs may also be seen *chronically* in other ongoing conditions such as drug addiction and autoimmune diseases and in ageing. In addition, positive serological tests are encountered in other treponemal infections such as yaws and pinta, and in other spirochaetal diseases such as Lyme disease.

The diagnosis of chancroid is made by culture of material from the base of an ulcer or from aspiration of a bubo. Gram stain of the material may reveal the small, pleomorphic Gram-negative coccobacilli in the 'school of fish' pattern (Fig. 15.16).

The diagnosis of LGV can be made by a positive chlamydial serology [21] or isolation of LGV from infected tissue. Donovanosis is usually diagnosed with histological examination of punch biopsy specimens or crush preparation made from granulation tissue. HSV lesions are diagnosed on clinical grounds, especially when lesions are seen later in the course of the outbreak. Culture confirmation for HSV is the diagnostic method of choice for suspect lesions; however, samples from these lesions can also be tested for herpes antigens by immunofluorescence and immunohistochemical techniques. Serological studies for HSV are often confusing and are less sensitive than viral culture confirmation in the acute setting [21].

In many instances, treatment is given before test results are available. Treatment for the most likely diagnosis is advised; if the diagnosis is uncertain, many experts recommend treatment for chancroid and syphilis [23]. This treatment strategy may also be necessary in cases where laboratory testing does not confirm or indicate any specific diagnosis.

The Centers for Disease Control (CDC) treatment guidelines [23] for these infections are shown in Table 15.5. Recommended treatments, as well as alternative choices, are provided. Of all the antimicrobials listed, acyclovir does not

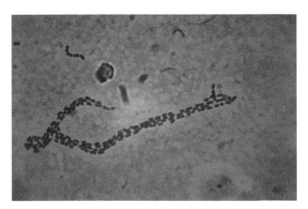

Figure 15.16. *The classic 'school of fish' arrangement of* Haemophilus ducreyi *on Gram stain. (Reproduced from ref. 55 with permission of Glaxo Wellcome Inc.)*

Table 15.5. *Recommended treatments and alternative regimens for genital ulcer diseases*

Clinical infection	Recommended treatments	Alternative regimens
Primary syphilis	Benzathine penicillin G, 2.4 million units i.m. in a single dose*	Doxycycline 100 mg orally twice a day for 2 weeks, **or** tetracycline 500 mg orally 4 times a day for 2 weeks
Chancroid	Azithromycin 1 g orally in a single dose, **or** ceftriaxone 250 mg i.m. in a single dose, **or** ciprofloxacin 500 mg orally twice a day for 3 days **or** erythromycin base 500 mg orally 4 times a day for 7 days	
Lymphogranuloma venereum	Doxycycline 100 mg orally twice a day for 21 days	Erythromycin base 500 mg orally 4 times a day for 21 days
First clinical episode of genital herpes[†]	Acyclovir 400 mg orally 3 times a day for 7–10 days, **or** acyclovir 200 mg orally 5 times a day for 7–10 days, **or** famciclovir 250 mg orally 3 times a day for 7–10 days, **or** valacyclovir 1 g orally twice a day for 7–10 days	
Recurrent episodes of genital herpes	Acyclovir 400 mg orally 3 times a day for 5 days, **or** acyclovir 200 mg orally 5 times a day for 5 days, **or** acyclovir 800 mg orally twice a day for 5 days, **or** famciclovir 125 mg orally twice a day for 5 days, **or** valacyclovir 500 mg twice a day for 5 days	
Herpes proctitis	Acyclovir 400 mg orally 5 times a day for 10 days **or** until clinically resolved[‡]	
HSV daily suppressive therapy	Acyclovir 400 mg orally twice a day, **or** famciclovir 250 mg orally twice a day, **or** valacyclovir 250 mg orally twice a day, **or** valacyclovir 500 mg orally once a day, **or** valacyclovir 1 g orally once a day	
HSV severe disease	Acyclovir 5–10 mg/kg body weight i.v. every 8 hours for 5–7 days or until resolved	
Granuloma inguinale[§]	Trimethoprim–sulfamethoxazole one double-strength tablet orally twice a day for a minimum of 3 weeks, **or** doxycycline 100 mg orally twice a day for a minimum of 3 weeks	Ciprofloxacin 750 mg orally twice a day, for a minimum of 3 weeks, **or** erythromycin base 500 mg orally 4 times a day for a minimum of 3 weeks

*Only penicillin regimens should be used to treat HIV-infected individuals in all stages of syphilis. Patients who report a history of penicillin allergy should be desensitized, then treated with penicillin.

[†]Treatment may be extended if healing is incomplete after 10 days of therapy.

[‡]Higher doses of acyclovir were used in treatment studies of first-episode herpes proctitis. It is unclear whether higher doses than used for genital herpes are required.

[§]The addition of an aminoglycoside (gentamicin I mg/kg every 8 hours) should be considered for any of these regimens if lesions do not respond within the first few days of therapy.

(Adapted from ref. 23.)

achieve clinical cure as the others do: it provides control of clinical signs and symptoms of initial and subsequent outbreaks only; viral latency still occurs. Regimens are also recommended as daily suppressive therapy in an attempt to reduce the frequency of recurrences [24].

Urethritis syndrome

Inflammation of the urethra can have various aetiologies. In most cases, urethritis is secondary to an infectious process. The relationship of certain chemicals, particularly alcohol, and the role of these agents in inducing or worsening urethral inflammation is often raised [25,26]. Clinically, the patient with urethritis experiences dysuria and symptoms such as pain, itching and urgency. Urethral discharge is the prominent presenting sign. The discharge can be thick and purulent or simply mucoid. At times it may be copious and at other times limited to a few drops of fluid noted in the morning or on the undergarments.

The infectious processes responsible for urethritis fall into two categories: the first category is gonococcal urethritis secondary to infection by *Neisseria gonorrhoeae*; the second category is the group of non-gonococcal urethritis (NGU) syndrome. NGU is caused primarily by *C. trachomatis*. *Ureaplasma urealyticum* is also a cause of NGU and *Mycoplasma genitalium* has been identified in some cases. HSV infections (Fig. 15.17) and *Trichomonas vaginalis* (Fig. 15.18) also produce signs and symptoms of urethritis.

Clinically, these two syndromes differ in that gonococcal urethritis is usually more acute in presentation than NGU: patients may recall the exact time that the symptoms of gonococcal urethritis began, whereas the onset of NGU is more insidious in nature, extending and increasing over a period of days. Incubation periods vary, with that of *N. gonorrhoeae* being 4 days and of NGU 7–14 days. Symptoms seen with NGU are usually milder. The discharge seen with gonococcal urethritis is more profuse and purulent (Fig. 15.19a), whereas it is often scant and watery with NGU (Fig. 15.19b).

Pharyngeal infection with these organisms can also occur following oral–genital sex. Many of these infections are asymptomatic. The sore throats and pharyngitis that occur following fellatio are thought to correlate with this sexual practice rather than infection with *N. gonorrhoeae*, *M. hominis* or *U. urealyticum* [27]. In other cases, however, a clinical picture of acute pharyngitis can be seen. Conjunctivitis may also be acquired with some of these entities as a result of auto-inoculation.

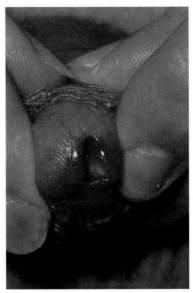

Figure 15.17. Herpes simplex *virus of the urethra. (Reproduced from ref. 45 with permission.)*

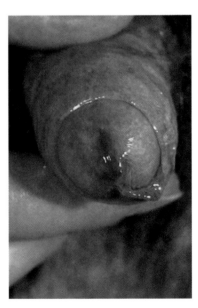

Figure 15.18. Trichomonas urethritis. *(Reproduced from ref. 56 with permission.)*

These symptoms will resolve if patients do not receive treatment. This can occur with either gonococcal urethritis or NGU, but is more likely with NGU because the symptoms may be so mild, or wax and wane, that they are ignored or overlooked. Asymptomatic infection is another possibility with either syndrome and can increase the chance and risk of transmission.

Although these syndromes may be classified by the differences noted, they are not sufficiently definite to establish the correct diagnosis clearly. In addition, many patients can be infected with more than one organism. Diagnosis requires culture or laboratory confirmation of infection.

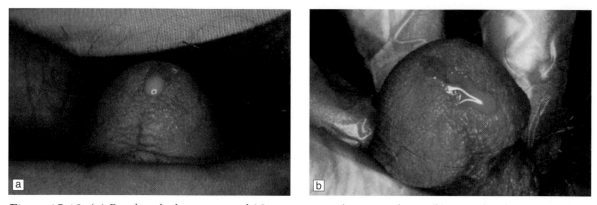

Figure 15.19. *(a) Purulent discharge seen with* Neisseria gonorrhoeae *urethritis; (b) mucoid and watery urethral discharge of non-gonococcal urethritis. (Reproduced from ref. 57 with permission.)*

Patients are examined as previously detailed. Discharge is usually available for analysis or can be obtained by 'stripping' the urethra or by insertion of a calcium alginate swab into the urethra. Cotton swabs are not used because of discomfort caused by their larger size and the toxicity to organisms of the wood and cotton that will hamper their recovery.

The material recovered from the urethra should be examined by Gram staining and inoculated onto growth media. The presence of polymorphonuclear neutrophils (PMNs) and intracellular Gram-negative diplococci on Gram staining is helpful in confirming *N. gonorrhoeae* (Fig. 15.20). The presence of PMNs without organisms is more suggestive of NGU (Fig. 15.21). Gram staining, however, cannot provide evidence for the existence of simultaneous infections. Culture confirmation for *N. gonorrhoeae* and non-culture tests for antigen detection of *C. trachomatis* or isolation in tissue culture are helpful in sorting this out. Trichomonads may be seen on a wet mount of the urethral discharge. Endo-urethral cultures or cultures of first-void urine are helpful for the diagnosis of trichomoniasis in men [28].

Because of the prevalence of *C. trachomatis* coexisting with *N. gonorrhoeae*, patients identified to have one of these infections are pre-emptively treated for the other as well [23]. Table 15.6 lists current treatment recommendations.

Disseminated gonococcal infection can result in response to an acute episode of infection with *N. gonorrhoeae*. It results in the dermatitis–arthritis syndrome, consisting of migratory polyarthralgias, frank arthritis and a characteristic rash of haemorrhagic papules. It is more common in women than in men and is also seen in patients who have a terminal component of complement deficiency. Other complications that can arise as

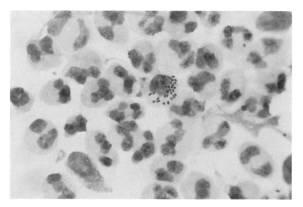

Figure 15.20. *Gram stain of urethral discharge secondary to infection with* N. gonorrhoeae *showing polymorphonuclear leucocytes and intracellular Gram-negative diplococci; 400×. (Courtesy of Eileen Burd, PhD, Henry Ford Hospital, Detroit, MI, USA.)*

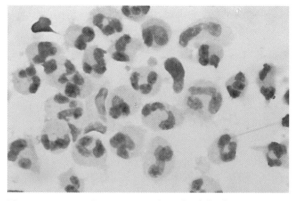

Figure 15.21. *Gram stain of urethral discharge in a patient with NGU showing polymorphonuclear leucocytes and no organisms; 400× (Courtesy of Eileen Burd, PhD, Henry Ford Hospital, Detroit, MI, USA.)*

Table 15.6. *Recommended treatments and alternative regimens for STDs presenting as urethritis [23]*

Infection	Recommended regimens	Alternative regimens
Uncomplicated infection of the urethra and rectum with *Neisseria gonorrhoeae**	Cefixime 400 mg orally in a single dose, **or** ceftriaxone 125 mg i.m. in a single dose, **or** ciprofloxacin 500 mg orally in a single dose, **or** ofloxacin 400 mg orally in a single dose	Spectinomycin 2 g i.m. in a single dose, **or** other single-dose cephalosporins, including ceftizoxime 500 mg i.m., cefotaxime 500 mg i.m., cefotetan 1 g i.m. **or** cefoxitin 2 g i.m. with probenecid 1 g orally, **or** other single-dose quinolones, including enoxacin 400 mg orally, lomefloxacin 400 mg orally, **or** norfloxacin 800 mg orally
Uncomplicated infection of the pharynx with *N. gonorrhoeae*†	Ceftriaxone 125 mg i.m. in a single dose, **or** ciprofloxacin 500 mg orally in a single dose, **or** ofloxacin 400 mg orally in a single dose	
Chlamydia trachomatis	Azithromycin 1 g orally in a single dose, **or** doxycycline 100 mg orally twice a day for 7 days	Erythromycin base 500 mg orally 4 times a day for 7 days, **or** erythromycin ethylsuccinate 800 mg orally 4 times a day for 7 days‡, **or** ofloxacin 300 mg orally twice a day for 7 days
Non-gonococcal urethritis (NGU)	Azithromycin 1 g orally in a single dose, **or** doxycycline 100 mg orally twice a day for 7 days	Erythromycin base 500 mg orally 4 times a day for 7 days, **or** erythromycin ethylsuccinate 800 mg orally 4 times a day for 7 days‡, **or** ofloxacin 300 mg twice a day for 7 days
Recurrent and persistent NGU	Metronidazole 2 g orally in a single dose **PLUS** erythromycin base 500 mg orally 4 times a day, **or** erythromycin ethylsuccinate 800 mg orally 4 times a day for 7 days	
Trichomonas vaginalis	Metronidazole 2 g orally in a single dose	Metronidazole 500 mg twice a day for 7 days

*Patients infected with *N. gonorrhoeae* are often co-infected with *C. trachomatis*. Therefore, treatment for both gonorrhoea and chlamydia is suggested.

†Although chlamydial co-infection of the pharynx is unusual, co-infection at genital sites sometimes occurs. Therefore, treatment for both gonorrhoea and chlamydia is suggested.

‡If only erythromycin can be used and a patient cannot tolerate high-dose erythromycin, one of the following can be used: erythromycin base 250 mg orally 4 times a day for 14 days, **or** erythromycin ethylsuccinate 400 mg orally 4 times a day for 14 days.

a result of urethritis are epididymitis and Reiter's syndrome. Reiter's syndrome is seen following NGU and manifests with reactive arthritis, uveitis and skin and mucous membrane lesions.

Papular lesions

Two different aetiologies are responsible for genital papular lesions: these are molluscum contagiosum, caused by the poxvirus, and HPV. Certain viral types of HPV are more likely to be associated with sexually acquired lesions. Of these, HPV types 6 and 11 are more likely to be associated with benign growths, whereas HPV types 16, 18, 31, 33 and 35 have a strong association with malignancy.

The lesions of molluscum contagiosum occur in the genital and pubic areas. The incubation period for the infection is 2–3 months. The lesions are usually asymptomatic and appear as skin-coloured, waxy, firm, umbilicated papules (Fig. 15.22). They can occur alone or in groups and are usually seen in the inguinal regions and on the thighs, buttocks and lower abdomen and, less commonly, on the external genitalia and in the perianal region. This is in sharp contrast to the distribution of HPV lesions. In addition to sexual acquisition, molluscum contagiosum can be spread through auto-inoculation. Diagnosis is usually made by clinical findings, but biopsy or examination of material from the lesion, which will reveal cytoplasmic inclusion bodies, can be performed in atypical cases. Treatment regimens include cryotherapy, electrodesiccation, and incision and curettage.

Molluscum contagiosum is seen frequently in patients with HIV, usually in those with lower CD4 counts. In these individuals it usually occurs on the face and the upper body and can have an unremitting course (Fig. 15.23).

The incubation period of HPV infections is long, ranging from 1 to 20 months. Lesions of HPV are flesh-coloured hyperkeratotic papules. In men they occur on the penis (Fig. 15.24), the urethral meatus, the distal urethra and the perianal areas. External anal lesions are often associated with internal lesions. The lesions of secondary syphilis — condylomata lata — which are seen in the perianal region, are sometimes confused with condylomata acuminata, the lesions of HPV. However, the lesions of condylomata lata are broad, moist and can be grey-white or erythema-

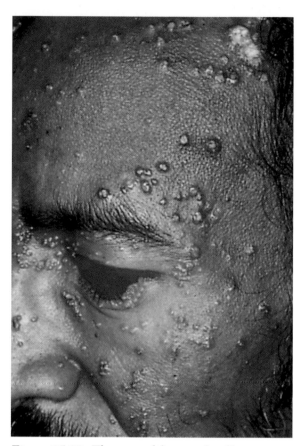

Figure 15.23. *The unusual feature of* molluscum contagiosum *in HIV infected patients is the large number of lesions and their occurrence on the face. (Reproduced from ref. 59 with permission of Glaxo Wellcome Inc.)*

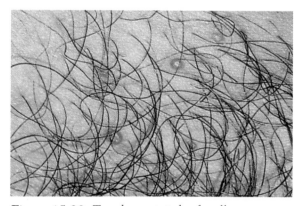

Figure 15.22. *Translucent papule of* molluscum contagiosum *with characteristic central umbilication. (Reproduced from ref. 58 with permission of Glaxo Wellcome Inc.)*

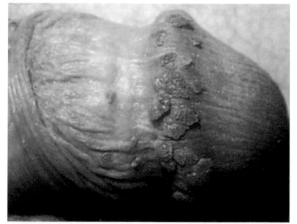

Figure 15.24. *Penile warts. (Reproduced from ref. 60 with permission of Glaxo Wellcome Inc.)*

tous (Fig. 15.25). HPV lesions can also be seen in the oral cavity (Fig. 15.26), possibly resulting from oral–genital contact or auto-inoculation.

Most lesions of HPV are asymptomatic, although non-specific symptoms such as pain and itching may occur. Diagnosis can be arrived at by the appearance of these lesions on clinical examination. Colposcopy following the application of 3–5% acetic acid for 3–5 minutes to demonstrate 'aceto-whitening' of

subclinical lesions may also be helpful [29]. Anoscopy is important to detect anal lesions in men with a history of receptive anal intercourse.

Therapy is not effective in eradicating HPV infection. Exophytic warts may be more infectious than subclinical infections and therapeutic 'debulking' has been suggested as a means of helping to reduce the risk for transmission. Recommended treatments [23] are listed in Table 15.7.

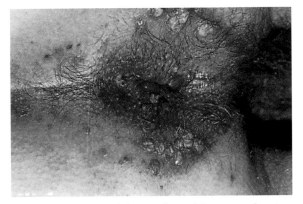

Figure 15.25. *Condylomata lata of the perianal region seen in secondary syphilis. (Reproduced from ref. 61 with permission.)*

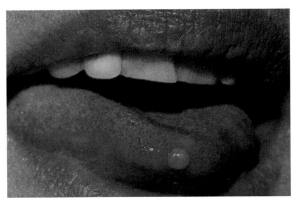

Figure 15.26. *Oral warts may appear as a result of oral genital contact. (Reproduced from ref. 62 with permission of Glaxo Wellcome Inc.)*

Table 15.7. *Recommended treatment considerations for HPV infections [23]*

Location of HPV infection	Treatment considerations
External genital/perianal warts	**Patient applied:** Podofilox 0.5% solution or gel for self-treatment of visible genital warts, **or** imiquimod 5% cream **Provider-administered:** Cryotherapy, **or** podophyllin resin 10–25% in compound tincture of benzoin, **or** trichloroacetic acid (TCA) **or** bichloroacetic acid (BCA) 80–90%, **or** surgical removal **Alternative treatments:** Intralesional interferon, **or** laser surgery
Urethral meatus warts	Cryotherapy, **or** podophyllin 10–25% in compound tincture of benzoin
Anal warts*	Cryotherapy, **or** TCA or BCA 80–90%, **or** surgical removal
Oral warts	Cryotherapy, **or** surgical removal

*Management of warts on rectal mucosa should be referred to an expert.

Because of the associated risk of anal cancer in those with HPV infection, particularly individuals also immunosuppressed by HIV, follow-up anal cytological examination and screening are recommended [30,31].

Proctitis, proctocolitis and enteritis syndromes

The list of pathogens that produce a picture of proctitis, proctocolitis and enteritis sheds a different light on the group of organisms referred to as STDs. These syndromes involve not only the classically identified STDs but also organisms traditionally not labelled as STDs. The organisms that produce proctitis and proctocolitis are acquired by receptive anal intercourse. Sexual practices that include oral–anal contact can also result in the transmission of these organisms. By virtue of these sexual practices, these syndromes are a prevalent feature of the STDs that are seen in MSM, and for this reason have often been referred to as 'the gay bowel syndrome'.

The anatomy of the perianal and rectal areas can lead to a better understanding of the above definitions as well as the organisms and the symptoms that produce these clinical pictures. Figure 15.27 is a basic sketch showing the anatomy of this region. The perianal region is the area up to the anal verge. The covering of this area is stratified squamous dermal epithelium similar in nature to other regions of the genital area. The anal canal is 2–3 cm in length and extends from the anal verge to the anorectal line. It is rich in sensory nerve endings and is surrounded by the anal sphincter muscle. The rectum begins above the anorectal line and extends for 15 cm to join the sigmoid colon.

Infection in the perianal region can occur with the organisms that cause infections in other genital areas. Because of the similarity of the epithelium, the presentation of these infections (i.e. ulcers, papules, etc.) is similar to that seen in the other areas. Proctitis is the inflammation produced within the 15 cm of the rectum. Because of the sensory nerve supply present in this area, this inflammation is associated with pain. Tenesmus and constipation can also occur because of spasm of the anal sphincter muscle. Purulent discharge may also be present. Proctocolitis occurs if there is involvement of the colonic muscosa in addition to the mucosa of the rectum. Diarrhoea and abdominal cramping are additional symptoms seen with proctocolitis. In enteritis, there is inflammation of the small intestine, resulting in diarrhoea. In cases of enteritis there is usually no involvement of the rectum or colonic mucosa.

The organisms responsible for perianal infections, proctitis, proctocolitis and enteritis differ as set out in Table 15.8. Examination, as previously discussed, should include inspection of the anus, digital examination of the rectum and anoscopy, with consideration of sigmoidoscopy and/or colonoscopy. Laboratory testing will be guided by the patient's symptoms and physical findings. External lesions of the perianal region should be evaluated in the same manner as for similar lesions in other genital regions. Any purulent material from the anus and rectum should be Gram stained and sent for culture. In addition, stool cultures and examination for ova and parasites are indicated with proctocolitis and enteritis.

Treatment will be directed by the specific diagnosis identified. If purulent material is identified on anorectal examination, or if PMNs are seen on Gram stain of anorectal sections, the CDC recommends the following empirical therapy pending test results [23]: ceftriaxone (or another agent effective against anal and genital gonorrhoea) 125 mg intramuscularly once a day, plus doxycycline 100 mg orally twice a day for 7 days (for *C. trachomatis*).

The treatment for some of the parasitic infections discussed is listed in Table 15.9 [32]. Treatment regimens for bacterial infections of

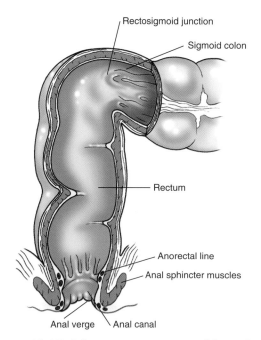

Figure 15.27. *Schematic representation of the anal, rectal and sigmoid colon regions.*

the gastrointestinal tract that can produce these symptoms are not completed established and must be individualized.

Ectoparasitic infections

Ectoparasites that are of concern as STDs are *Phthirus pubis*, or pubic lice, and *Sarcoptes scabiei*,

Table 15.8. *Infectious aetiologies associated with perianal infections, proctitis, proctocolitis and enteritis*

Infection	Possible aetiologies
Perianal infections	*T. pallidum, H. ducreyi*, granuloma inguinale, HSV, HPV
Proctitis	*N. gonorrhoeae, C. trachomatis*, LGV serovars of *C. trachomatis, T. pallidum*, HSV
Proctocolitis	*Campylobacter* spp., *Shigella* spp., *Entamoeba histolytica*
Enteritis	*Giardia lamblia, Salmonella* spp.*, *Cryptosporidium* spp.*, *Isospora belli*, *Microsporidium* spp.*, CMV*, HIV

*In patients infected with HIV.

HSV (herpes simplex virus); HPV (human papillomavirus); LGV (lymphogranuloma venereum); CMV (cytomegalovirus); HIV (human immunodeficiency virus).

T. pallidum (Treponema pallidum); H. ducreyi (Haemophilus ducreyi); N. gonorrhoeae (Neisseria gonorrhoeae); C. trachomatis (Chlamydia trachomatis).

Table 15.9. *Treatment recommendations in selected parasitic infections [32]*

Infection	Treatment recommendations
Amoebiasis (*Entamoeba histolytica*) asymptomatic	Iodoquinol* 600 mg 3 times a day for 20 days, **or** paromomycin 25–35 mg/kg/day in 3 doses for 7 days, **or** diloxanide furoate† 500 mg 3 times a day for 10 days
mild to moderate intestinal disease	Metronidazole 750 mg 3 times a day for 10 days, **or** Tinidazole‡ 2 g/day for 3 days
severe intestinal disease, hepatic abscess	metronidazole 750 mg 3 times a day for 10 days, **or** tinidazole 600 mg‡ twice a day or 800 mg 3 times a day for 5 days
Cryptosporidium species	Paromomycin 500–750 mg 4 times a day
Giardia lamblia	Metronidazole 250 mg 3 times a day for 5 days, **or** tinidazole‡ 2 g once, **or** furazolidone 100 mg 4 times a day for 7–10 days, **or** paromomycin 25–35 mg/kg/day in 3 doses for 7 days
Isospora belli	Trimethoprim 160 mg /sulfamethoxazole 800 mg 4 times a day for 10 days, then twice a day for 3 weeks
Microsporidium [Enterocytozoon bieneusi, Septata (Encephalitozoon) intestinalis]	Albendazole 400 mg twice a day may be effective for *S. intestinalis* infections and may be helpful for *E. bieneusi* infections. Octreotide (Sandostatin) has provided relief in some patients with large-volume diarrhoea

*Dosage and duration of administration should not be exceeded because of the possibility of causing optic neuritis; maximum dose is 2 g/day.

†In the USA this drug is available from the CDC Drug Service, Centers for Disease Control and Prevention, Atlanta, Georgia 30333; telephone 404-639-3670 (evenings, weekends, and holidays 404-639-2888).

‡A nitro-imidazole similar to metronidazole, but not marketed in the USA; tinidazole appears to be at least as effective as metronidazole and better tolerated.

or scabies. These organisms live either on or in the skin of the infected individual and draw nourishment from their host. Pruritus is the major symptom that will usually bring infected patients to medical attention. These parasites are transmitted by close contact, which includes sexual activity. Scabies may also be transmitted by sharing contaminated clothing and bedding. Scabies may require more than a brief encounter to be transmitted and is more often seen in partners who spend the night together [33].

Pubic lice usually live in the pubic hair but in some instances can be seen in the scalp hair, the eyebrows, eyelashes, axillary hair, and hair on the chest and back of men [34]. Eggs that are laid by these lice are attached to body hairs. These eggs, which can be found at the base of body hair, are referred to as 'nits'. Nymphs emerge from these deposited eggs and need to obtain a blood meal. While doing so, they pierce the skin and inject saliva into it to prevent blood clotting. This area of injection also becomes intensely pruritic because of hypersensitivity to antigens in the saliva. Small blue spots, also known as 'maculae caeruleae', may appear on the skin secondary to the anticoagulant that is injected in the saliva [34]. During feeding, pubic lice may deposit dark red faeces on the skin.

Pubic lice are diagnosed by finding nits attached to the base of the body hair where they were deposited (Fig. 15.28), or by finding the lice (Fig. 15.29). These should be plainly visible on examination. Recommended treatments for pubic lice [23] are given in Table 15.11.

Scabies burrow into the skin of humans where eggs are laid and from which larvae emerge. The classic linear burrow (Fig. 15.30) is pathognomonic for the infection. These linear burrows often cross skin lines and are usually seen in the interdigital spaces (Fig. 15.31), the wrists and ankles, elbows, anterior axillary folds, abdomen, genitals and buttocks. The penis and scrotum can be infested. The pruritus seen with scabies characteristically occurs at night. Erythematous papules, nodules and vesicles may be seen in these areas as well.

A more severe form of scabies, known as crusted or Norwegian scabies, also occurs and more recently has been seen in individuals infected with HIV. Patients are heavily infested with mites and this form of scabies is highly contagious. Hyperkeratotic crusted plaques are noted on the hands and feet (Fig. 15.32). Treatment of Norwegian scabies is more difficult because of the heavy mite infestation.

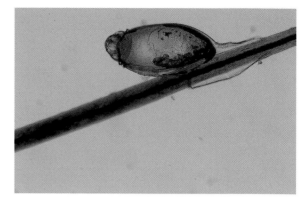

Figure 15.28. *Magnification of hair with 'nit', 16×. (Courtesy of Eileen Burd, PhD, Henry Ford Hospital, Detroit, MI, USA.)*

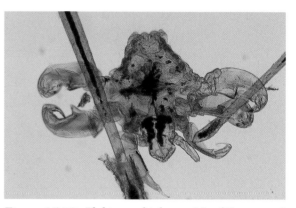

Figure 15.29. *Phthirus pubis louse; 16×. (Courtesy of Eileen Burd, PhD, Henry Ford Hospital, Detroit, MI, USA.)*

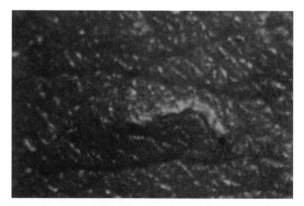

Figure 15.30. *Thready tortuous gray lesion of scabies; this is a picture of the classic diagnostic burrow of the scabies mite as seen through a magnifying glass. (Reproduced from ref. 63 with permission of Glaxo Wellcome Inc.)*

Scabies is diagnosed by finding the organism, eggs or faeces. These are identified (Fig. 15.33)

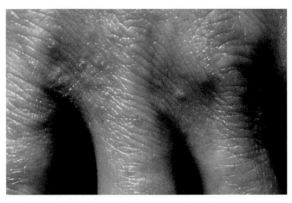

Figure 15.31. *Interdigital lesions of scabies. (Reproduced from ref. 63 with permission of Glaxo Wellcome Inc.)*

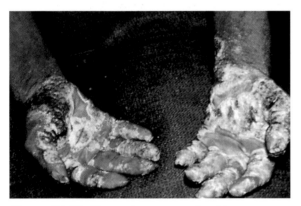

Figure 15.32. *Norwegian or crusted scabies. (Reproduced from ref. 64 with permission of Glaxo Wellcome Inc.)*

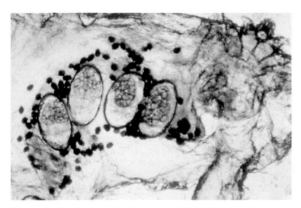

Figure 15.33. *Scabies burrow (40×) showing four eggs, an adult female mite and numerous dark specks which are faeces. (Reproduced from ref. 63 with permission of Glaxo Wellcome Inc.)*

by obtaining skin scrapings or biopsies to examine under the microscope [33]. Recommended

treatments for scabies [23] are listed in Table 15.10.

Mononucleosis syndrome

The Epstein–Barr virus (EBV) produces the classical picture of infectious mononucleosis, which consists of sore throat, fever and lymphadenopathy. Cytomegalovirus (CMV) can present in a similar fashion. EBV is most often transmitted by oropharyngeal secretions; CMV is found in semen and cervical secretions; both are transmitted by close personal contact, which includes sexual activity. Viral hepatitis, secondary to infection with HAV or HBV, is also a part of the differential diagnosis and can also be sexually transmitted. Today, acute HIV infection is included in the differential diagnosis because it, too, can present a picture of infectious mononucleosis. These viral infections must be separated from non-STDs that present in a similar manner, such as toxoplasmosis, rubella and drug reactions [35].

The prominent clinical features seen with a 'mononucleosis-like' syndrome are a combination of fever, sore throat, generalized malaise, an exudative pharyngitis, lymphadenopathy, hepatosplenomegaly and rash. Atypical lymphocytosis is the hallmark finding on laboratory investigation. Mild anaemia and thrombocytopenia may also be present. A rise in serum transaminases also occurs.

EBV is diagnosed most often in adolescents. The finding of lymphadenopathy and splenomegaly on examination of someone with sore throat and fever will often raise the possibility of EBV. The diagnosis is made by serological testing and a positive heterophile antibody test is confirmatory. If specific EBV serological testing is performed, the diagnosis of acute EBV is made by demonstrating the presence of immunoglobulin M (IgM) viral capsid antibodies. This is the only serological titre indicative of an acute infection.

Acute CMV infection in the normal host is usually asymptomatic. It tends to be seen in patients slightly older than those with EBV. When CMV presents symptomatically, the picture is similar to that described for EBV. CMV is confirmed with serological testing for a positive IgM titre.

Viral hepatitis can present symptomatically, which is usually the case with HAV; HBV, however, can be asymptomatic, and many patients are often unaware that they have been infected with HBV. The degree of liver dysfunction seen with viral hepatitis is more marked than that seen with EBV or CMV and the diagnosis can be

Table 15.10. *Recommended treatments and alternative regimens for ectoparasitic infections [23]*

Ectoparasitic infection	Recommended treatment	Alternative regimen
Pediculosis pubis	Permethrin 1% creme rinse applied to affected areas and washed off after 10 minutes, **or** lindane 1% shampoo applied for 4 minutes to the affected area, and then thoroughly washed off, **or** pyrethrins with piperonyl butoxide applied to the affected area and washed off after 10 minutes	
Scabies	Permethrin cream 5% applied to all areas of the body from the neck down and washed off after 8–14 hours	Lindane 1%, 1 fluid ounce of lotion or 30 g of cream applied thinly to all areas of the body from the neck down and washed off thoroughly after 8 hours*, or sulphur 6% precipitated in ointment applied thinly to all areas nightly for 3 nights. Previous application should be washed off before new applications are applied. Thoroughly wash off 24 hours after the last application

*Lindane should not be used following a bath, nor by persons with extensive dermatitis.

assumed with less difficulty. The diagnosis of both is made with serological studies. The presence of IgM antibodies to HAV provides evidence of acute infection. Hepatitis B is diagnosed with the clinical findings of liver dysfunction together with the presence of positive serological studies for the HBV surface antigen.

Infection with EBV, CMV and HAV is usually self-limiting. Therapy is supportive and resolution of symptoms is seen over 2–6 weeks. Infection with HBV may take on a more prolonged course and in some cases becomes chronic, leading eventually to cirrhosis.

Most patients with an acute HIV infection may be seen by their family physician or in other acute care clinics for symptoms similar to those discussed above; they may remain undiagnosed because HIV is not considered at the time of presentation [36]. This presentation of HIV as an STD is seen 2–4 weeks after exposure and has become known as the acute retroviral syndrome. Of patients who become infected, 53–93% will be symptomatic, possibly as a result of a larger viral inoculum and the particular route of administration. Symptoms may last for 1–2 weeks.

The onset is usually abrupt. On examination, distinctive oral mucocutaneous ulcerations that are rounded and sharply demarcated may be seen. Lymphadenopathy is detected in up to 70% of cases and it may be generalized in some. A characteristic non-pruritic erythematous maculopapular rash of the face and trunk is seen in 40–60% of cases (Fig. 15.34).

Lymphopenia is detected early with a significant decrease in the number of CD4+ cells; later, atypical lymphocytosis can occur. Testing for HIV antibodies by the ELISA or Western blot methods is negative at this time because immunity has not yet developed (Fig. 15.35). To arrive at the diagnosis, testing for viral presence should be performed and includes *p24* antigen testing, a determination of plasma HIV RNA or a qualitative HIV-DNA assay.

Antiretroviral therapy is currently advised for the acute retroviral syndrome [36,37]. Regimens with two nucleoside analogues in combination

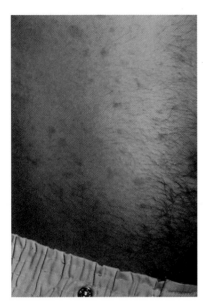

Figure 15.34. *Exanthem associated with acute HIV infection: multiple erythematous macules and papules on the trunk. (Reproduced from ref. 65 with permission.)*

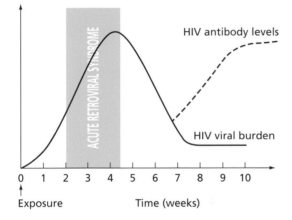

Figure 15.35. *Schematic representation of HIV viral burden and antibody levels during the acute retroviral syndrome. Viral burden is measurable during the acute syndrome, whereas antibody levels are not detectable as early. (—) Detectable as p24 antigen or viral RNA/ DNA assays. (---) Serologically-detectable antibody.*

with a protease inhibitor are currently recommended [38]. Therapy with the three drugs should be instituted simultaneously to avoid the development of resistance. The length of time that treatment should be continued is still undetermined.

Prevention

There are many facets to the prevention of STDs. Until vaccines are discovered that will help limit the number of STDs, the best means

to control their number is to prevent them from occurring. This is particularly important for infections such as HSV (where there is no cure), for HPV (which is associated with the development of malignancies) and for HIV (which becomes chronic and fatal). Strategies available as a means of prevention include (a) changing all sexual behaviour that places a patient at increased risk of the development of an STD and (b) the use of barrier contraception, which physically prevents their transmission. Certain physical and biological factors have been identified that facilitate transmission: these include the presence of genital ulcers and lack of circumcision [39]. Infectivity is also higher when the inoculum is greater. This is seen, for example, in the acute retroviral syndrome where larger quantities of virus are present.

In the area of STDs there is an emphasis on certain types of behaviour and sexual practice that place individuals at risk of acquiring an STD: activity that increases the number of exposures, activity with many different partners and activity with anonymous partners all increase the risk of disease transmission. Additionally, certain forms of sexual behaviour carry more risk of disease transmission than others. When these forms of sexual activity occur in an 'unprotected' manner, the chances of disease transmission are even higher.

One report [40] demonstrated that HIV transmission was a function of the number of sexual partners and the practice of receptive anal intercourse. Anal mucosa that is compromised because of frequent contact can increase the chance of infection. Additionally, other sexual practices such as oral–anal contact allow for exposure to pathogens that might not be acquired through other forms of behaviour. As a result of the AIDS epidemic, attention has become focused on those sexual activities that are more likely to facilitate disease transmission (Table 15.11). It is essential that patients at risk of STD acquisition are aware of the dangers of such practices.

Education and knowledge are the primary focus for changing sexual behaviour. Interventions to reduce high-risk behaviour have been shown to work at both the individual and community-based levels [41]. This was clearly demonstrated at the beginning of the AIDS epidemic, when the gay community was effective in promoting such education and change to prevent acquisition of the disease.

Not all infections are symptomatic and many of these are transmitted unknowingly. Disease

Table 15.11. *Guidelines on safer sexual practices*

Safe	Possibly safe	Unsafe
Hugging, massage	'Wet' kissing	Oral–genital contact with ejaculation
Body-to-body rubbing	Vaginal intercourse with a condom	Oral–anal contact
Mutual masturbation	Receptive anal intercourse with a condom	Vaginal intercourse without a condom
Social 'dry' kissing	Contact with urine	Digital or manual contact inside the rectum
Using one's own sex toys		Insertive anal intercourse without a condom
		Receptive anal intercourse without a condom
		Sharing sex toys

transmission can be prevented with the use of both physical and chemical barrier contraceptive methods [42]. Condoms, when properly used (Table 15.12), are capable of preventing STDs. Spermicides, such as nonoxynol-9, have documented activity against a number of sexually transmitted pathogens. To achieve additive effects, a barrier method and spermicide are frequently used together.

Interrupting the cycle of disease transmission is important: for those who are already infected, follow-up monitoring and evaluation are crucial; for those who have been exposed, evaluation for the presence of disease and treatment are advised.

Conclusions

STDs continue to be a major health problem and a significant cause of morbidity and mortality. This has been highlighted most recently by the AIDS epidemic. Men who have sex with other men demonstrate a higher incidence of STDs than their strictly heterosexual counterparts and lesbian women; this is due to a variety of sexual behaviours with many, often anonymous, partners. Because of these sexual practices, many pathogens, not traditionally considered to be sexually transmitted, are acquired and labelled as STDs. Prevention of these diseases is important: in some instances it is the only available means of controlling their spread and of preventing the complications associated with them.

Table 15.12. *Guidelines for correct condom use*

▨ Store condoms in a cool, dry place* where damage to the condom is unlikely to occur

▨ A new condom should be used with each intercourse. DO NOT REUSE CONDOMS

▨ If the condom appears to be brittle or sticky upon opening the package, do not use it

▨ Avoid tearing or damaging the condom

▨ The condom should be inserted over an erect penis before there is ANY genital contact with the partner

▨ Unroll the condom to the base; leave an empty space at the end of the condom to collect semen

▨ Squeeze the tip of the condom to remove all air trapped inside

▨ Proper lubricant should be ensured; if additional lubricant is needed, use only water-based lubricants; DO NOT use oil-based lubricants such as petroleum jelly, mineral oil or cold cream

▨ The penis should be withdrawn while erect to prevent the condom from slipping off and to prevent spillage of semen; the base of the condom should be held firmly during withdrawal

*Wallets, glove compartments and similar places with the possibilities of warmer temperatures and physical damage are best avoided.

References

1. McNeill WH. Plagues and peoples. New York: Doubleday, 1976

2. Fleming DT, McQuillan GM, Johnson RE *et al.* Herpes Simplex Virus Type 2 in the United States, 1976 to 1994. *N Engl J Med* 1997; 337: 1105–1111

3. Catchpole MA, Mercey DE, Nicoll A *et al.* Continuing transmission of sexually transmitted diseases among patients infected with HIV-1 attending genitourinary medicine clinics in England and Wales. *Br Med J* 1996; 312: 539–542

4. Frisch M, Glimelius B, Adriaan JC *et al.* Sexually transmitted infection as a cause of anal cancer. *New Engl J Med* 1997; 337: 1351–1358

5. Gordon SM, Carlyn CJ, Doyle LJ *et al.* The emergence of *Neisseria gonorrhoeae* with decreased susceptibility to ciprofloxacin in Cleveland, Ohio: epidemiology and risk factors. *Ann Intern Med* 1996; 125: 465–470

6. Centers for Disease Control and Prevention. Fluoroquinolone resistance in *Neisseria gonorrhoeae* — Colorado and Washington, 1995. MMWR 1995; 44: 761–764

7. Centers for Disease Control and Prevention. Decreased susceptibility of *Neisseria gonorrhoeae* to fluoroquinolones — Ohio and Hawaii, 1992–1994. MMWR 1994; 43: 325–327

8. William DC. Editorial: Sexually transmitted diseases in gay men: an insider's view. *Sex Transm Dis* 1979; 6: 278–280

9. Owen WF. Sexually transmitted diseases and traumatic problems in homosexual men. *Ann Intern Med* 1980; 92: 805–808

10. Ostrow DG. Homosexual behavior and sexually transmitted diseases. In: Holmes KK, Mardh P, Sparling PF *et al.* (eds) Sexually transmitted diseases. New York: McGraw-Hill, 1990: 61–69

11. Seidman SN, Rieder RO. A review of sexual behavior in the United States. *Am J Psychiatry* 1994; 151: 330–341

12. Robertson R, Schachter J. Failure to identify venereal disease in a lesbian population. *Sex Transm Dis* 1981; 8: 75–76

13. Ostrow DG. Sexually transmitted diseases and homosexuality. *Sex Transm Dis* 1983; 10: 208–215

14. Owen WF. The clinical approach to the male homosexual patient. *Med Clin North Am* 1986; 70: 499–535

15. Council on Scientific Affairs, American Medical Association. Health care needs of gay men and lesbians in the United States. JAMA 1996; 275: 1354–1359

16. Lewis CE. Sexual issues: are physicians addressing the issues? *J Gen Intern Med* 1990; 5: S78–S81

17. Boekeloo BO, Marx ES, Kral AH *et al.* Frequency and thoroughness of STD/HIV assessment by physicians in a high-risk metropolitan area. *Am J Public Health* 1991; 81: 1645–1648

18. Briggs LP, Patnaude P, Scavron J *et al.* The importance of social histories for assessing sexually transmitted disease risk. *Sex Transm Dis* 1995; 22: 348–350

19. Tramont EC. Treponema pallidum (syphilis). In: Mandell GL, Bennett JE, Dolin R (eds). Principles and practice of infectious diseases. New York: Churchill Livingstone, Inc, 1995: 2117–2133

20. Weller PF. Syphilis and nonvenereal treponematoses. In: Dale DC, Federman DD (eds) Scientific American medicine 1997. *Scientific American* 1997; 7: (VI): 1–12

21. Thomas DL, Quinn TC. Serologic testing for sexually transmitted diseases. *Infect Dis Clin North Am* 1993; 7: 793–824

22. Juardo RL. Syphilis serology: a practical approach. *Infect Dis Clin Pract* 1996; 5: 351–358

23. Centers for Disease Control and Prevention. 1998 Guidelines for treatment of sexually transmitted diseases. *MMWR* 1998; 47 (no. RR-1)

24. Goldberg LH, Kaufman R, Kurtz TO *et al.* Long-term suppression of recurrent genital herpes with acyclovir. *Arch Dermatol* 1993; 129: 582–586

25. Bowi WR. Urethritis in Males. In: Holmes KK, Mardh P, Sparling PF *et al.* (eds) Sexually transmitted diseases. New York: McGraw-Hill, 1990: 627–639

26. McCormack WM, Rein WF. Urethritis. In: Mandell GL, Bennett JE, Dolin R (eds) Principles and practice of infectious diseases. New York: Churchill Livingstone, 1995: 1063–1074

27. Sackel SG, Alpert S, Fiumara NJ *et al.* Orogenital contact and the isolation of *Neisseria gonorrhoeae*, *Mycoplasma hominis*, and *Ureaplasma urealyticum* from the pharynx. *Sex Transm Dis* 1979; 6: 64–68

28. Krieger JN, Jenny C, Verdon M *et al.* Clinical manifestations of trichomoniasis in men. *Ann Intern Med* 1993; 118: 844–849

29. Bonnez W, Reichman RC. Papillomaviruses. In: Mandell GL, Bennett JE, Dolin R (eds) Principles and practice of infectious diseases. New York: Churchill Livingstone, 1995: 1387–1400

30. Palefsky JM, Gonzales J, Greenblatt RM *et al.* Anal intraepithelial neoplasia and anal papillomavirus infection among homosexual males with group IV HIV disease. *JAMA* 1990; 263: 2911–2916

31. Palefsky JM, Holly EA, Hogeboom CJ *et al.* Anal cytology as a screening tool for anal squamous intraepithelial lesions. *J Acquir Immune Defic Syndr Hum Retrovirol* 1997; 14: 415–422

32. Drugs for parasitic infections. *Med Lett Drugs Ther* 1995; 37: 99–108

33. Orkin M, Maibach H. Scabies. In: Holmes KK, Mardh P, Sparling PF *et al.* (eds) Sexually transmitted diseases. New York: McGraw-Hill, 1990; 473–479

34. Wilson BB. Lice (pediculosis). In: Mandell GL, Bennett JE, Dolin R (eds) Principles and practice of infectious diseases. New York: Churchill Livingstone, 1995; 2558–2560

35. Al-Hajjar S, Hussain Qadri SM. Epstein–Barr virus. *Infectious Disease Practice for the Clinician* 1996: 41–44

36. Rosenberg E, Cotton DJ. Primary HIV infection and the acute retroviral syndrome. *AIDS Clin Care* 1997; 9: 22–25

37. Quinn TC. Grand rounds at the Johns Hopkins Hospital: acute primary HIV infection. *JAMA* 1997; 278: 58–62

38. Panel on Clinical Practices for Treatment of HIV Infection. Guidelines for the use of antiretroviral agents in HIV-infected adults and adolescents, 1997

39. Moses S, Plummer FA, Bradley JE *et al.* The association between lack of male circumcision and risk for HIV infection: a review of the epidemiological data. *Sex Transm Dis* 1994; 21: 201–210

40. Winkelstein W, Lyman DM, Padian N *et al.* Sexual practices and risk of infection by the human immuno-deficiency virus. *JAMA* 1987; 257: 321–325

41. Kelly, JA. Sexually transmitted disease prevention approaches that work: interventions to reduce risk behavior among individuals, groups, and communities. *Sex Transm Dis* 1994; 21: S73–S75

42. Stratton P, Alexander NJ. Prevention of sexually transmitted infections, physical and chemical barrier methods. *Infect Dis Clin North Am* 1993; 7: 841–859

43. Centers for Disease Control and Prevention. Sexually transmitted disease surveillance 1995. Atlanta, GA: Division of STD Prevention, Centers for Disease Control and Prevention, 1996

44. Korting GW. Practical dermatology of genital region. Philadelphia: Saunders, 1980: 48

45. Korting GW. Practical dermatology of genital region. Philadelphia: Saunders, 1980: 49

46. Kaminester LH. Sexually transmitted diseases: an illustrated guide to differential diagnosis. Research Triangle Park, NC: Burroughs Wellcome Co, 1991: 19

47. Korting GW. Practical dermatology of genital region. Philadelphia: Saunders, 1980: 32

48. Korting GW. Practical dermatology of genital region. Philadelphia: Saunders, 1980: 33

49. US Department of Health, Education and Welfare. Syphilis: a synopsis. Public Health Service Publication No. 1660. Washington, DC: US Government Printing Office, 1968: 49

50. Fitzpatrick TB, Johnson RA, Polano MK *et al.* Color atlas and synopsis of clinical dermatology. New York: McGraw-Hill, 1992: 391

51. Fitzpatrick TB, Johnson RA, Polano MK *et al.* Color atlas and synopsis of clinical dermatology. New York: McGraw-Hill, 1992: 395

52. US Department of Health, Education and Welfare. Syphilis: a synopsis. Public Health Service Publication No. 1660. Washington, DC: US Government Printing Office, 1968: 51

53. Felman YM, Hoke AW. Wellcome atlas of sexually transmitted diseases. Research Triangle Park, NC: Burroughs Wellcome Co, 1984: 14

54. Fitzpatrick TB, Johnson RA, Polano MK *et al.* Color atlas and synopsis of clinical dermatology. New York: McGraw-Hill, 1992: 399

55. Felman YM, Hoke AW. Wellcome atlas of sexually transmitted diseases. Research Triangle Park, NC: Burroughs Wellcome Co, 1984: 32

56. Korting GW. Practical dermatology of genital region. Philadelphia: Saunders, 1980: 165

57. Fiumara NJ. Pictorial guide to sexually transmitted diseases. New York: Cahners, 1989: 11

58. Kaminester LH. Sexually transmitted diseases: an illustrated guide to differential diagnosis. Research Triangle Park, NC: Burroughs Wellcome Co, 1991: 14

59. Fitzpatrick TB, Johnson RA, Polano MK *et al.* Color atlas and synopsis of clinical dermatology. New York: McGraw-Hill, 1992: 439

60. Kaminester LH. Sexually transmitted diseases: an illustrated guide to differential diagnosis. Research Triangle Park, NC: Burroughs Wellcome Co, 1991: 16

61. Korting GW. Practical dermatology of genital region. Philadelphia: Saunders, 1980: 177

62. Kaminester LH. Sexually transmitted diseases: an illustrated guide to differential diagnosis. Research Triangle Park, NC: Burroughs Wellcome Co, 1991: 17

63. Felman YM, Hoke AW. Wellcome atlas of sexually transmitted diseases. Research Triangle Park, NC: Burroughs Wellcome Co, 1984: 44

64. Felman YM, Hoke AW. Wellcome atlas of sexually transmitted diseases. Research Triangle Park, NC: Burroughs Wellcome Co, 1984: 45

65. Fitzpatrick TB, Johnson RA, Polano MK *et al.* Color atlas and synopsis of clinical dermatology. New York: McGraw-Hill, 1992: 417

CHAPTER 16

Men and suicide: assessment and management in a primary care setting

D. P. Sugrue

Incidence

Suicide is a significant problem in Western culture, especially for men. In the USA in 1994, more than 32 000 people committed suicide (12.4 per 100 000 population) [1] and more than 300 000 people made a suicide attempt [2]. One in four Americans have given suicide serious consideration on at least one occasion in their past [3]. Despite women attempting suicide at least three or four times more frequently than men [4], four times as many men than women die from suicide each year [1]. Although the rate of suicide differs dramatically from country to country, this relationship of male to female suicides remains consistent.

Owing to a reporting bias, the reported incidence of suicide of 1–1.5% of all deaths in the USA grossly underestimates the magnitude of the problem. Some authorities suggest that as many as 30% of suicides go unrecognized or unreported [5]. In all likelihood, a significant number of fatal car crashes, accidental falls, and alcohol-related mishaps are, in actuality, acts of self-destruction.

Age
Adolescent suicide
Between the ages of 15 and 65, the rate of male suicides in the USA is relatively stable, ranging between 22 and 25 suicides per 100 000 population [1]. What these statistics fail to underscore is the growing epidemic of adolescent suicides. In 1950, the suicide rate for 15- to 19-year-old adolescents (both males and females) was 2.7 per 100 000, compared with 10.9 per 100 000 in 1993 [6]. The tragic magnitude of this increase is highlighted by the fact that suicide today is the third leading cause of death for 15- to 24-year-old males, outnumbering combined deaths due to cancer, heart disease, HIV infection, birth defects, chronic lung problems, pneumonia, influenza and stroke.

Adolescents face numerous developmental tasks, including separating from parents, reassessing childhood values and beliefs, redefining their self-concept, coming to terms with physical and sexual maturation and facing pending decisions about their career paths. These developmental tasks can overwhelm an adolescent and leave him (or her) vulnerable to normal life-stressors. Another reason why adolescent suicides often come as a surprise is the frequent absence of blatant warning-signs: whereas the overwhelming majority of adults who commit suicide are identifiably depressed prior to their suicide attempt, many adolescents fail to display overt signs of depression. For some, depression may be present but is masked by the moodiness, boredom and restlessness that is often observed and assumed to be part of a normal adolescent phase. For others, there is no predisposing depression: rather, the suicide is an impulsive over-reaction to a disappointment. Unlike adults, adolescents lack the life experience necessary to place disappointment and failure into proper context.

Risk factors for adolescent suicide include a family history of suicide; a family history of a psychiatric or substance-abuse disorder; family turmoil due to separation or divorce; family violence including emotional, physical and sexual abuse; an unwanted pregnancy; a previous suicide attempt; incarceration; presence of a firearm in the household; and exposure to the suicidal behaviour of others (e.g. classmate or teen icon) [7–11]. Teenagers who are impulsive and display symptoms of a conduct disorder [9] and those who are overachieving and perfectionist [12] are at higher risk of attempting suicide.

The elderly
The incidence of suicide increases significantly after the age of 65. Men between 75 and 84 years are twice, and men over 85 years are almost three times more likely to commit suicide than men

aged 35–44 years [1]. These rates probably under-represent the frequency of elderly suicide because they miss chronic, passive suicidal behaviour — the wilful slowing-down of eating, increasing alcohol consumption, or altering the use of medications in the hopes of dying [13]. The high rate of suicide among elderly men is probably due to fear of debilitating illness, determination to not burden loved ones and growing public acceptance of terminal patients ending their lives. Of elderly men who commit suicide, 50% suffer from chronic physical illness [14]. Divorced and widowed men in this age group are almost three times more likely to commit suicide than are married men [15]. Other risk factors for elderly men include alcohol abuse, depression and social isolation [16].

Ethnicity and nationality

The rate of male suicides differs dramatically from country to country. During the late 1980s, Hungary averaged 52.1 male suicides annually per 100 000 population. A number of Central European countries had equivalent annual rates in the low to mid 30s, whereas the USA, Canada, Australia, New Zealand and Western European countries ranged between 15 and 25 male suicides per 100 000 population per annum. Suicide mortality was low in the UK, southern Europe, Latin America and reporting African nations (2–10 male suicides per 100 000). Likewise, reporting Asian nations had low suicide mortality rates, with the exception of the more industrialized nations (Japan, Hong Kong and Singapore), which had rates comparable with those of North America and Western Europe [17].

Rates within a country can vary according to ethnicity and geography. For example, in the USA, the rate of suicide mortality for males in 1993 was 19.9 per 100 000; African-American males, however, were less likely to take their own lives, with a suicide mortality rate of 12.5 compared with 21.4 for White Americans [1]. The western mountain region of the USA had a suicide rate more than double that of males in the mid-Atlantic states.

There is no clear consensus when considering explanations for these differences between countries, nationalities, and geographic regions. Some countries with low suicide mortality rates, especially underdeveloped countries, may under-report suicides owing to limited reporting mechanisms. In addition, in countries with a strong religious influence, there may be pressure on public officials to misclassify suicides to avoid national scandal. Nevertheless, reporting bias cannot fully account for the dramatic differences reported above, nor can variations in economic and political stability account for these differences. Instead, it appears that more enduring cultural factors have a persistent influence that is passed along from generation to generation. This persistence of cultural influence is demonstrated in a study of ethnic groups that migrated to Australia. The suicide rate for each group was more similar to the rate in the country of origin than to Australia's national rate of suicide, regardless of how long the migrants had been separated from their place of birth [18].

Suicide method

In 1993, 14% of male suicides in the USA used overdosing or poisoning and 66% used a firearm. In the USA, a firearm in the household increases the chances of suicide five-fold [19]. This apparent association between firearms and the risk of suicide may be specific to the American culture, as many other countries with strict gun control policies have higher rates of suicide than are found in the USA.

Motives for suicidal behaviour

What can possibly prompt a person to take his or her own life? For some, suicide is the result of an impulsive act during intoxication, when thinking is blurred, options are lost and consequences are not fully comprehended. For others, suicide is the result of psychotic thinking — obedience to internal voices or desperate attempts to escape imagined demons. For most, however, neither drugs nor psychosis fuel suicide; instead, it is the result of rage, hopelessness, guilt and misery.

In trying to understand the phenomenology of suicide it is helpful to make a distinction between people who truly attempt to die (attempters), people who act not to die but to make a point (gesturers), and people who think about suicide but fail to act on these thoughts (ideators).

Attempters

A true attempter is someone who has made up their mind that they want to die. If they happen to survive the attempt, it was by accident and they are enraged by their failure. For some of these people, suicide is an act of self-loathing, which does not typically occur spontaneously or solely in response to failure but is often planted and nurtured in early childhood. Other true attempters, via a tragically twisted logic, use their own destruction to punish other people. They harbour the fantasy that an insensitive spouse or disinterested parent will suffer horrific pangs of guilt upon learning of their suicide [20]. The victim finds comfort in the final thought, 'Now they'll finally know how much they've hurt me', or, 'Now they'll feel guilty every day for the rest of their lives'. Perhaps the most common motivation, however, is hopelessness. Overwhelmed by unbearable psychic or physical pain and convinced that there is no possibility of respite, some individuals commit suicide, not to make a statement, not to punish themselves or others, but simply to end the suffering.

Gesturers

Of the hundreds of thousands of suicide attempts in the USA each year, the vast majority are more likely to be gestures, or parasuicides [21], than true attempts. Unlike the true attempter, who wants to die, the gesturer wishes to manipulate others or achieve some end other than death. As with true attempters, there are many possible reasons prompting gesturers to engage in potentially lethal behaviour. For some, actions like slashing their wrists or overdosing may serve as a cry for help. For others, suicidal gestures are intended to gain attention, perhaps from an inattentive spouse or indifferent parents. Some gesturers use suicidal behaviour as a means to be admitted into inpatient care, a place they perceive as a safe haven during times of stress.

Even though the gesturer does not intend to die, such actions should not be dismissed or minimized. As many as 10–15% of people who make suicidal gestures will eventually succeed [22]. Whereas many of the gesturers who successfully commit suicide have died by accident, some became true attempters — they finally gave up and opted to die.

Ideators

In addition to true attempters and gesturers, there are many people who think about suicide but fail to act on the ideation. Suicidal ideation is quite common and reflects a person's desperation to find a solution to what appears to be a hopeless situation. Whatever the challenge or crisis they are facing, the ideator is at a loss on how to resolve the dilemma. Ideators are ambivalent about dying and are typically receptive to assistance in finding a non-lethal solution for their problem. As with the gesturer, if the ideator is left to his or her own devices, their ambivalence about dying could deteriorate into despair, hopelessness and, ultimately, suicide.

Contributing factors

There is no single cause of suicide. Although we have no definitive answer about what prompts a human being to take his or her own life, research highlights multiple factors that are associated with increased suicide rates, including the following:

- Gender (males more often than females) [1];
- Age (increased risk for the elderly) [1];
- Race (Native Americans at greater risk than Whites [23], Whites at greater risk than African-Americans [1]);
- Nationality [16];
- Place of residence (the larger the urban area, the higher the suicide rate) [24];
- Health status (35–40% of all suicides have some significant physical illness) [25];
- Relationship status (increased risk for men who are single, widowed or divorced) [26,27];
- Occupation (physicians, farmers and law-enforcement personnel have elevated suicide rates) [28];
- Religion (church attendance is inversely related to the rate of suicide) [29].

Five additional factors warrant close attention when considering causes for suicidal behaviour, namely psychosocial stressors, psychiatric illness, substance abuse, genetics and personality style.

Psychosocial stressors

A major disappointment can often be identified in a person's life preceding a suicide attempt. In a study of 19 consecutive hospital suicides, clinicians judged 18 of them as being influenced by family loss (divorce, death or estrangement) [30]. Diagnosis of a terminal illness, financial ruin and public scandal are other common stressors associated with suicidal behaviour. However, for every person who commits suicide following a break-up, bankruptcy or scandal, there are tens of thousands of other people who experience the same stressors and survive. When attempting to understand a suicide, rather than being satisfied with merely identifying a major stressor it is necessary to look for other factors that may have left the victim so vulnerable. In most cases, suicide is the result of the unfortunate convergence of multiple factors at a time when the person is least capable of adapting.

Psychiatric illness

Psychiatric illness can significantly compromise a person's ability to cope with major life stressors.

When emotionally incapacitated and rendered defenceless, the person becomes susceptible to feelings of hopelessness and despair.

Affective disorders

Although estimates vary widely, research findings clearly indicate that a significant majority of adult suicides suffer from major depression or a bipolar disorder [31]. When an adult becomes clinically depressed, the risk of suicide increases dramatically: whereas suicide accounts for less than 2% of all deaths in the USA, it accounts for 15% of the deaths of people diagnosed with a major mood disorder [32].

Schizophrenia

About 20% of schizophrenic patients will attempt suicide during their lifetime, and 5–10% of all schizophrenics will eventually die by suicide [32,33]. For some, suicidal behaviour is not an intentional attempt to die but, rather, is a response to a delusional belief or an attempt to comply with demands coming from auditory hallucinations. Under such circumstances, one could argue that death was due not to suicide but to natural causes — that is, the result of a disease process. Other schizophrenic suicides may occur, not when the person is in a psychotic state but when he or she has sufficiently compensated to understand their dismal prognosis. This latter pattern has been observed in young schizophrenic patients following their first or second decompensation.

Anxiety disorders

Although suicidal behaviour is often associated with depression, research has suggested a high incidence of suicidal ideation associated with panic and general anxiety disorders [34]. These disorders often coexist with affective disorders but probably contribute independently to the emergence of suicidal behaviour.

Substance abuse

Alcohol or illegal drugs may be involved in as many as 80% of all adult suicides [35]. Twenty per cent of suicide victims are alcohol dependent [22]. In a large sample of male alcoholics, 17% had made at least one suicide attempt [36]. Alcoholics are at the greatest risk of committing suicide either when their drinking leads to a personal crisis — such as marital break-up, arrest, or loss of employment — or after they have achieved sobriety for a number of months. In the latter case, upon sobriety, the alcoholic loses alcohol's natural anaesthetizing effect on psychic pain, leaving him vulnerable to the ravages of major life stressors.

Genetics

In a study of the Pennsylvania Amish, it was found that 16% of the extended families accounted for 73% of the community's suicides [37]. A family history of suicide has long been noted as a risk factor for suicide, associated with as much as a fourfold increase in the suicide rate for surviving relatives [38]. Many dismiss any genetic link but argue, instead, that an increased incidence of suicide within certain families occurs because the family milieu is toxic (i.e. it spawns impulsive, violent responses to crises). Others suggest that, once the boundary prohibiting self-destruction has been breached in the family system, the unthinkable — suicide — suddenly becomes more than a theoretical possibility. There are data, however, that suggest that the relationship between a family history of suicide and increased suicidal risk goes beyond pure psychosocial explanations. This is exemplified by the observation that the rate of identical twins both committing suicide is more than six times greater than the rate for fraternal twins [39].

Is there a 'suicide gene'? This appears unlikely. Part of the concordance rate among family members is probably due to the inheritance of vulnerability to affective disorders and substance abuse. In addition, there may be an inheritable defect associated with the neurotransmitter serotonin that may compromise a person's capacity to control impulses in the presence of acute stress. Serotonin deficiencies have been noted not only in depressed patients but also in individuals prone to impulsive, violent behaviour. Depressed patients with low serotonin levels appear to be more prone to suicidal behaviour — especially to violent, highly lethal suicidal behaviour — than are depressed patients with normal serotonin levels [40]. In one study of patients hospitalized following violent suicide attempts, those with low cerebrospinal fluid levels of a serotonin derivative were 10 times more likely to kill themselves during the following year [41]. In post-mortem studies of suicides, excess serotonin receptors have been found, perhaps reflecting the brain's attempt to compensate for low serotonin levels [42].

Personality type

Personality styles are the product of both biology and early experiences in the family of origin. As a result of these influences, each person develops his or her own characteristic way of interacting with people and coping with stress. In reference to suicide, research and clinical experience have suggested that some personality styles are particularly ill-suited for dealing with major life crises. When people with these personality styles encounter a significant psychosocial stressor, and at the same time are burdened with a coexisting risk factor such as substance abuse or an affective disorder, the possibility of suicidal behaviour is increased.

Compulsive personalities

Many theorists have described suicide as a violent act against oneself — the ultimate act of self-loathing. It would follow, therefore, that self-esteem is a critical factor when assessing suicide potential. The core of self-esteem develops early; it is largely shaped by how parents react to the child. Ideally, each child experiences unconditional positive regard, which leads to an internalized message that the child is worthwhile and valued regardless of mistakes or failures. Some children, however, receive praise and encouragement only when they please the parent; at other times, they are shamed and made to feel worthless. Their parents are often highly controlling, insistent on compliance, intolerant of failure, and withholding of affection unless the child pleases them. Desperate for acceptance, many of these children learn to please by striving for perfection — anything less brings the threat of criticism and rejection. When they become adults, failure and rejection make them feel worthless because they never learned that they had fundamental value independent of accomplishments or success. It is, therefore, not surprising that if these individuals fail miserably they may resort to self-loathing and, ultimately, self-destruction.

Borderline and antisocial personalities

For many people with compulsive features, self-esteem is scripted as: 'Your worth is what you achieve'. For people with borderline and antisocial personalities, there is no such ambiguity about self-worth: 'You're worthless, you do not deserve to live'. Such individuals are often raised in physically and emotionally abusive households. Being the constant targets of abuse, such children can conclude only that they are somehow worthless and deserving of such abuse. Some will survive by dissociating, i.e. learning to depart emotionally and intellectually from the situation and retreat into fantasy. Others will learn to lessen the pain of being abused by striking out at others. Consistent with the adage, 'Misery loves company', in a perverted way, lashing out and hurting others lessens — albeit momentarily — the pain that comes from self-loathing.

People with antisocial or borderline personalities are largely defenceless when encountering trauma. Programmed with the message that they are intrinsically worthless, they have few skills and little confidence when facing what appears to be an insurmountable challenge. Since early childhood they have been scripted to die; a crisis can serve as their cue.

Constricted personalities

The ability to deal with feelings is an important skill in life: it allows a person to form intimate relationships and cope with problems and disappointments. As with self-esteem, the ability to contend with strong emotions, both positive and negative, comes from early childhood experience. Ideally, children are able to express excitement, fear, anger, happiness and love without fear of reprisal. They learn from parental example and teaching how to respond to a spectrum of emotions in an adaptive fashion. For the emotionally constricted individual, however, emotionality is stifled throughout childhood. Family secrets often exist — terrible secrets such as physical, sexual or substance abuse taking place in the household. The child learns not to discuss family problems, but to keep secret his or her own inner struggles, worries and concerns. In this dysfunctional system, one parent is often an enabler, a person who makes excuses for the abusive partner. The child is not allowed to verbalize his or her horror or fear, but is admonished to keep secret the family problems and to love the abusive parent.

As an adult, this person has little ability to recognize, express or cope with strong emotions. This person will suppress feelings and approach life on a cognitive plane. Unfamiliar with strong emotions, this individual will be ill equipped to cope with overwhelming stress. If his or her world begins to crumble, the response will probably be an intolerable anxiety — so intolerable that, in a moment of desperation, death may seem to be the only respite.

Why men?

As stated earlier, men are four times more likely than women to commit suicide, even though the incidence of affective disorders is higher for women than for men. One possible explanation for this discrepancy is how gender roles in our society leave men less equipped for dealing with trauma. Starting early in life, men in our culture are scripted to be strong, independent, self-sufficient and in control of their emotions. Tearful little girls are swept up into a parent's arms and the tears are wiped away. Tearful little boys are admonished that 'Men don't cry'. Little boys are told, 'Take charge', 'Win', and 'Act like a man', whereas little girls are often discouraged from competing in sporting or academic pursuits, or from group leadership. As a result, men are at a distinct disadvantage when experiencing overwhelming stresses in their life. Failure is inconsistent with how manhood has been defined. Displaying emotions is not an option, unless they are willing to allow themselves to be emasculated further. They ultimately have neither the experience nor the permission to deal as readily and openly with emotional trauma as do women.

There may also be biological factors that put men at greater risk for lethal suicide. As discussed earlier, the presence of impulsive aggression significantly increases the chances of a lethal suicide attempt. The relationship between aggression and androgens has been well documented in both animal and human studies [43]. Although evidence is sparse, some authorities also suspect that serotonin deficiencies associated with impulsive aggression are more common in men than women [44]. If this is accurate, it would help to explain how women can have a higher incidence of affective disorders, yet depressed men are at greater risk for suicide.

In sum, it appears that dysphoric men are more likely to have the lethal combination of the hopelessness of depression, emotional constriction and the impulsive aggressiveness that can lead to highly lethal, suicidal behaviour.

Identification of risk in a primary care practice

The primary care provider is in a unique position to identify and assist suicidal patients. More than 80% of suicide victims visit a doctor within 6 months of their suicide, half within a month, and 40% during the week prior to their death [45–47]. Yet in one survey of physicians caring for patients prior to suicide, only one of six doctors was aware of their patient's suicidal ideation [45]. Research findings suggest that suicide rates can be reduced by as much as 30% if primary care providers are trained in risk identification and intervention [48].

It has been suggested that all patients should be screened for suicidal ideation as part of a general health workup. Certainly, if symptom checklists are administered as part of a medical workup, questions regarding suicidal ideation should be included. If, however, suicidal screening is not a standard part of a medical workup, at a minimum, every patient with symptoms of depression, anxiety or substance abuse should be questioned about suicidal ideation and monitored during the course of treatment for their condition. Research shows that patients in a primary care setting with suicidal ideation may not necessarily appear to be depressed: many of these patients present instead with symptoms of panic disorders, generalized anxiety disorders and substance abuse [49].

Some physicians have expressed concern that asking about suicide might highlight an option that the patient might have otherwise not considered. There is no evidence, however, to suggest that raising the issue of suicide will prompt a person suddenly to act upon the suggestion. On the contrary, many patients report a sense of relief once the topic has been raised — they feel that the physician has given them permission to discuss what they felt to be an unspeakable thought.

The goals for assessment of suicide are simple and straightforward. First of all, it is necessary to know whether the patient is, indeed, having thoughts about suicide. By asking, not only is the physician alerted to a possible risk but also the patient is being provided with an essential outlet to discuss his pain and desperation. Secondly, by asking about suicidal intent, the physician can assess the degree of risk and determine whether the patient's suicidal ideation can be managed as part of his medical care, warrants a referral to a mental health professional, or requires immediate hospitalization.

The following series of questions can help the primary care physician to detect suicidal risk and to assess lethality.

'Have you recently been thinking about dying or taking your life?' Depressed patients will often have thoughts about dying, either fearing death or deciding that they would be better off dead. Typically, by themselves, these thoughts are not indicative of imminent suicidal risk, but should be noted and monitored during the patient's course of treatment for depression or anxiety.

If the patient denies suicidal ideation but is depressed, permission to discuss such thoughts in the future can be helpful. For example, the physician might say, 'For some people when they're under a lot of pressure, there can be periods of time when suicide might seem like a solution. If that should ever happen to you, don't hesitate to call me.' This, or a similar message, not only can communicate the physician's acceptance and support but also can provide hope in the event that the patient later finds himself feeling more desperate.

If, on the other hand, the patient acknowledges that he not only is thinking about death but also has had thoughts about taking his life, further questions are indicated.

'Have you thought about how you would take your life?' The presence of a well-developed plan not only is a warning of imminent risk but also provides clues on the potential lethality of the attempt and preventative steps that should be taken. For example, a plan involving a firearm suggests a much higher risk of a successful suicide than slashing or overdose. Making sure that all firearms are removed from the household would be a potentially important intervention. Even if the patient does not have a well-formed plan, further assessment and ongoing monitoring are still indicated.

'Have you ever attempted suicide in the past?' If the patient has made previous attempts, it can be helpful to learn how the attempt was made, why it failed and how the patient feels about the failure. Previous attempts serve as a powerful predictor of future attempts — over 80% of those who successfully commit suicide had made a previous suicidal attempt [50]. The risk is particularly acute when the patient fails to express ambivalence about past failures, but instead clearly communicates disappointment and anger over not succeeding.

'Do you have any family members who have committed suicide?' As discussed earlier in this chapter, a family history of suicide serves as another strong predictor of risk [51]. The relationship between family history and suicide may be due to genetic factors, to a toxic emotional environment, or to a precedent set by the earlier suicide which made the unthinkable thinkable. When interviewing an adolescent patient, an additional variant of this question would be, 'Do you know anyone who has recently committed suicide?' The phenomenon of copycat suicides, or suicide contagion, has been well documented for adolescents [11] and should be carefully assessed.

'What do you think your death would accomplish?' For some people, suicide represents a desperate last attempt to resolve what otherwise seems to be an insurmountable problem. When a patient answers, 'It's the only way I can stop feeling guilty over the arrest', or 'It'll stop the hurt from my wife leaving me', there is a fairly good prognosis. The patient is looking for a solution to a problem and is open to any help that can provide him a solution other than dying. When a person answers, 'It'll put me out of my misery', or 'I'll finally be at peace', the prognosis is much worse. For this patient, hopelessness goes beyond any one stressor or conflict; life in general has lost meaning, and death appears to be the only way of ending the pain.

'Who besides you would be most affected by your death?' A favourable prognostic sign is when a suicidal person has concerns about his survivors. Answers such as, 'I feel bad about my parents, this will be difficult for them', or even a response like, 'My kids, but they'll be better off without me', are hopeful because they suggest continued attachments to living people, attachments that can be used to help dissuade the person from dying. On the other hand, when a person views the impact of his death on others as being desirable, this indicates imminent risk. For example, a patient might answer, 'My wife, it'll serve her right having to support herself when I'm gone', or 'All you damn doctors who wouldn't listen to me when I told you how sick I am'. The fantasy that one's death will be the ultimate punishment for survivors, as distorted as this logic is, can be a powerful motivator for suicide [20].

'What would you like to see for your future?' When a person with suicidal ideation can still envisage a future, still have hope for a better life, he has not yet psychologically severed himself from the world. An example of such a response would be, 'I wish I could meet someone and fall in love', or 'If only I could get a job and support my family'. Indicative of greater risk, on the other hand, would be a response like, 'I can't even imagine the future; I'll have nothing but misery until I die'.

'Are there any guns at home?' Because accessibility to a gun increases the risk of successful suicide, learning of the presence of firearms not only is a warning about a possible method but also prompts an intervention — removal of all firearms from the household.

'**Are you living alone?**' Social isolation increases the risk of suicidal behaviour and makes management more challenging. It is helpful for the physician to know what kind of social support the patient has and who might be contacted in the event of a crisis.

With the information derived from the questions above, as well as knowledge of epidemiological findings summarized earlier in this chapter, the physician can assess the risk of lethality. Special attention should be paid to the presence of the following factors:

- Previous suicide attempts;
- Family history of suicide;
- Existence of a well-formed plan;
- Hopelessness — no sense of a future;
- Inability to identify circumstances responsible for distress;
- Motivated by a need to 'get even';
- Abusing alcohol or other substances;
- Lack of social support;
- Psychosis.

If any of the above features are present, there is at least a moderate risk of suicide and, at the very least, a referral to a mental health clinician should be considered. When hopelessness is coupled with a well-formed plan, a history of past attempts, substance abuse or psychosis, the risk is severe and the intervention needs to be aggressive and immediate.

Office interventions

When a patient acknowledges suicidal ideation, the first decision facing the physician is whether it is safe to let the patient leave the office. When intoxication, psychosis, rage or despair prevents the patient from offering reassurance that he will resist the impulse to act, immediate hospitalization should be considered. The key issue here is that no contract can be made with the patient — he is 'non-contractible' in that he cannot or will not enter into an agreement to work with the physician and other care providers to address the current crisis. Hospitalization should also be considered when the physician suspects that the patient is 'pseudo-contractible' — when the patient's hopelessness is dramatic and his agreement to seek help appears to be an effort to put off the physician. Finally, if a patient presents immediately following an unsuccessful suicide attempt,

regardless of whether or not he is contractible, at least 24 hours of observation should be considered.

Some may question whether not only the high-risk patients described above but all patients who seriously consider suicide should be hospitalized. Indeed, before the days of managed care and national health-care programmes, suicidal patients were more readily hospitalized and spent longer periods of time in inpatient treatment than is the case today. This change is due not merely to fiscal attempts to decrease inpatient utilization but also to awareness that patients most often benefit from care provided in the least restrictive environment. Unfortunately, hospitalization carries the risk of possible iatrogenic effects [52,53]. For patients who can be managed on an outpatient basis, hospitalization creates an unnecessary social stigma: it can subtly communicate the belief that the patient is incapable of coping, which further assaults the patient's already beleaguered self-esteem. It can foster passivity and encourage some patients to resort to manipulative behaviours in order to gain readmission each time they feel the need to avoid conflict. In the absence of imminent risk, outpatient management of suicidal risk is usually preferable. When there is imminent danger of self-destructive behaviour, however, hospitalization is a critical intervention because it provides a secure environment within which treatment can be initiated.

If the physician determines that the suicidal risk does not warrant hospitalization, the next decision is whether the patient can be managed in a primary care setting or should be referred to a mental health professional. If a patient denies suicidal intent and does not display any of the risk factors listed in the preceding section, the risk of suicide is less imminent and often can be managed in a primary care setting as part of the treatment for depression or an anxiety disorder. Important considerations when making this decision, however, include the physician's level of comfort about managing suicidal risk and his or her availability to monitor closely any change in the risk of lethality.

Regardless of whether the physician decides to assume sole responsibility for the patient's treatment or to work in conjunction with a mental health professional, there are a number of treatment interventions critical for effective care.

Outline contingency plan
If a patient with suicidal ideation denies intent, it is important to remind him that if this situation changes (i.e. if he begins to consider suicide as a possible solution) he should let the physician

know immediately. Providing every patient with a 24-hour emergency telephone number and detailed instructions on steps to be taken if self-destructive impulses intensify not only serves as a valuable safeguard in the event of a crisis but also helps to underscore the physician's concern for the patient's well-being.

Secure the environment

If firearms are present in the home, the physician should encourage the patient to transfer them to a friend or relative for safe keeping. If the patient's plan is to overdose, removing or limiting lethal substances should be suggested. If the patient is not addicted and therefore not at risk of going into withdrawal, recommending abstention from alcohol can diminish the possibility of impulsive acting-out.

Mobilize support

The patient should be encouraged to avoid social isolation and to disclose his current circumstances to someone whom he trusts. The physician should obtain from the patient the name and telephone number of at least one friend or family member who can provide support in the event of a crisis. If the physician later suspects that the patient's condition is deteriorating, the friend or family member can provide valuable information and can be enlisted to help monitor the patient's behaviour until additional safeguards can be put in place.

Initiate pharmacotherapy

Pharmacotherapy is often a critical intervention for the suicidal patient, especially if a clinical depression is present. When treating suicidal patients, some physicians prescribe subclinical doses of antidepressants because they fear that the patient may try to overdose. Unfortunately, subclinical dosages often lack efficacy [54]. The use of selective serotonin re-uptake inhibitors (SSRIs) offers important advantages over tricyclic antidepressants. SSRIs are less toxic than tricyclics [55] and offer the additional advantage of having a more favourable tolerance profile. Because patients tend to experience fewer side effects on SSRIs, therapeutic levels can be achieved quickly, thereby allowing the patient to benefit more rapidly from the therapeutic action of the medication than is often the case with other antidepressant agents.

When SSRIs first became available, some researchers expressed concern that they might increase suicidal risk [56]. Sufficient data have subsequently emerged, however, to demonstrate that suicidal risk is not exacerbated by SSRI administration [57,58]; on the contrary, numerous studies have demonstrated that suicidal ideation decreases following administration of SSRIs [59].

If the patient fails to respond to an adequate trial of antidepressant medication, a psychiatric referral should be considered. The psychiatrist can assess indications for other treatment options, including alternative medications, thyroid hormones to augment medication effect, electroconvulsive therapy and phototherapy.

Consider referral for psychotherapy

Most suicidal patients can benefit from psychotherapy. Cognitive–behavioural therapy in particular has been shown to be effective in both the treatment of depression and the management of suicidal risk [60,61].

Co-ordinate care with other professionals

Even when another professional becomes involved in the care of a suicidal patient, the primary care provider often continues to participate in treatment, especially if the therapist is a non-physician. Ongoing communication between the physician and therapist will be important for monitoring the patient's progress and co-ordinating care.

Redirect the patient's thinking

Perhaps the most important message for a patient to hear in the midst of a crisis is that there is hope. Challenging the magnitude or importance of the patient's problems is not effective — it will not alter the patient's interest in dying and will only make it easier to dismiss the physician as being uncaring and uninformed. Instead, the following points need to be made to the patient:

- The physician is aware that the patient is struggling;
- Suicidal thinking is symptomatic of an underlying psychiatric problem that requires treatment;
- Effective treatment exists;
- The most dangerous aspect of a suicidal crisis is that the person concerned is temporarily blinded from seeing any hope for the future;
- The vast majority of people who survive a suicidal attempt are later thankful that they survived. They readily admit that, in time, the world and their problems can look very different.

Continue to monitor risk

It is important to note that initial improvement of a patient's depression does not necessarily mean a diminution of suicidal risk. In some cases, the risk of suicidal behaviour is greatest when a patient first shows improvement in his depressive symptoms. The improved mood can be due to the patient finally making the decision to die — the improved affect is a reflection of the peace that comes at the conclusion of a tortuous decision-making process. After making the decision, all that is left for the patient to do is to put his affairs in order and then carry out his plan. In other cases, there can be legitimate — albeit tenuous — improvement early in treatment but, in the face of new disappointments or failure, these gains can crumble and the patient can drop into an even deeper despair. Ongoing assessment, therefore, even after initial signs of improvement, is essential.

Conclusions

Because of differences in social scripting and biological makeup, men are three to four times more likely than women to commit suicide. Because almost 50% of people who commit suicide will visit a physician within 4 weeks of their death, physicians are in a unique position to reduce the incidence of suicide. By developing a further understanding of self-destructive behaviour, physicians can better identify suicidal patients, assess their risk of lethality and determine the appropriate level of care.

Acknowledgements

The author gratefully acknowledges helpful comments and suggestions from C. Edward Coffey, MD, and Richard Heavenrich, PhD.

References

1. United States Department of Commerce. Statistical Abstract of the United States, 116th edn. Washington, DC: US Government Printing Office, 1996: 94–102
2. Berman AL. Self-destructive behavior and suicide: epidemiology and taxonomy. In: Roberts AR (ed) Self-destructive behavior. Springfield, IL: Charles C. Thomas, 1975: 5–20
3. Lineham M, Laffaw J. Suicidal behaviors among clients at an outpatient psychology clinic versus the general population. *Suicide Life Threat Behav* 1982; 12: 234–239
4. Moscicki EK, O'Carroll P, Reiger DA *et al.* Suicide attempts in the Epidemiologic Catchment Area Study. *Yale J Biol Med* 1988; 61: 259–268
5. Jacobson J, Jacobson DM. Suicide in Brighton. *Br J Psychiatry* 1972; 121: 369–377
6. Diekstra RF. The epidemiology of suicide and parasuicide. *Acta Psychiatr Scand* 1993; 371: 9–20
7. Pfeffer CR. The family system of suicidal children. *Am J Psychother* 1981; 35: 330–341
8. Green AH. Self destructive behavior in battered children. *Am J Psychiatry* 1978; 135: 579–582
9. Gould MS, Shaffer MD, Fisher P *et al.* The clinical prediction of adolescent suicide. In: Maris RW, Berman AL *et al.* (eds) Assessment and prediction of suicide. New York: Guilford, 1992: 130–143
10. Bukstein OG, Brent DA, Perper JA *et al.* Risk factors for completed suicide among adolescents with a lifetime history of substance abuse: a case–control study. *Acta Psychiatr Scand* 1993; 88: 403–408
11. Robbins D, Conroy RC. A cluster of adolescent suicide attempts: is suicide contagious? *J Adolesc Health Care* 1983; 3: 253–255
12. Shaffer D, Garland A, Gould M *et al.* Preventing teenage suicide: A critical review. *J Am Acad Child Adolesc Psychiatry* 1988; 27: 675–687
13. Butler RN, Lewis MI, Sunderland T. Aging and mental health: positive psychosocial and biomedical approaches, 4th edn. New York: Macmillan, 1991
14. Gatter K, Bowen D. A study of suicide autopsies 1957–1977. *Med Sci Law* 1980; 20: 37–47
15. Stack S. New micro level data on the impact of divorce on suicide, 1959–1980: a test of two theories. *J Marr Fam* 1990; 52, 119–127
16. Osgood NJ, Brant BA, Lipman A. Suicide among the elderly in long term care facilities. New York: Greenwood Press, 1991
17. La Vecchia C, Lucchini F, Levi F. Worldwide trends in suicide mortality, 1955–1989. *Acta Psychiatr Scand* 1994; 90: 53–64
18. Burvill PW, Woodings TL, Stenhous NS *et al.* Suicide during 1961–70 migrants to Australia. *Psychol Med* 1982; 12: 29–308
19. Kellerman AL, Rivara FP, Somes G *et al.* Suicide in the home in relation to gun ownership. *N Engl J Med* 1992; 327: 467–472
20. Litman RE. Suicide as acting out. In: Shneidman ES, Farberow NL, Litman RE (eds) The psychology of suicide. New York: Science House, 1970: 293–304
21. Kreitman N. Parasuicide. London: John Wiley and Sons, 1977
22. Murphy G. Suicide and attempted suicide. In: Michaels R (ed) Psychiatry. Philadelphia: J.B. Lippincott, 1985: 1–15
23. Berlin I. Suicide among American Indian adolescents: an overview. *Suicide Life Threat Behavior* 1987; 17: 218–232
24. Sainsbury P. The epidemiology of suicide. In: Roy A (ed) Suicide. Baltimore: Williams and Wilkins, 1986; 181–195
25. Whitlock FA. Suicide and physical illness. In: Roy A (ed) Suicide. Baltimore: Williams and Wilkins, 1986; 151–170

26. Monk M. Epidemiology for suicide. *Epidemiol Rev* 1987; 9: 51–69

27. Smith JC, Mercy JA, Conn JM. Marital status and the risk of suicide. *Am J Public Health* 1988; 78: 78–80

28. Boxer PA, Burnett C, Swanson N. Suicide and occupation: a review of the literature. *J Occup Environ Med* 1995; 37(4): 442–452

29. Martin WT. Religiosity and United States suicide rates, 1972–1978. *J Clin Psychol* 1984; 40(5): 1166–1169

30. Conroy RW, Smith K. Family loss and hospital suicide. *Suicide Life Threat Behav* 1983; 13: 179–194

31. Black DW, Winokur G. Prospective studies of suicide and mortality in psychiatric patients. *Ann N Y Acad Sci* 1986; 487: 106–113

32. Kreitman N. The clinical assessment and management of the suicidal patient. In: Roy A (ed) Suicide. Baltimore: Williams and Wilkins, 1986: 181–195

33. Drake RE, Gates C, Cotton PG. Suicide among schizophrenics: a review. *Compr Psychiatry* 1985; 26: 90–100

34. Hirchfeld RMA. Etiology, diagnosis and course of panic disorder. 17th CINP Congress, Kyoto, Japan

35. Alcohol, Drug Abuse and Mental Health Administration. Alcohol and Health: Fifth Special Report to the US Congress. Serial # 017-024-01199-1. Washington DC: US Government Printing Office, 1983

36. Schuckit MA. Primary men alcoholics with histories of suicide attempts. *J Stud Alcohol* 1986; 47: 78–81

37. Egeland J, Sussex J. Suicide and family loadings for affective disorders. *JAMA* 1985; 254: 915–918

38. Tsuang M. Risk of suicide in the relatives of schizophrenics, manics, depressives, and controls. *J Clin Psychiatry* 1983; 44: 396–400

39. Roy A, Segal N, Centerwall B *et al.* Suicide in twins. *Arch Gen Psychiatry* 1991; 48: 29–32

40. Asberg M, Traskman L, Thoren P. 5HIAA in the CSF: a biochemical suicide predictor. *Arch Gen Psychiatry* 1976; 33: 1193–1197

41. Traskman L, Asberg M, Bertilsson L, Sjostrand L. Monoamine metabolites in CSF and suicidal behavior. *Arch Gen Psychiatry* 1981; 38: 631–636

42. Stanley M, Mann J, Cohen S. Serotonin and serotonergic receptors in suicide. In: Mann J, Stanley M (eds) Psychobiology of suicidal behavior. New York: New York Academy of Science Annals, 1986: 122–127

43. Archer J. The influence of testosterone on human aggression. *Br J Psychol* 1991; 82: 1–28

44. Harvard Medical School. Suicide — Part I. *Harv Ment Health Lett* 1996; 13(5): 1–5

45. Murphy G. The physician's responsibility for suicide, II: Errors of omission. *Ann Intern Med* 1975; 82: 305–309

46. Barraclough B, Bunch J, Nelson B *et al.* A hundred cases of suicide: clinical aspects. *Br J Psychiatry* 1974; 125: 355–373

47. Van Casteren V, Van der Vekan J, Tafforeau J *et al.* Suicide and attempted suicide reported by general practitioners in Belgium, 1990–1991. *Acta Psychiatr Scand* 1993; 87: 451–455

48. Rutz W, Von Knorring L, Walinder W. Frequency of suicide on Gotland after systematic postgraduate education of general practitioners. *Acta Psychiatr Scand* 1989; 80: 151–154

49. Lish JD. Suicide screening in a primary care setting at a Veterans' Affairs medical center. *Psychosomatics* 1996; 37: 413–424

50. Dowart RA, Chartock L. Suicide: A public health perspective. In: Jacobs D, Brown H (eds) Suicide — understanding and responding. Madison, CN: International University Press Inc., 1989: 41

51. Roy A. Risk factors for suicide in psychiatric patients. *Arch Gen Psychiatry* 1982; 39: 1089–1095

52. Zinberg NE. The threat of suicide in psychotherapy. In: Jacobs D, Brown H (eds) Suicide — understanding and responding. Madison, CN: International University Press Inc., 1989: 295–325

53. Litman RE. Predicting and preventing hospital and clinic suicides. In: Maris RW, Berman AL *et al.* (eds) Assessment and prediction of suicide. New York: Guilford, 1992: 448–466

54. Isacsson G, Boethius G, Bergman U. Low level of antidepressant prescription for people who later commit suicide: 15 years of experience from a population-based drug database in Sweden. *Acta Psychiatr Scand* 1992; 85: 444–448

55. Andrews JM, Nemeroff CB. Contemporary management of depression. *Am J Med* 1994; 67: 24–32

56. Fava M, Rosenbaum JF. Suicidality and fluoxetine: is there a relationship? *J Clin Psychiatry* 1991; 52: 108–111

57. Beasley CM Jr, Dornseif BE, Bosomworth JC *et al.* Fluoxetine and suicide: a meta-analysis of controlled trials of treatment for depression. *Br Med J* 1991; 303: 685–692

58. Montgomery SA, Dunner DL, Dunbar GC. Reduction of suicidal thoughts with paroxetine in comparison with reference antidepressants and placebo. *Eur Neuropsychopharmacol* 1995; 5: 513

59. Mann JJ, Kapur S. The emergence of suicidal ideation and behavior during antidepressant pharmacotherapy. *Arch Gen Psychiatry* 1991; 48: 1027–1033

60. Ellis T. Toward a cognitive therapy for suicidal individuals. *Prof Psychol Theory Res* 1986; 17: 125–130

61. Lineham M. Dialectical behavior therapy: a cognitive behavioral approach to parasuicide. *J Pers Assess* 1987; 1: 328–333

CHAPTER 17

Office treatment and prevention of common sports injuries

J. B. Ryan

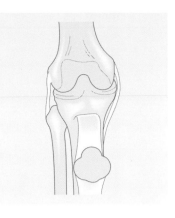

Introduction

This chapter details the various types of common sports injuries that can occur and how they are diagnosed and treated following presentation to an office practice in the USA.

Injuries to the pelvis, hip and thigh

Anatomy

The pelvis is composed of several large flattened bones jointed anteriorly at the symphysis pubis and posteriorly at the sacro-iliac joints, firmly attaching the lower extremities to the spine (Fig. 17.1). The pelvis supports the abdominal contents and back and abdominal musculature, and is an intricate component of locomotion, being the origin of many of the muscles of the lower extremity. The hip joint is a ball-and-socket joint. The femur (thigh bone) is the longest bone in the body and has a thickened cortical wall in response to the forces placed through this region. The biceps femoris, semitendinosus, semimembranosus, gracilis and rectus femoris muscles have origins and insertions in the lower extremity that cross both the hip joint and the knee joint.

Epidemiology

A study of sports injuries in 4551 athletes indicated that pelvis, hip and thigh injuries accounted for 6.2% of cases [1], 4.6% being in male and 1.6% in female athletes. Contact and collision sports were associated with most injuries to the pelvis and thigh. Stress fractures of the femur, although rare, are seen in military recruits. The cumulative incidence of femoral stress fractures is between 2.8 and 3.5% of all fractures reported in all athletes. The incidence of stress fractures in female athletes with eating disorders or history of amenorrhoea is 2–3 times higher than in male athletes [2,3]. Muscle strains are common (7–12% of injuries) in the thigh because of the forces involved and number of muscles crossing the hip and knee joint [4]. Hamstring strains are twice as common as quadriceps strains and there are no gender differences in hamstring injuries.

Initial presentation

Pain over the iliac crest may represent an avulsion of the abdominal musculature, avulsion of the iliac hypophysis in teenagers or haematoma from local bleeding following a contusion of the iliac crest with the ground or hard surface. Anterior hip pain (inguinal pain) may indicate a femoral neck stress fracture, inguinal hernia, inflammation of the iliopsoas bursa, or a groin strain. Lateral hip pain may occur with proximal snapping of the iliotibial band over the greater trochanter, greater trochanteric bursitis, or bone contusion. Posterior hip pain may involve contusion to the ischial tuberosity, avulsion of proximal hamstring muscle or irritation to the sciatic nerve.

Physical examination and diagnostic tests

The presence of a large subcutaneous haematoma in the area of the iliac crest or posterior thigh indicates a bony avulsion or significant tearing of the musculotendinous junction (Fig. 17.2). The hip should be placed through a full and normal range of motion, first active then passive. Muscle strength in flexion, extension, adduction and abduction should be quantified. Occasionally, injuries in or around the pelvis can present as distal thigh pain or knee pain. By checking hip motion and strength, pelvic pathology can be identified as the source of this referred knee pain. Routine radiographs in the anteroposterior (AP) and lateral planes of the pelvis, hip and thigh will identify most traumatic injuries. Magnetic resonance imaging (MRI) of the soft tissue musculature has proved to be successful in localizing

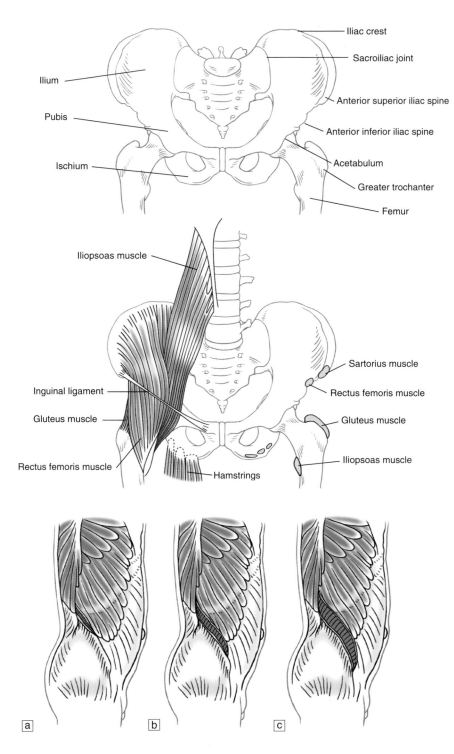

Figure 17.1. *Anterior view of the pelvis and hip illustrating bony structures (top) and muscle attachments (bottom).*

Iliac crest

Sacroiliac joint

Ilium

Anterior superior iliac spine

Pubis

Anterior inferior iliac spine

Ischium

Acetabulum

Greater trochanter

Femur

Iliopsoas muscle

Sartorius muscle

Rectus femoris muscle

Inguinal ligament

Gluteus muscle

Gluteus muscle

Rectus femoris muscle

Iliopsoas muscle

Hamstrings

Figure 17.2. *Degrees of detachment of the aponeurosis at the iliac crest: (a) mild (first degree), a small tear; (b) moderate (second degree), an appreciable tear with bare bone exposed; and (c) severe (third degree) avulsion of the caput.*

a b c

muscle tears; however, treatment and outcome are rarely affected by this diagnostic test [5].

Treatment and prevention
Contusions of the bony prominences of the pelvis are treated with ice, rest and gradual return to sports. Quadriceps contusions should initially be immobilized in patient-tolerated knee flexion (90–120 degrees) as soon as possible after the injury [6]. Rehabilitation should include gradual return of active motion, avoiding any additional soft tissue bleeding. Athletes may return to activity following complete return of range of motion and strength, but should be protected with extra padding for 6 months to avoid a second injury to the region. Occasionally, calcification forms in the region of the haematoma (myositis ossificans), limiting the return of range of motion and

strength. Patients with myositis ossificans should be referred to the orthopaedic department for serial evaluation.

Avulsion injury of the iliac crest, ilium, pubic ramus, ischial tuberosity, or the greater or lesser tuberosity of the femur should be referred for orthopaedic consultation. The vast majority of these injuries are treated non-operatively; however, if there is significant bony avulsion and displacement of the bony fragment, operative reattachment can be considered.

Muscle strains are quite common in the pelvis and thigh region. Initial treatment includes ice, compressive elastic wrap and rest. Ambulation with crutches may be necessary initially. As tenderness resolves, gradual pain-free stretching may begin. Full range of motion and muscle strength should be present prior to any return to sports. Evidence of early degenerative arthritis should prompt referral for orthopaedic consultation. Inflammation to the soft tissue in the regions of the greater trochanteric bursa and the iliopsoas bursa is common (bursitis); however, traumatic injuries or stress fractures must be ruled out. Once the diagnosis of an inflamed bursa is made, treatment is usually with anti-inflammatory medications (NSAIDs), rest and partial weight bearing.

Prevention of injuries to the pelvis, hip, and thigh is sports specific. Collision or contact sports require appropriate padding to bony prominences. Overuse injuries can be prevented by muscle stretching and appropriate warm-up in activities.

Knee injuries

Anatomy

The curved bicondylar distal portion of the femur articulates with the proximal flat plateau of the tibia stabilized by ligaments that allow flexion, extension inward, outward motion and inward and outward rotation (Fig. 17.3). The medial and lateral menisci of the knee provide cushioning between the femur and tibia and also stability. The patella articulates with the anterior femur in a groove and is stabilized by capsular ligamentous and muscle attachments. The patella provides a mechanical aid for the quadriceps musculature as it crosses the knee and is distally attached to the patellar tendon.

Epidemiology

Knee injuries comprise 6% of all injuries to the extremities presenting to emergency rooms [7]. In skiing, 30% of all injuries involve the knee; 16%

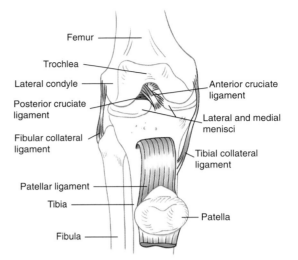

Figure 17.3. *Formation of the knee joint from the articulation of the condyles of the femur with the condyles of the tibia.*

involve damage to the anterior cruciate ligament and 18% involve damage to the medial collateral ligament [8]. There is a higher incidence of female than male injuries in basketball and soccer, especially of injury to the anterior cruciate ligament [9]. Overuse injuries to the knee presenting to the primary care physician include tendinitis (20%), apophysitis (10%) and joint cartilage injuries (10%) [10].

Frequently, athletes with knee injuries can pinpoint the exact location of pain, which should then be correlated with underlying pathology. Ligament structures can be painful at the area of failure or partial failure (Fig. 17.4). These structures should be palpated at their origins on the femur or tibia and throughout the substance of the ligament. Although joint-line tenderness has been shown not to be diagnostic of meniscal tears, it may indicate irritation of the synovial lining of the knee, consistent with underlying meniscal tears and articular cartilage damage. Muscle tendons attaching in the region of the knee medially (gracilis, semimembranosus, sartorius and semitendinosus) and laterally (biceps femoris) are occasionally associated with overuse tendon pain (tendinosis). Inflammation in the region of the medial hamstring (bursa) can promote pain.

A twisting injury to the knee can occasionally cause tearing of the intraarticular structures (anterior cruciate ligament, posterior cruciate ligament, meniscus) (Fig. 17.5) or shearing fractures of the joint surface and subchondral bone (osteochondral fractures), resulting in rapid onset, large, tense effusions of the knee secondary to local bleeding

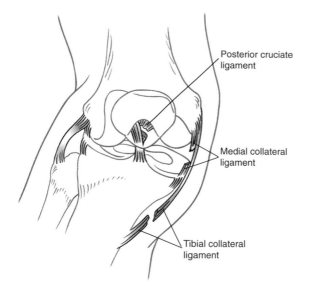

Figure 17.4. *Multiple disruptions of the ligamentous structures due to sudden external forces.*

into the joint. These acute effusions (haemorrhagic) should alert the examiner to significant injuries.

Occasionally, athletes have gradual onset of swelling, which is probably due to irritation of the synovial lining associated with degenerative arthritis, chronic instability or tears to the menisci in the avascular region (central two-thirds). Loss of motion of the knee may be due to swelling, which makes the joint capsule tense and gives the patient the sensation of a tight balloon. Swelling in the anterior knee limiting full flexion may be caused by acute haemorrhage into the prepatellar bursa. Limitation of flexion may also be due to swelling inside the knee. Occasionally there is a mechanical block to extension or flexion caused by a torn, trapped meniscus. Some athletes present with intermittent locking or decreased range of motion that is relieved by wiggling the knee, followed by periods of normal activity. These finding are most suggestive of a torn meniscus or loose body.

Significant ligament injuries can be caused by direct blows to the knee or non-contact injuries. Direct lateral blows to the knee can injure the medial collateral ligament and the anterior cruciate ligament. Direct anterior blows most frequently injure the posterior cruciate ligament. Direct medial blows to the knee cause injury to the lateral collateral ligament. Planting the foot and cutting vigorously without any contact can occasionally cause injury to the anterior cruciate ligament. Patients with this presentation frequently feel a 'pop' in the knee followed by a large effusion. Athletes occasionally complain of instability of the kneecap, most frequently associated with lateral subluxation or dislocation of the kneecap. This can be due to direct blunt trauma or to muscle contracture during vigorous activity. Manual or spontaneous reduction allows return of motion and is frequently associated with the tenderness and swelling in the region of the partial or compete capsular tear in a patellofemoral joint.

Physical examination of the knee

The knee should be scrutinized for areas of ecchymosis and swelling. It should be determined whether the swelling is extra-articular (outside the knee joint, traumatic prepatellar bursitis), Baker's cyst in the posterior aspect of the knee, meniscal cyst in the medial or lateral area of the knee, or in the pes bursa. Intra-articular effusions cause the patella to float away from the anterior aspect of the femur and are best tested by feeling if the patella is floating anterior to the femur. The range of motion of the knee should be checked: even a small intra-articular effusion will prevent the knee from coming into full extension when compared with the

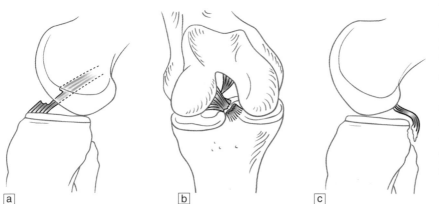

Figure 17.5. *Tibial attachments of the anterior and posterior cruciate ligaments in relationship to the synovial cavity: (a) partial tear of the anterior cruciate ligament; (b) mop-end tear of the anterior cruciate ligament; (c) bony avulsion of the posterior cruciate ligament.*

opposite side. Holding the feet by the heels and placing the great toes at the same level allows the examiner to determine the extension of both knees. If one knee is higher than the other, there is a flexion contracture or limitation to extension on that side indicative of an effusion or mechanical block to full extension. While placing the patient with both hips and knees at 90 degrees of flexion and supporting the heels, the physician will note sagging of the tibia when looking at the tibia tubercle if the posterior cruciate is torn. Flexing the knee to 30 degrees and attempting to translate the tibia anteriorly on the femur (Lackman test) is the best test for anterior cruciate stability.

Muscle strength of the major extensors and flexors of the knee is tested to rule out strain injuries. If the patient is not able to extend the knee actively from a flexed position and there is anterior knee pain, injury to the quadriceps mechanism must not be ruled out: the quadriceps tendon can be torn proximal to the patella and the patellar tendon can be ruptured from the tibial tubercle or the distal pole of the patella, or the tendon may be ruptured in its mid-substance. Palpation in the region proximal and distal to the patella will indicate the most likely cause. Palpation in and around the knee, associated with tenderness, must be correlated with underlying anatomy and pathological processes.

Diagnostic radiography can frequently demonstrate fractures, loose bodies and degenerative arthritis. Ultrasonography has been demonstrated to diagnose tendinous injuries to the quadriceps mechanism accurately and is economical. Although MRI studies accurately demonstrate soft tissue and bone injuries in and about the knee, several studies have demonstrated that history and physical diagnosis can accurately pinpoint acute and chronic problems in and around the knee. Before MRI of the knee is requested, orthopaedic consultation should be considered.

Treatment and prevention

Patients presenting with acutely swollen and painful knees should receive a thorough history and physical examination, along with routine radiographs. Aspiration of the effusion may demonstrate blood or yellow synovial fluid. Acute haemarthrosis of the knee indicates significant traumatic injury and has been shown to be associated with treatable interarticular pathology. These patients should be considered for orthopaedic consultation. Most injuries can be treated with a compressive dressing and crutch ambulation. Occasionally, splinting with a removable brace or knee immobilizer for the patient's

comfort is appropriate. If the aspiration demonstrates clear synovial fluid, consideration can be given to a single dose of corticosteroid to decrease the synovial inflammation. If symptoms persist or swelling recurs, orthopaedic consultation should be obtained to rule out meniscal pathology, condylar flap tears of the hyaline cartilage, or early degenerative changes of the hyaline cartilage not demonstrated on routine radiography.

If, during the course of the physical examination, the patient is found to have acute instability of the anterior, posterior, medial or lateral collateral ligament, appropriate consultation should be obtained. Initial treatment is primarily directed to comfort the patient, with immobilization with a removable splint and protected ambulation. Younger, more active patients or athletes committed to returning to collision, contact, or high-energy sports frequently require reconstruction following acute knee injuries. Chronic instability, if symptomatic, should also be considered as an indication for reconstruction. Isolated medial collateral ligament injuries frequently require only symptomatic treatment. In patients with markedly swollen knees with two or more major ligament injuries, a partial knee dislocation should be suspected and treated urgently.

Anterior knee pain can be due to repetitive microtrauma to the patellar tendon associated with degenerative changes of the tendon. Treatment is primarily palliative with non-steroidal anti-inflammatory drugs (NSAIDs) and rest. Ultrasonography may demonstrate areas of degenerative tissue in the inner substance of the tendon. If symptoms do not resolve, consultation with an orthopaedic surgeon is appropriate. Occasionally, these areas of degenerative change can be excised and symptoms resolved (Fig. 17.6).

Patellofemoral pain is usually due to an imbalance of the quadriceps muscle strength and hyperpronation of the foot. Muscle training and rehabilitation are the keystone of treatment. Occasionally, arch supports preventing hyperpronation of the foot can be beneficial in partially relieving symptoms. A prolonged rehabilitation programme should be undertaken before consideration of surgical intervention.

Instability of the patellofemoral joint is more frequently treated with immobilization and rehabilitation. Acute or chronic quadriceps tendon or patellar tendon (ligament) ruptures require immediate orthopaedic consultation. The vast majority of these injuries require surgical reattachment to ensure maximal return of quadriceps function. Patients with degenerative arthritis of

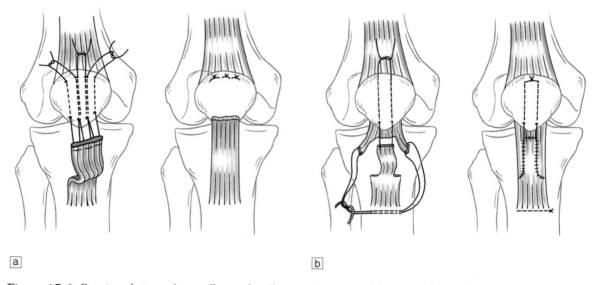

Figure 17.6. *Repair techniques for patellar tendon (ligament) rupture: (a) neat avulsion of entire tendon from the inferior patella; (b) technique for repair of more irregular rupture within the body of the tendon.*

the knee who do not respond to appropriate treatment with anti-inflammatory medications and rehabilitation should be considered for consultation to identify problems treatable by diagnostic arthroscopy, anatomical realignment or total joint replacement.

Prevention of knee injuries is controversial. In a prospective randomized study of intramural football players playing eight-man contact football, knee injuries were reduced by the use of a lateral knee brace in a population of athletes averaging under 180 lb ($\approx$81 kg) [11]. Additional research is necessary to demonstrate the effectiveness of this brace in larger individuals. Many sports have instituted rule changes to prevent intentional blows to the knee. Patellar instability has been treated in the past with bracing and taping.

Injuries of the leg, foot and ankle

Anatomy

The leg, foot and ankle are uniquely designed to provide shock absorption and propulsion during jumping, walking and running. The tibia and fibula articulate with the ankle joint at the talus. In the proximal half of the leg, the muscle bellies are ensheathed by firm connective tissue creating four muscle compartments. The ankle is stabilized medially and laterally by firm ligamentous attachments. In addition, the distal articulations of the tibia and fibula are stabilized by the anterior and posterior tibio/fibular ligament. The mid-

foot and forefoot are firmly reinforced by ligamentous structures that support the concave arch of the foot (Fig. 17.7). Leg muscles that are attached to the foot provide plantar flexion, dorsiflexion and inward (inversion) and outward (eversion) movement.

Epidemiology

Ankle sprains are the most common sports-related injury. In a population of 4000 cadets, over 400 ankle sprains were experienced annually; the vast majority of these were inversion injuries causing damage to the lateral ligamentous structure [12]. Over 95% were mild or moderate sprains. In 14% of tendon injuries the ankle is involved, with injuries to the Achilles tendon (24%), anterior tibial muscle (7%), posterior tibial tendon (3%) and flexor hallucis longus (2%).

Fractures in the lower extremities involving the tibia, fibula, ankle and metatarsals accounted for 40% of all fractures in a male population of college, professional, high-school and recreational athletes [1]. Women have a slightly higher incidence of tibial and metatarsal fractures, especially associated with eating disorders and amenorrhoea [2]. No gender differences in acute ankle injuries or acute traumatic fractures in the lower extremities have been recorded.

Initial presentation

Pain in the leg, ankle and foot must be correlated with the underlying anatomy. Diffuse leg pain along the anterior shin is indicative of 'shin

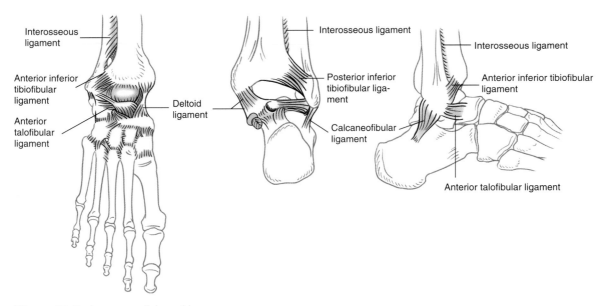

Figure 17.7. *Anatomy of the ankle.*

splints'. Aching pain in the muscle and leg, especially with activity, may indicate exertional compartment syndrome. Isolated pinpoint tenderness in the area of the leg may represent a localized stress fracture. Pain, especially in the region of the musculotendinous junction of the gastrocnemius and soleus, is consistent with a partial tear of the fibres. Chronic pain localized to the anterior ankle is most likely to be due to synovitis, associated either with old scar tissue or with early or advanced degenerative arthritis.

Medial or lateral ankle pain directly over ligaments usually indicates a lateral ligament injury. Inversion (turning foot and ankle inward) injuries stretch or tear the anterior talofibular and calcaneofibular ligament. External rotation injuries of the ankle cause sprains to the medial ligament (deltoid ligament) and the syndesmosis. Overactivity or abnormal underlying biomechanics of the foot can lead to insertional pain of tendons in the region of the calcaneus (Achilles tendon), midfoot (posterior tibialis and anterior tibial tendons) or lateral foot (peroneal brevis tendon). Lateral foot pain in the region of the base of the fifth metatarsal may be due to a partial tendon avulsion or a stress fracture (Jones). Gradual onset of pain is more indicative of overuse injury and stress fracture than acute pain associated with a traumatic event.

Occasionally, patients present with chronic instability (giving way) of the ankle associated with recurrent episodes of ankle sprains. Patients have difficulty in walking on uneven terrain because the foot cannot accommodate to the changing angle. Some ankle pain may be due to subluxation of the tendons around the lateral or medial malleolus.

Acute tendon ruptures can occur in and around the leg, foot and ankle and often are associated with running or jumping sports. Athletes present with the complaint that something 'snapped' in their leg, with localized pain, and weakness in plantar flexion (Achilles tendon rupture) (Fig. 17.8). Similar complaints can be

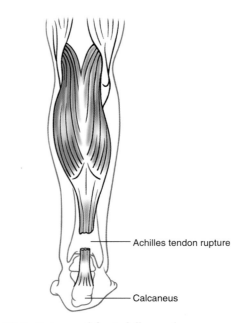

Figure 17.8. *Rupture of the Achilles tendon.*

203

present with injuries to the anterior or posterior tibial tendon. The anterior tibial tendon causes decreased strength in dorsiflexion, whereas damage to the posterior tibial tendon causes decreased ability to turn the foot inward and the appearance of loss of the physiologic arch (traumatic flat foot); injury to the peroneal tendons causes decreased ability to turn the foot outward.

Physical examination

Physical examination of the leg, ankle and foot initially begins with observation and inspection. Areas of ecchymosis are noted along with areas of increased swelling and maximal tenderness. With the patient prone, squeezing the mid-calf causes plantar flexion of the foot (Thompson squeeze test); if this is absent, then the Achilles tendon is probably torn. With active muscle testing, tenderness along the entire anterior aspect of the tibia indicates possible periosteal irritation secondary to shin splints. A localized tenderness in the tibia or foot is much more likely to be due to stress fracture. Occasionally, there is tenderness over the medial aspect of the foot in the region of the great toe tarso/metatarsal joint, consistent with a bunion. A similar process can occur in the lateral aspect of the foot at the junction of the tarsometatarsal joint of the small toe (Taylor's bunion). A bunion is due to a bursal swelling and irritation over the region of the bony prominence. Swelling along any tendon sheath may indicate irritation of the tendon secondary to partial injury or localizing stenosing tenosynovitis. Plantar pain can be associated with irritation of the thick subcutaneous tissue (plantar fasciitis), causing pain over the entire plantar aspect of the foot starting with the distal tip of the calcaneus.

Radiographic evaluation of the leg, ankle and foot require AP, lateral and, occasionally, oblique views of the ankle for optimum visualization of the bone and joint surfaces. Rarely is advanced diagnostic study warranted for common leg, ankle and foot injuries.

Treatment and prevention

The vast majority of leg, ankle and foot problems are due to overtraining. Suspected stress fractures are initially treated with decreased activity and protected ambulation. If symptoms do not improve, additional studies to include repeat radiographs every 3 weeks are warranted. Diffuse muscular leg pain, especially associated with running, may be due to high compartment pressures in the region of the muscle bellies associated with decreased blood flow in the small nutrient blood vessels (exertional compartment syndrome). Treatment again consists of decreased activity. Referral is necessary if symptoms do not resolve.

Complete rupture of any musculotendinous unit in the leg, ankle or foot requires consultation with an orthopaedic surgeon. A first-time ankle sprain is best treated with compression, ice and elevation, followed by rigorous physiotherapy. Taping and bracing can be beneficial. If symptoms of instability persist (recurrent sprains, giving way on uneven terrain), referral is warranted. Pain in the area of the plantar fascia is initially treated with anti-inflammatory medication. Arch supports may be beneficial in reducing symptoms. If symptoms persist for more than 3–6 months, consultation should be obtained.

Most spurs in the region of the Achilles tendon insertion on the posterior aspect of the calcaneus and the undersurface of the calcaneus are associated with bursitis. These complaints are treated symptomatically with NSAIDs. Corticosteroid injection should be avoided in this region because of significant complications. Symptomatic relief can be obtained with heel cups and shoe modification. If symptoms persist for more than 6 months, referral is necessary.

Prevention of injuries to the leg, ankle and lower extremities primarily involves training techniques. Adequate stretching and warm-up should be allowed; cross-training activities to rest overused areas is also encouraged. Acute ankle sprains can be prevented by the use of ankle braces and semi-rigid bimalleolar orthotics.

Shoulder injuries

Anatomy

The shoulder is a complex musculoskeletal unit. The scapula articulates with the chest wall and the clavicle, stabilized by muscles. The humerus firmly articulates with the glenoid of the scapula through the capsular ligaments (Fig. 17.9). The acromioclavicular joint has anterior, superior and inferior ligaments. The clavicle is also secured to the scapula by the coracoclavicular ligaments. The glenohumeral capsule acts as a hammock to support the humerus in the shallow glenoid. The ligaments of this joint are designed to prevent anterior, inferior and posterior translation primarily. The musculature of the glenohumeral joint is in two layers: the rotator cuff muscles (teres minor, infraspinatus, supraspinatus and subscapularis) glide underneath the arch of the acromion and attempt to keep the humeral head centred in the glenoid: the large deltoid provides gross motor function for the arm in forward flexion, abduction, adduction and extension.

Epidemiology

In football, 10% of injuries are localized to the shoulder. Athletes younger than 35 years present primarily with instability, whereas those above 35 years of age present with complaints associated with degenerative changes of the rotator cuff (Fig. 17.10), acromioclavicular joint and glenohumeral joint. There are no well-documented studies indicating a gender difference in shoulder pain or instability, although women do have a greater incidence of increased joint laxity.

Initial presentation

A patient under the age of 35 complaining of pain with activity must be evaluated for underlying instability with secondary irritation of the subacro-

mial region or rotator cuff. Patients over the age of 35, without history of previous shoulder instability, should be evaluated for degenerative changes of rotator cuff tendon, subacromial bursitis, and acromioclavicular and glenohumeral arthrosis.

Indirect force applied through the upper extremity (e.g. a fall on an outstretched hand) can injure the acromioclavicular ligament, without placing stress on the coracoclavicular ligament (Fig. 17.11). Falling directly on the tip of the shoulder can cause acute pain and elevation of the distal clavicle. Some athletes present with acute, traumatic glenohumeral instability; such patients should be immobilized for three weeks following reduction of the shoulder joint. Some athletes present with recurrent instability. Shoulder laxity that is gradual in onset, and not associated with an isolated traumatic event, is associated with multidirectional instability (anterior, inferior and posterior). Vague diffuse shoulder pain and lateral arm pain can be associated with referred pain from a subacromial inflammation of the bursa or injury to the rotator cuff muscles. Some athletes present with a decreased range of motion that may be associated with a traumatic event. These patients should be evaluated for early adhesive capsulitis, which is an inflammatory process involving the anterior and superior aspect of the shoulder, increased scar formation and decreasing range of motion. Clicking or locking, with range of motion of the shoulder may be associated with a tear of the glenoid labrum or partial tear of the biceps tendon.

Physical examination

Patients should be asked to pinpoint where the pain is maximal, to facilitate appropriate correla-

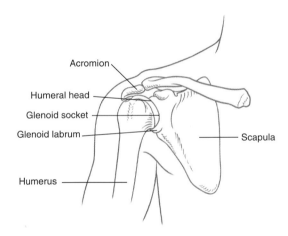

Figure 17.9. *The glenohumeral joint.*

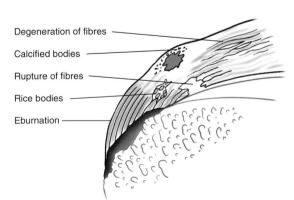

Figure 17.10. *Differential rotator cuff changes.*

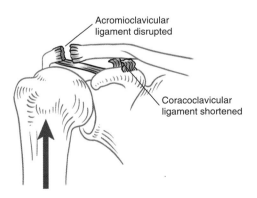

Figure 17.11. *Displacement of the acromion superiorly from the clavicle by an indirect force applied through the upper extremity.*

tion to underlying pathology. The patient's active and passive range of motion should be documented in forward flexion, abduction, and internal and external rotation at 0 degrees of abduction and 90 degrees of abduction (Fig. 17.12). The patient should demonstrate the maximal capacity for touching the spinous processes by placing the hand over the affected shoulder and behind the back. This scratch test can be compared with the opposite unaffected side, demonstrating the limitation of forward flexion, extension and internal rotation. Tenderness in the region of the acromioclavicular joint may indicate acute ligamentous sprain. Instability is tested in the anterior plane by abduction and external rotation of the arm and with anterior pressure applied to the humerus. The examiner is warned that this manoeuvre can cause acute dislocation if performed too vigorously. Posterior instability is tested with the patient supine with the arm forward-flexed to 90 degrees and with gentle posterior pressure applied to the arm. Passive forward flexion of the humerus may demonstrate pain (Neer test) associated with

subacromial pathology (bursitis, rotator cuff problems).

Radiographic evaluation of the shoulder should rule out any chronic unreduced dislocation. Because of the orientation in the acromioclavicular joint, a special AP view is obtained with the tube of the radiographic equipment oriented 10 degrees cephalad (Zanca view). Ultrasound is a valuable tool to document partial or complete rotator cuff tears. Rarely is MRI indicated in the initial evaluation and treatment of shoulder injuries.

Treatment and prevention

Athletes presenting after acute initial dislocation of the glenohumeral joint should be immobilized for 3 weeks in a shoulder immobilizer. Subsequently, they should receive physiotherapy to increase their range of motion and muscle strength. Return to sports can be considered after 4 months of treatment. Those participating in violent collision or contact sports can be protected with a brace that limits abduction and external rotation for acute anterior instability. Athletes

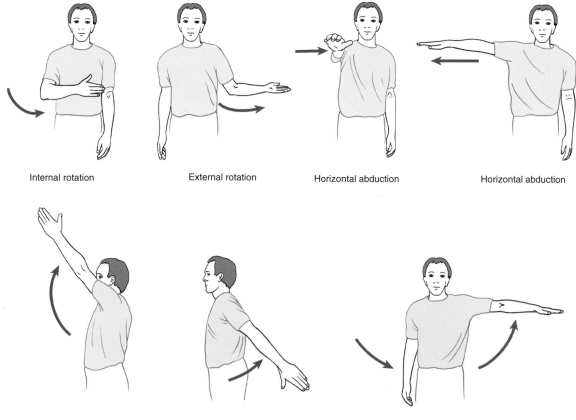

Internal rotation   External rotation   Horizontal abduction   Horizontal abduction

Shoulder flexion   Shoulder extension   Adduction   Abduction

Figure 17.12. *Movements of the shoulder.*

who present after recurrent dislocations should be placed in rehabilitation almost immediately. After full and normal range of motion is obtained, consultation with an orthopaedic surgeon is warranted. If the patient is under 30 years of age and is participating in a regular athletic activity or having symptoms with daily activities, consideration should be given to surgical stabilization of the shoulder. The recurrence of shoulder instability, as demonstrated by redislocation or subluxation (incomplete dislocation), in a young patient population of military cadets was over 90% following an initial acute dislocation, despite a rigorous rehabilitation programme [12]. Such patients in a high-risk population for redislocation should consider early stabilization. Athletes who present with instability without a history of a traumatic event should have an initial course of prolonged physical therapy for muscular strengthening and protected return to sports. These patients should be considered for orthopaedic consultation early in the course of their disease.

A direct fall on the acromioclavicular joint causes complete or incomplete dislocation of that joint. After radiographs have ruled out fracture or posterior translation, the vast majority of these injuries can be treated with initial immobilization in a sling, followed by gradual return to normal activity. Return to sports is allowed when the patients are pain free and have a normal range of motion and strength. Acromioclavicular arthritis can be treated with anti-inflammatory medications. If this is not successful, then surgical excision of the distal clavicle can be considered. Orthopaedic consultation is advised if there is severe superior translation of the distal clavicle with tenting of the skin, posterior or subcoracoid translation or a possible fracture of the distal clavicle.

If a rotator cuff tear is identified, physical therapy is warranted to obtain normal range of motion and to maximize functional return of strength. A single subacromial injection of corticosteroid may decrease the patient's pain and improve strength. Younger patients (less than 50 years old) with rotator cuff tears, and older athletes with significant complaints of pain or weakness, should be evaluated at an early stage by an orthopaedic surgeon. Frequently, these tears can be repaired and good-to-excellent motion and strength can be obtained. Incomplete or complete injuries of the biceps tendon can be treated with anti-inflammatory medications. If symptoms persist, diagnostic arthroscopy and débridement of the tendon may be indicated. Supination strength and elbow flexion power of the forearm

may be increased by stabilizing the tendon to the lateral humerus. Patients with decreased range of motion without evidence of fracture or instability should be evaluated for adhesive capsulitis. This disease has a prolonged course, requiring gradual return of range of motion and strength. Supervised physiotherapy is frequently required. If prolonged therapy and treatment with NSAIDs are unsuccessful, arthroscopic release and surgical manipulation may be considered.

Prevention of shoulder injuries deals primarily with appropriate training. Muscle imbalance can cause significant distortion of the normal motion in and about the shoulder. Rehabilitation and training should strive to maintain the normal strength of all relevant major muscle groups.

Injuries to the elbow

Anatomy

The elbow joint is primarily a hinged joint. The bicondylar shape of the distal humerus articulates with the concaved proximal ulna, creating a stable hinged joint (Fig. 17.13). The radius has a flat surface which articulates with the capitulum (laterally) and rotates sufficiently to allow pronation/supination of the hand and wrist. The joint is stabilized anteriorly and posteriorly by the joint capsule and by the bony architecture of the proximal ulna. The joint is stabilized medially and laterally by ligamentous structures. During throwing, the medial side of the joint is markedly stretched while the lateral side of the joint is compressed. The biceps tendon crosses the glenohumeral joint and the elbow joint to insert on the radius. The distal humerus is the origin for several muscles that flex and extend the wrist and digits.

Epidemiology

In an office study by Dehaven and Lintner, 3.9% of elbow injuries occurred in male and 4.1% in female patients [1]. Of 136 joint dislocations in male patients, seven were elbow dislocations; of 53 dislocations in female patients, one was an elbow dislocation. Elbow fractures are rare in athletic events; however, 33% of elbow fractures involve the radial head, which accounts for 1.7–5.9% of all fractures [1]. Lateral epicondylitis (tennis elbow) occurs in 39.7–50% of tennis players; it is usually seen in players 30 years of age or older and occurs equally in men and women [13]. Medial epicondylitis (medial tennis elbow, golfer's elbow) occurs about one-fifth as often as

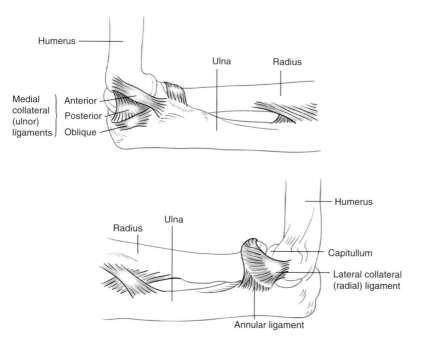

Figure 17.13. *Medial and lateral aspects of the collateral ligaments.*

lateral epicondylitis, and more frequently in men than in women.

Presentation

Elbow problems initially present as pain associated with grasping an object or swinging a racket or club; this pain may be associated with a decreased range of motion. Lateral epicondylitis is associated with lateral elbow pain, made worse with forward pronation and wrist dorsiflexion (Fig. 17.14). Lateral elbow pain can infrequently be caused by instability due to laxity of the radial (lateral collateral) ligaments.

Medial epicondylitis (medial tennis elbow, golfer's elbow) is associated with scar tissue of the pronator teres or flexor carpi radialis. Medial elbow pain may also be associated with instability of the ulnar (medial) collateral ligament, primarily from high loading of the arm during pitching, and is seen frequently in baseball players. Few non-athletes can generate forces of the magnitude necessary to stretch or avulse this ligament. A reduced range of motion is occasionally seen as an initial presenting complaint of patients following a traumatic dislocation. These patients develop calcification of the soft tissue of the elbow region, which may limit the range of motion. Other causes of a decreased range of motion as a presenting complaint include small interarticular loose bodies and traumatic avulsion of the biceps tendon from its insertion on the radius. Some patients also experience decreased range of motion with early inflammation of the olecranon bursa, which prevents normal elbow flexion. Flexion can also be inhibited by tendinitis of the triceps surae muscle.

Physical examination

Patients are usually helpful in pointing to the exact location of the origin of their pain. Knowledge of underlying anatomy can assist in establishing the diagnosis. Areas of haemorrhage, ecchymosis and swelling should be noted. The patient's range of motion should be tested (flexion, extension, pronation and supination). Muscle strength should be tested in the course of the evaluation. The elbow joint should be stressed medially and laterally in approximately 30 degrees of flexion because the joint loses some

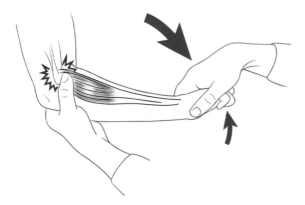

Figure 17.14. *The tennis elbow test: lateral elbow pain, which is made worse with forward pronation and wrist dorsiflexion.*

of its bony stability at that angle. The ligamentous structure should be palpated for tenderness. The ulnar nerve, which lies in a prominent position on the medial aspect of the posterior elbow, should be gently palpated and percussed to determine whether elbow pain is secondary to instability of the nerve or to local constriction.

Radiographic evaluation of the elbow should include AP and lateral radiographs. Oblique views of the posterior aspect of the elbow will occasionally demonstrate a pathological osteophyte of the olecranon or a loose body in the olecranon fossa. Ultrasound and MRI have been helpful in demonstrating soft tissue pathology in difficult cases, but are rarely indicated in the initial diagnosis and treatment.

Treatment

Medial and lateral instability can be treated with bracing; however, return of high-intensity athletics usually requires reconstruction. Symptomatic loose bodies and interarticular calcification usually require surgical excision.

The vast majority of elbow problems (epicondylitis, neuritis, ligament sprains and olecranon bursitis) are all treated with rest, anti-inflammatory medications and rehabilitation to stretch constricted soft tissue and improve muscle strength. Heterotopic ossification is best treated by a gentle active range of motion and rarely by surgical excision. Ulnar nerve neuritis and ulnar nerve subluxation can be treated by anti-inflammatory medications and padding; if this is unsuccessful, anterior transposition of the nerve is possible.

Counterforce bracing with a tennis elbow strap can relieve the symptoms of medial and lateral epicondylitis.

Injuries of the wrist and hand

Anatomy

The distal portion of the radius and ulna articulate with the carpal bones of the wrist. The motion of these bones allows for significant dorsiflexion and volar flexion, together with modest radial and ulnar deviation. The thumb has significant motion across the palm, improving grasp and pinch. Each digit has a long and a short tendon flexor which, when combined with the intrinsic muscles of the hand, allows strong grasp and flexion at the metacarpophalangeal, proximal inner phalangeal and distal phalangeal joints. Extensor tendons provide balance to the flexors.

Epidemiology

Injuries to the wrist and hand comprise 3–9% of all athletic injuries [14] and 14% of all football injuries. Younger athletes involved in collision and contact sports have a higher frequency of such injuries. In skiing, the ulnar collateral ligament of the thumb is involved in 7% of all injuries [8].

Presentation

Injuries to the hand frequently cause pain to the bone or soft tissue. This acute or soft tissue inflammatory process is consistent with general injuries to bone, ligaments or tendons. Loss of motion of the digits requires the physician to evaluate the function of individual tendons, which may become avulsed from their bony insertion (Fig. 17.15). Gliding tunnels attached to the bone in the region of the joints may become avulsed leading to secondary (palm side) instability of that joint (volar plate injuries). Acute injury to ulnar collateral ligaments of the thumb may present with the initial complaint that the athlete is unable to grasp objects without significant pain.

Physical examination

Documented areas of swelling, ecchymosis and haemorrhage are noted, as is the range of motion for the wrists and digits. Gross and fine motor strength of the digits are assessed. Because sensation is so important in the hand, neurovascular status is routinely checked: two-point discrimination should be 5 mm or less. Anterior and posterior radiographic evaluation of the wrist and hand should demonstrate no evidence of fracture or bony avulsions.

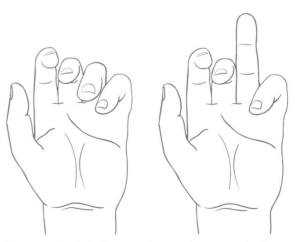

Figure 17.15. *Indication of cut or damage to the flexor tendon: extension of one finger while remaining digits are flexed.*

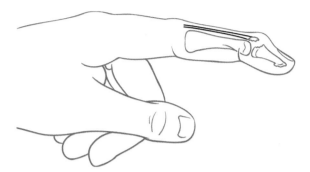

Figure 17.16. *A mallet finger with bony avulsion.*

Treatment and prevention

The vast majority of bony fractures of the digits heal with minimal immobilization (3 weeks) in functional casting or bracing. If there is evidence of instability, loss of motion across a joint or there are radiographic changes suggestive of an avulsion fracture (Fig. 17.16), orthopaedic consultation should be sought. Any acute tendinous, neural or vascular injury should be immediately referred to an orthopaedic or hand specialist. Interarticular fractures of the digits are frequently best treated by percutaneous pinning or open reduction and internal fixation.

Prevention of wrist and hand injuries can benefit from state-of-the-art equipment: for example, changes in ski-pole grips have reduced ulnar collateral ligament injuries over the last several years.

References

1. Dehaven K, Lintner DM. Athletic injuries: comparison by age, sport, and gender. Am J Sports Med 1986; 14(3): 218–224

2. Jones B, Bovee MW, Harris JM, Cowan DN. Intrinsic risk factors for exercise-related injuries among male and female army trainees. Am J Sports Med 1993; 21: 705–710

3. Bennell K, Malcolm SA, Thomas SA et al. Risk factors for stress fractures in track and field athletes: a 12-month prospective study. Am J Sports Med 1996; 24: 810–818

4. DeLee L, Drez D Jr. Orthopaedic Sports Medicine. Philadelphia: Saunders, 1994

5. Speer K, Lohnes J, Garrett WE. Radiographic imaging of muscle strain injury. Am J Sports Med 1993; 21: 89–95

6. Ryan J, Wheeler JH, Hopkinson WJ, Arciero RA. Quadriceps contusions: West Point update. Am J Sports Med 1991; 19: 299–304

7. Nielsen A, Yde J. Epidemiology of acute knee injuries: a prospective hospital investigation. J Trauma 1991; 31: 1644–1648

8. Warme W, Feagin JA, King P, Lambert KL. Ski injury statistics, 1982 to 1993, Jackson Hole Ski Resort. Am J Sports Med 1995; 5: 597–600

9. Arendt E, Dick R. Knee injury patterns among men and women in collegiate basketball and soccer: NCAA data and review of literature. Am J Sports Med 1995; 23: 694–701

10. Birrer R. Sports medicine for the primary care physician, 2nd edn. Boca Raton, FL: CRC Press, 1994

11. Sitler M, Ryan J, Hopkinson W, Wheeler J. The efficacy of a prophylactic knee brace to reduce knee injuries in football: a prospective randomised study at West Point. Am J Sports Med 1990; 18: 310–315

12. Wheeler J. Ryan J, Arciero R. Arthroscopic versus nonoperative treatment of acute shoulder dislocations in young athletes. Arthroscopy 1989; 5: 213–217

13. Nirschl R. Sports and overuse injuries to the elbow. In: Morrey B (ed) The elbow and its disorders. Philadelphia: Saunders, 1993: 537–552

14. Brown M. The older athlete with tennis elbow: rehabilitation considerations. Clin Sports Med 1995; 14: 267–275

CHAPTER 18

Osteoporosis in men

A. C. Scane

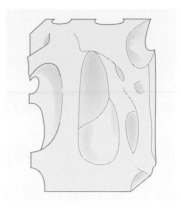

Introduction

Osteoporosis is characterized by a reduction in the amount of normal mineralized bone in the skeleton, leading to increased fragility and risk of fracture, and is now recognized as a major health problem throughout the world. There are over 150 000 osteoporosis-related fractures in the UK each year and the cost of these has been estimated to be at least £750 million. (This cost has been estimated to relate to direct treatment costs, as well as indirect costs related to such items as patients entering nursing homes.) Fracture of the hip in both sexes is associated with a 15–20% mortality. Vertebral fractures are also associated with an excess mortality over the subsequent 5 years of about 17%, although this is likely to be due to coexisting conditions rather than a direct effect of the fracture. Although osteoporosis is more common in women, increasingly it is being diagnosed in men, owing to both greater awareness and a rising age-specific incidence.

Prevalence

The three commonest sites of fracture in patients with osteoporosis are the forearm, the vertebral body and the femoral neck. The incidence of these fractures rises with age in both sexes (Fig. 18.1). By the age of 60, about 7% of women and 3% of men have sustained a fracture at one of these sites, rising to 25% and 8%, respectively, at the age of 80. The future lifetime risk of clinically diagnosed vertebral fracture for a 50-year-old white male in the USA has been estimated to be 5%, compared with 15.6% for a woman of the same age. The prevalence of vertebral deformity may be higher in younger men than women, owing to trauma sustained earlier in life [1,2]. The incidence of vertebral fractures in men varies widely across Europe, which may reflect differences in physical activity and other lifestyle factors [2]. The number of osteoporotic fractures is likely to rise further, owing to an increase in the age-specific incidence of fracture and to the demographic changes toward an ageing population. Reasons underlying this rise include the sur-

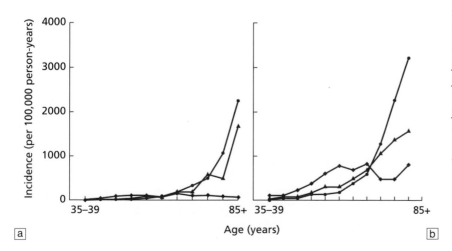

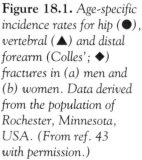

Figure 18.1. *Age-specific incidence rates for hip (●), vertebral (▲) and distal forearm (Colles'; ◆) fractures in (a) men and (b) women. Data derived from the population of Rochester, Minnesota, USA. (From ref. 43 with permission.)*

vival of more frail individuals and secular changes in smoking, alcohol consumption, diet and physical activity. The risk of fracture is influenced by bone mass, trabecular architecture and the frequency and severity of trauma applied to the skeleton. The difference in fracture rate between men and women is due to differences between the sexes in the above factors and is explored in more detail below.

Development of bone mass

Bone mass rises steeply in adolescence and is followed by a plateau phase before a period of bone loss. The bone mass in later life is clearly influenced by the peak mass achieved in early adult life, the age at which bone loss begins and the rate of bone loss thereafter. By the age of 18, 95–99% of the ultimate peak bone mass has been attained [3]. The adolescent rise in bone mass occurs at a younger age in females, because of their earlier onset of puberty [3]. Peak bone mass is influenced by the following factors: race, with Negroids having greater bone mass than Asians or Caucasians; heredity, which has been estimated to account for 80% of the variance; hormonal factors; and calcium intake and physical activity during childhood and adolescence [4,5].

The timing of hormonal influences on the skeleton, in particular the effect of testosterone, may be of importance. Young men with constitutionally delayed puberty who underwent bone density measurements in their mid-20s were shown to have reduced bone density in the forearm and lumbar spine when compared with normal men matched for duration of exposure to post-pubertal levels of testosterone [6]. There was a correlation between radial and spinal bone mineral measurements in normal men, but not in those individuals with delayed puberty, suggesting differential effects on cortical and trabecular bone.

Bone loss

Trabecular bone loss begins at about the age of 35 in both sexes, whereas the onset of cortical bone loss commences about 10 years later [7]. Men lose less bone than women: they lose 15–45% of trabecular bone compared with 35–50% in women, and 5–15% of cortical bone compared with 25–30% in women [7,8]. Age-related bone loss is the result of several factors, although it is not known whether these act equally in both sexes [7]. Trabecular architecture is better preserved during bone loss in men than women [9,10].

Factors implicated in the pathogenesis of age-related bone loss in men include heredity, hormonal factors, physical inactivity, tobacco and alcohol consumption, nutrition and decreased calcium absorption [4,5]. When considering family history as a risk factor for reduced bone density, both parents should be considered rather than just the female relatives. The Rancho Bernado study showed that men with a family history of osteoporosis had a reduced bone density at the hip; furthermore, bone mass decreased in a stepwise manner with increasing numbers of affected relatives [11].

At the time of the menopause in women there is a marked reduction in the circulating concentrations of oestradiol and progesterone, which leads to increased bone loss over the next few years. Although there is no endocrine counterpart of the menopause in middle-aged men, a fall in testosterone levels occurs in some men over the age of 70. Free testosterone index (ratio of serum testosterone to sex-hormone-binding globulin) was reported to correlate with bone mineral density (BMD) in the distal and ultradistal radius in a group of Australian men [12]. Parathyroid hormone is negatively correlated with bone mass at the hip in healthy older men, but no association was found with 25-hydroxy-vitamin D levels [13]. In a cross-sectional study of 137 Australian men, there was a positive relation between physical activity and bone density at the lumbar spine and femoral neck in those under 50 years of age, but there was no relation in the elder subjects [14]. However, a UK study has shown body weight, muscle bulk and physical activity to be significant determinants of bone mass in normal elderly men [15]. Current smokers have significantly reduced BMD at the lumbar spine in both sexes compared with those who have never smoked; BMD was reduced by 7.3% in men and 7.7% in women when adjusted for confounding variables. Furthermore, each decade of smoking was associated with a deficit in spinal bone density of 1.5% and hip bone density of 1.1% [16]. Alcohol has a direct toxic effect on the osteoblast; in addition, excessive consumption is often associated with malnutrition. Dietary calcium is a significant predictor of bone density in men, explaining 24% of the variance at the lumbar spine and 42% of the variance at the hip [12].

Osteoporosis

The World Health Organization has now defined osteoporosis as a bone mass more than two and a half standard deviations below that of a young adult of the same sex. In the very elderly, many will have become osteoporotic owing to age-related bone loss. In younger individuals, however, additional factors will have been necessary to cause bone mass to be reduced to this level. As bone is lost, the risk of fracture rises: it has been estimated that a reduction in bone density of one standard deviation is associated with an increase in the risk of fracture of 50%.

Osteoporosis may be classified as either primary or secondary, depending on the presence or absence of conditions known to cause bone loss. [7,8]. An underlying secondary cause of osteoporosis may be detected in up to 55% of men with symptomatic vertebral fractures [10,17,18] compared with approximately 40% in women.

Primary osteoporosis

Men with vertebral crush fractures due to primary osteoporosis have reduced cortical and trabecular bone mass, decreased trabecular number and biochemical evidence of increased bone turnover compared with age-matched controls [10]; bone formation may also be reduced. Osteoporosis in men may be associated with hypercalciuria, with or without renal stone disease. Although the cause of the increased urinary calcium remains uncertain, it is associated with increased calcium absorption and impaired bone formation [19].

Secondary osteoporosis

The major secondary causes identified in men presenting with symptomatic vertebral fractures are: steroid therapy, hypogonadism, excess alcohol consumption, skeletal metastases, multiple myeloma, gastric surgery and anticonvulsant treatment. More than one cause may be detected in up to 10% of cases (Fig. 18.2). In a case–control study of men presenting with vertebral crush fractures, smoking, alcohol consumption and medical conditions known to affect bone or calcium metabolism were shown to be significant risk factors, with relative risks of 2.3, 2.4 and 5.5, respectively. In contrast, obesity was marginally protective, with a relative risk of 0.3 [17].

The prevalence of secondary osteoporosis in men presenting with other osteoporotic fractures is uncertain, although a reduction in serum

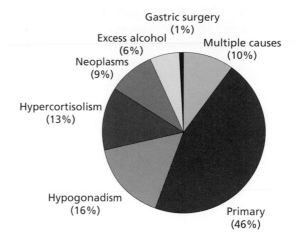

Figure 18.2. *Causes of osteoporosis in a cohort of men with symptomatic vertebral fractures. (From ref. 18 with permission.)*

testosterone may be a risk factor for femoral fracture in men. Low serum testosterone levels were reported in 58% of elderly men presenting with hip fracture after minimal trauma, compared with 18% in control subjects [20]. A UK case–control study of femoral neck fractures in men indicates that physical inactivity and low dietary calcium intake are significant risk factors, although the effect of calcium intake disappears when allowance is made for confounding variables [21].

Hypogonadism has been demonstrated in several studies to be a major cause of osteoporosis in males. The prevalence varies between studies, but is present in up to 30% of men with vertebral crush fractures. The diagnosis of hypogonadism may not always be clinically apparent: one study reported that half of patients with biochemical evidence of hypogonadism had no clinical features to suggest this diagnosis [18]. The underlying causes of hypogonadism in men with osteoporosis include Klinefelter's syndrome, idiopathic hypogonadotrophic hypogonadism, hyperprolactinaemia, haemochromatosis and primary testicular failure [22].

Orchiectomy used for the treatment of prostate cancer has been followed by severe osteoporosis. Gonadotrophin analogues, used in the treatment of both benign and malignant prostatic disease, have been associated with a reduction in bone density. In a study of 17 men treated with D-Trp^6-luteinizing hormone-releasing hormone (LHRH), there was a reduction in serum testosterone from a mean of 20.3 + 7.1 to 1.7 + 0.8 nmol/l within 1 month of commencing treatment. BMD decreased significantly in five individuals within 6 months of commencing treatment and was reduced in a further five men after 1 year [23]. In a retrospective review of 224 men treated with LHRH analogues for prostatic cancer, 20 subjects (9%) had developed a fracture. Duration of treatment varied from 1 month to 96 months with a mean of 22.2 months. However, only seven of these fractures would be regarded as osteoporotic in origin (i.e. vertebral or hip fracture after a simple fall). Eight had associated significant trauma, five were of mixed aetiology and two were thought to be pathological fractures [24]. Fractures due to osteoporosis in this cohort were much more common than pathological fractures or those due to major trauma [25].

The pathogenesis of bone loss in hypogonadal men is likely to be multifactorial in origin and several mechanisms have been proposed, including the direct effects of androgen or oestrogen deficiency, low plasma 1,25-dihydroxy-vitamin D concentrations, malabsorption of calcium [26] and reduced circulating calcitonin levels [27]. Cortical and trabecular bone are both lost, owing to reduced mineralization and increased bone resorption. All these metabolic changes may be reversed by treatment with testosterone.

Osteoporotic fractures

In a prospective epidemiological study from Australia, 820 men over the age of 60 were assessed for potential risk factors for osteoporotic fractures. Higher risk of fracture was associated with lower bone density at the femoral neck, quadriceps weakness, higher body sway, falls in the preceding 12 months, a history of fractures in the previous 5 years, lower body weight and shorter current height. Use of thiazide diuretics, higher physical activity and moderate alcohol intake were protective against fracture [28].

It is important to remember that only one-third of vertebral fractures cause symptoms that bring them to medical attention at the time. Many crush fractures will thus be asymptomatic or cause only mild symptoms initially, but subsequently other sequelae will develop. Classically, crush fractures will give rise to acute back pain, which usually subsides after 6–8 weeks. Multiple vertebral fractures lead to progressive loss of height which may amount to 200 cm or more. A kyphosis often ensues, with a consequent reduction in lung volume and a tendency to an increased incidence of respiratory infection.

When the loss of vertebral height has been substantial, the lower ribs may descend on to the pelvic brim, producing discomfort and pain.

In a study of 70 patients with vertebral fractures, which included 19 men, Leidig et al. demonstrated that 64% of individuals had pain on standing, walking or bending, and 30% had pain at rest [29]. Assistance with activities of daily living was necessary in some subjects: for instance, help with dressing was required in 19% and almost all had difficulty with lifting and carrying. There were no statistical differences between the men and women in this series, but the numbers included were quite small: 47% of female patients were dependent on extra help compared with 26% of male patients. The questions used in this study had not been validated, however, making interpretation of the results difficult.

Well-recognized tools for assessing patients include the Sickness Impact Profile [30], Arthritis Impact Scale [31], or the Nottingham Health Profile (NHP) [32]. One study using the NHP as a measure of the patient's perceived health found that men with vertebral fractures had evidence of increased morbidity when compared with previously published control data [33]. In a group of 63 men with symptomatic vertebral crush fractures, half reported some loss of height and 54% had developed a kyphosis. When responses to individual statements on the NHP were analysed, high levels of morbidity were identified (Fig. 18.3): 30% admitted to having unbearable pain and 11% thought life was not worth living. Not surprisingly, 52% of these men were using analgesics on a daily basis and 24% used tablets to help them sleep. The individual statements in the NHP were weighted and summated to give scores out of 100 for six areas or domains. Results showed that men with vertebral fracture had substantially less energy, poorer sleep, and more emotional problems, pain, immobility and social isolation than expected [33]. More recently, the NHP has been used in a case–control study of men with symptomatic vertebral crush fracture and their responses compared with age-matched community control subjects recruited from local general practitioners [34]. Results indicated statistically significant differences in all domains other than social isolation (Fig. 18.4).

There is also considerable morbidity among patients who survive femoral neck fracture, with over 50% having pain at the fracture site 6 months after surgery and only 32% being fully mobile. Of those patients who were previously living in their own homes, 5% subsequently

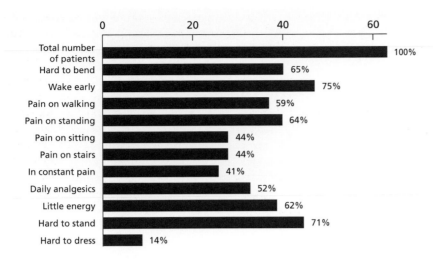

Figure 18.3. *Percentage of men with vertebral fractures agreeing with particular statements on the Nottingham Health Profile (n = 63) [33].*

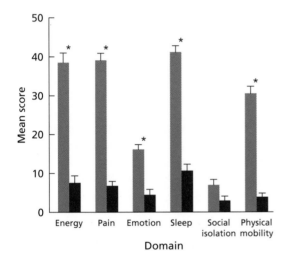

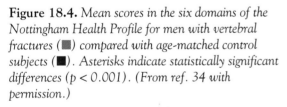

Figure 18.4. *Mean scores in the six domains of the Nottingham Health Profile for men with vertebral fractures (■) compared with age-matched control subjects (■). Asterisks indicate statistically significant differences (p < 0.001). (From ref. 34 with permission.)*

Table 18.1. *Recommended initial investigations in men with osteoporosis*

Full blood count

Erythrocyte sedimentation rate

Biochemical profile

Thyroid function tests

Serum testosterone, sex-hormone-binding globulin

Luteinizing hormone, follicle-stimulating hormone

Serum and urine immunoelectrophoresis

Chest radiograph

moved to live with relatives and a further 18% required institutional care. Of patients who were discharged back to their own homes, 11% required greater provision of services. Sex differences in the degree of morbidity have not been reported, and length of hospital stay does not differ significantly between men and women.

Investigations

Investigations should be used to confirm a diagnosis of osteoporosis and to look for secondary causes of excessive bone loss (Table 18.1). Spinal radiographs are frequently performed; these may demonstrate vertebral deformation indicating osteoporosis, provided that there is no history of significant trauma, or reduced bone density but no fracture. Bone densitometry should normally be performed to confirm the diagnosis and to allow monitoring of subsequent treatment. Currently, the modality of choice is dual energy X-Ray absorptiometry (DEXA), as this involves a relatively small dose of radiation and will measure the lumbar spine and the femoral neck with a precision of about 1%. However, there can occasionally be difficulties in the interpretation of the results of DEXA scanning: if there has been marked vertebral deformation or if there are osteophytes present, bone mass may be falsely elevated; this may also occur in patients who have had previous gold treatment.

As mentioned earlier, secondary causes of osteoporosis occur in approximately 55% of men presenting with vertebral fractures. It is important to identify patients with secondary osteoporosis, as treatment of the underlying condition may reduce the rate of bone loss. Investigations should include full blood count, erythrocyte sedimentation rate, plasma biochemical profile, serum testosterone with sex-hormone-binding globulin, thyroid function tests, gonadotrophins (luteinizing hormone and follicle-stimulating hormone), serum and urine immunoelectrophoresis and a chest radiograph. Further investigations may be necessary in the light of the results, such as bone marrow examination and isotope bone scan. In some cases of hypogonadism, more extensive endocrine investigations may be needed to exclude underlying conditions. In most cases where steroids are thought to be a risk factor, this will be due to exogenous steroids given therapeutically for other pathological conditions. If Cushing's syndrome is suspected, a 24-hour urinary free-cortisol estimation is the best initial screening test. Transiliac bone biopsy and histomorphometry has been recommended in men with apparently idiopathic osteoporosis; in order to look for evidence of increased bone turnover, however, this would not be considered by most clinicians as a routine investigation. Markers of bone formation and resorption are currently regarded as research tools but, when followed serially, may give early indications of therapeutic success.

Treatment

In patients who have sustained a fracture, treatment should be twofold: first, to alleviate symptoms resulting from the injury; secondly, to reduce subsequent bone loss. In particular, analgesia is often necessary and its adequacy needs to be monitored. Non-pharmacological treatment, such as transcutaneous electronic nerve stimulation (TENS), is useful in a proportion of patients. A full explanation of the condition should be given, as it is still widely believed that osteoporosis affects only women. It should be explained that any underlying causes need to be identified and a future management plan drawn up. Details on other sources of information and support, such as the National Osteoporosis Society, should be made available.

If a secondary cause — such as hypogonadism, thyrotoxicosis or myeloma — is discovered on clinical assessment or investigation, then initial treatment should be directed at the underlying condition. Hypogonadal osteoporosis is associated with low plasma 1,25-dihydroxy-vitamin D levels, malabsorption of calcium, and reduced androgen, oestrogen and calcitonin concentrations [26,27]. Treatment with testosterone reverses these changes [26], leading to decreased bone resorption, stimulation of bone mineralization and an increase in bone density in the forearm and lumbar spine. Testosterone should be used with caution in men with benign prostatic hyperplasia or ischaemic heart disease, and is contraindicated in patients with prostatic cancer. Patients should also be warned of possible changes in their libido.

In patients with hyperprolactinaemia, medical or surgical treatment that leads to normal testosterone levels leads to a significant increase in radial bone density, with only a minimal rise in lumbar spine bone mass. No change in bone mass is seen at either site in patients who remain hypogonadal despite the correction of hyperprolactinaemia [35]. In a small cohort of men with haemochromatosis and hypogonadism who were treated with venesection and intramuscular testosterone over 2 years, Diamond et al. reported increases in forearm and lumbar spine bone density of 4.7 and 13.1%, respectively [36].

In patients on oral steroids, the lowest possible dose should be used and consideration given to an alternative route of administration. Unfortunately, high-dose inhaled steroids have been shown to reduce serum osteocalcin, suggesting reduced bone formation. Reid et al. [37] reported on the use of monthly intramuscular testosterone injections in a group of asthmatic men requiring long-term oral steroids, which had resulted in mild biochemical hypogonadism. Testosterone treatment (mean dose 9 mg) over a 12-month period resulted in a 5% increase in bone density and smaller rises at several sites around the hip [37]. Adachi et al. [38] have recently demonstrated that intermittent cyclical etidronate (400 mg daily for 14 days) and calcium (500 mg daily for 76 days) given concurrently to patients starting on oral steroids, led to an increase in bone density. Patients who received calcium alone while on steroids had a reduction in bone density of 3.72% at the lumbar spine and 4.14% at the trochanter after 12 months [38]. Alternatively, steroids that have less detrimental effects on bone could be used, such as deflazocort, which, at equivalent anti-inflammatory doses, has been shown to produce less impairment of calcium absorption than other steroids [39].

There is little information on the treatment of men without a demonstrable secondary cause of osteoporosis, as few men have been included in the published studies. An early observational study on the effects of intramuscular testosterone given over 3 years to eugonadal men showed an increase in bone density of 6.1%. More recently, Anderson *et al.* showed a 5% increase in bone density over 6 months in men given fortnightly intramuscular testosterone [40]. There was no overall adverse effect on cardiovascular risk factors. Because of the small numbers of men treated in these studies, there are no data on any possible reduction in fracture incidence. To date, most studies have used intramuscular testosterone in the form of mixed testosterone esters: 30 mg proprionate, 60 mg phenylproprionate, 60 mg isocaproate and 100 mg decanoate (Sustanon, 250 mg) given every 2–4 weeks [36,37,40]. The optimum dose and route of administration of testosterone is not clear, but replacement with subcutaneous pellets lasting 4 months produced a greater fall in gonadotrophins than fortnightly intramuscular testosterone, which in turn was superior to twice-daily oral testosterone.

Bisphosphonates, such as disodium etidronate and alendronate, are well-established treatments for postmenopausal osteoporosis in women, but as yet there are no randomized controlled trials in men. An observational study involving 42 men with primary osteoporosis showed an annual increase in lumbar spine bone mass of 3%, with a small non-significant rise of 0.7% at the hip when treated with intermittent cyclical disodium etidronate and calcium (Didronel PMO) for a median of 31 months [41]. Although bisphosphonates and testosterone appear to be effective treatments, confirmation is required in formal clinical trials, together with other promising agents, such as calcitonin, fluoride and vitamin D. As the number of men with osteoporotic fractures is rising, it is essential that studies are performed to determine the optimal treatment for these patients.

Prevention of osteoporosis in men

As treatment of established osteoporosis in men is currently empirical, emphasis should be placed on preventative strategies that are effective, safe, inexpensive and acceptable to the individual. Prevention of osteoporotic fractures could include measures to achieve an optimal peak bone mass, to reduce subsequent bone loss and to decrease the rate of falls.

Approximately 80% of the variance in peak bone mass is due to genetic factors; the remaining 20% may be modifiable and involves lifestyle factors, such as diet and exercise. Skeletal growth is maximal during adolescence and requires an abundance of calcium. An intake of 1600 mg calcium daily may have a beneficial effect on peak bone mass [42]. Calcium supplementation in one of a pair of twins of both sexes has been shown to lead to a rise in bone density of 5.1% in the midshaft radius, 3.8% in the distal radius and 2.8% in the lumbar spine over the 3-year study period [42]. Children and young adults of both sexes who are physically active have a bone mass 5% greater than that in more sedentary individuals.

Age-related bone loss in men is multifactorial, owing to a combination of genetic, endocrine, mechanical and nutritional factors, some of which may be modified. Maintaining physical activity reduces bone loss and may decrease the risk of falls. Moderation of tobacco and alcohol consumption may be beneficial to the skeleton, as both suppress osteoblast function and new bone formation. A balanced diet rich in calcium should be recommended, and patients should be encouraged to go out of doors several times a week during the summer months, to ensure adequate production of vitamin D by the skin. In housebound individuals, vitamin D supplementation should probably be given, although there is little information on its use in men. Thiazide diuretics should be considered in hypertensive individuals, as their use is associated with a reduced rate of bone loss. This needs to be monitored, however, as postural hypotension may ensue, leading to an increased risk of falls.

Falling is clearly a risk factor for fractures, although only 6% of falls will lead to any fracture and only 1% of falls lead to hip fracture. The incidence of falls rises with age: approximately 20% of community-dwelling individuals over the age of 60 will have a fall in 12 months. Attempts to reduce the risk of falls should include clinical assessment, review of medication and advice on environmental hazards. Hip protectors, which reduce the impact of a fall, are now available and reduce the rate of hip fracture. They are cumbersome at present, which reduces compliance, but their use should be encouraged in those who remain at high risk of falls despite intervention.

Follow-up

To date, there are no randomized controlled trials in men with osteoporosis that have shown a significant reduction in the rate of fractures. It is, therefore, desirable for men with osteoporosis to be referred to a specialist service to facilitate a multicentre study in the future. In the meantime, any empirical therapy should be monitored for its efficacy and safety. Biochemical markers of bone turnover may give early indications of improvement, but follow-up bone density measurements are more useful. The optimum interval is unknown but annual scanning is probably justified. Patients being treated with testosterone require a regular full blood count to monitor the rise in haemoglobin and haematocrit. It has also been recommended that men over the age of 50 should have serial digital prostate examination and estimation of serum prostate-specific antigen.

Shared care and evidence-based guidelines

There is very little definitive evidence on which to base guidelines in the management of male osteoporosis at present. Shared care between the primary care team and a specialist is particularly relevant if empirical treatment is being given. This would allow regular review of analgesia, early identification of difficulty with daily living activities and close monitoring for any adverse events. Osteoporosis nurse specialists are employed in some centres to assist with these tasks. They are also able to disseminate information on osteoporosis and its management to the primary care team and the general public. Prospective interventional trials on the treatment of male osteoporosis are now urgently needed and should allow evidence-based guidelines to be formulated in the future.

References

1. O'Neill TW, Varlow J, Felsenberg D et al. Variation in vertebral height ratios in population studies. J Bone Miner Res 1994; 9: 1895–1907
2. O'Neill TW, Felsenberg D, Varlow J et al. Influence of sex and geography on the prevalence of vertebral deformity. J Bone Miner Res 1996; 11: 1010–1018
3. Bonjour JP, Thientz G, Buchs B et al. Critical years and stages of puberty for spinal and femoral bone mass accumulation during adolescence. J Clin Endocrinol Metab 1991; 73: 555–563
4. Compston JE. Risk factors for osteoporosis. Clin Endocrinol 1992; 36: 223–224
5. Scane AC, Francis RM. Risk factors for osteoporosis in men. Clin Endocrinol 1993; 38: 15–16
6. Finkelstein JS, Neer RM, Biller BMK et al. Osteopenia in men with a history of delayed puberty. N Engl J Med 1992; 326: 600–604
7. Riggs BL, Melton LJ III. Involutional osteoporosis. N Engl J Med 1986; 314: 1676–1684
8. Francis RM. Pathogenesis of osteoporosis. In: Francis RM (ed) Osteoporosis: pathogenesis and management. Lancaster: Kluwer, 1990: 51–80
9. Aaron JE, Makins NB, Sagreiya K. The microanatomy of trabecular bone loss in normal aging men and women. Clin Orthop 1987; 215: 260–271
10. Francis RM, Peacock M, Marshall DH et al. Spinal osteoporosis in men. Bone Miner 1989; 5: 347–357
11. Soroko SB, Barrett-Connor E, Edelstein SL, Kritz-Silverstein D. Family history of osteoporosis and BMD at the axial skeleton: the Rancho Bernado Study. J Bone Miner Res 1994; 9: 761–769
12. Kelly PJ, Pocock NA, Sambrook PN, Eisman JA. Dietary calcium, sex hormones, and bone mineral density in men. Br Med J 1990; 300: 1361–1364
13. Murphy S, Khaw KT, Prentice A, Compston JE. Relationships between parathyroid hormone, 25-hydroxy-vitamin D, and bone mineral density in elderly men. Age Ageing 1993; 22: 198–204
14. Need AG, Wishart JM, Scopacasa F et al. Effect of physical activity on femoral bone density in men. Br Med J 1995; 310: 1501–1502
15. Francis RM, Johnson FJ, Rawlings D. The determinants of bone mass in normal elderly men. In: Ring EFJ (ed) Current research in osteoporosis and bone mineral measurement II. London: British Institute of Radiology, 1992: 54–55
16. Egger P, Duggleby S, Hobbs R et al. Cigarette smoking and bone mineral density in the elderly. J Epidemiol Community Health 1996; 50: 47–50
17. Seeman E, Melton LJ III, O'Fallon WM, Riggs BL. Risk factors for spinal osteoporosis in men. Am J Med 1983; 75: 977–983
18. Baillie SP, Davison CE, Johnson FJ, Francis RM. Pathogenesis of vertebral crush fractures in men. Age Ageing 1992; 21: 139–141
19. Zerwekh JE, Sakhaee K, Breslau NA et al. Impaired bone formation in male idiopathic osteoporosis: further reduction in the presence of concomitant hypercalciuria. Osteoporosis Int 1992; 2: 128–134
20. Stanley HL, Schmitt BP, Poses RM, Deiss WP. Does hypogonadism contribute to the occurrence of a minimal trauma hip fracture in elderly men? J Am Geriatr Soc 1991; 39: 766–771
21. Cooper C, Barker DJP, Wickham C. Physical activity, muscle strength, and calcium intake in fracture of the proximal femur in Britain. Br Med J 1988; 297: 1443–1446

22. Jackson JA, Kleerekoper M. Osteoporosis in men: diagnosis, pathophysiology and prevention. *Medicine* 1990; 69: 137–152

23. Goldray D, Weisman Y, Jaccard N *et al.* Decreased bone density in elderly men treated with the gonadotrophin-releasing hormone agonist decpeptyl (D-Trp⁶ -GnRH). *J Clin Endocrinol Metab* 1991; 76: 288–290

24. Townsend MF, Sanders WH, Northway RO, Graham SD. Bone fractures associated with luteinizing hormone-releasing hormone agonists used in the treatment of prostate carcinoma. *Cancer* 1997; 79: 545–550

25. Daniell HW. Osteoporosis after orchiectomy for prostate cancer. *J Urol* 1997; 157: 439–444

26. Francis RM, Peacock M, Aaron JE *et al.* Osteoporosis in hypogonadal men: role of decreased plasma 1,25-dihydroxyvitamin D, calcium malabsorption and low bone formation. *Bone* 1986;7:261–268

27. Foresta C, Busnardo B, Ruzza G, Zanatta G *et al.* Lower calcitonin levels in young hypogonadic men with osteoporosis. *Horm Metab Res* 1983; 15: 206–207

28. Nguyen TV, Eisman JA, Kelly PJ, Sambrook PN. Risk factors for osteoporotic fractures in elderly men. *Am J Epidemiol* 1996; 144: 255–263

29. Leidig G, Minne HW, Sauer P *et al.* A study of complaints and their relation to vertebral destruction in patients with osteoporosis. *Bone Miner* 1990; 8: 217–219

30. Bergner M, Bobbitt RA, Kressel S *et al.* The sickness impact profile: conceptual formulation and methodology for the development of a health status measure. *Int J Health Serv* 1976; 6: 393–415

31. Meenan RF, Gertman PM, Mason JH. Measuring health status in arthritis: the arthritis impact measurements scales. *Arthritis Rheum* 1980; 23: 146–152

32. Hunt SM, McEwen J, McKenna SP. Measuring health status: a new tool for clinicians and epidemiologists. *J R Coll Gen Pract* 1985; 35: 185–188

33. Scane AC, Sutcliffe AM, Francis RM. The sequelae of vertebral crush fractures in men. *Osteoporosis Int* 1994; 4: 89–92

34. Scane AC, Francis RM, Sutcliffe AM *et al.* A case control study of pathenogenesis and sequelae of symptomatic vertebral fractures in men. *Osteoporosis Int* 1999; 9: 91–97

35. Greenspan SL, Neer RM, Ridgway EC, Klibanski A. Osteoporosis in men with hyperprolactinaemic hypogonadism. *Ann Intern Med* 1986; 104: 777–782

36. Diamond T, Stiel D, Solomon P. Effects of testosterone and venesection on spinal and peripheral bone mineral in six hypogonadal men with haemochromatosis. *J Bone Miner Res* 1991; 6: 39–43

37. Reid IR, Wattie DJ, Evans MC, Stapleton JP. Testosterone therapy in glucocorticoid-treated men. *Arch Intern Med* 1996; 156: 1173–1177

38. Adachi JD, Bensen WG, Brown J *et al.* Intermittent etidronate therapy to prevent corticosteroid-induced osteoporosis. *N Engl J Med* 1997; 337: 382–387

39. Villareal DT, Civitelli R, Gennari C, Avioli LV. Is there an effective treatment for glucocorticoid-induced osteoporosis? *Calcif Tissue Int* 1991: 49: 141–142

40. Anderson FH, Francis RM, Faulkner K. Androgen supplementation in eugonadal men with osteoporosis: effects of six months treatment on bone mineral density and cardiovascular risk factors. *Bone* 1996; 18: 171–177

41. Anderson FH, Francis RM, Bishop JC, Rawlings DA. Effect of intermittent cyclical etidronate therapy on bone mineral density in men with vertebral fractures. *Age Ageing* 1997; 26(5): 359–365

42. Johnston CC Jr, Miller JZ, Slemenda CW *et al.* Calcium supplementation and increases in bone mineral density in children. *N Engl J Med* 1992; 327: 82–87

43. Cooper C, Melton LJ. Epidemiology of osteoporosis. *Trends in Endocrinology and Metabolism* 1992; 3: 224–229

CHAPTER 19

Disorders of the head and neck

M. S. Benninger and G. M. Gardner

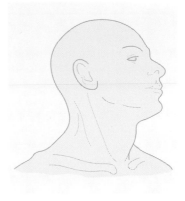

History

When a man presents with a complaint referable to the upper airway or head and neck, the first and perhaps most critical part of the assessment is obtaining a thorough history. Information regarding the time from onset, the severity of the symptoms, whether the symptoms vary by time of day or exposure to certain environments or conditions, and any previous treatment for this condition should be obtained. A general review of other head and neck symptoms follows, as well as details of general health, medications being taken, and history of previous diseases or surgery. Particular habits that are important with regard to the head and neck should be considered, such as tobacco or alcohol use.

Physical examination

The head and neck physical examination usually begins during the history. At that time speech and voice, gross hearing and any abnormalities of facial movement or skin conditions or masses can be assessed. The skin and scalp are usually evaluated first followed by an examination of the ears.

The ear
The external ear and ear canal are assessed with an otoscope to identify inflammation or skin conditions. The middle ear is visualized for normal landmarks and absence of infection, masses, fluid or retraction of the eardrum. Air insufflation (pneumatic otoscopy) is particularly useful in evaluating middle ear function, negative pressure or fluid. If any concerns are raised during otoscopy, a microscope can be used to delineate better any potential abnormalities. Hearing can be assessed with the use of tuning forks, followed by a formal audiogram if necessary.

The nose
A nasal examination is generally obtained with a head mirror, indirect light and a nasal speculum. Decongesting the nose will allow improved visualization into the more posterior aspects of the nose. An otoscope may give an adequate view for most disorders in primary care clinics. If concerns are raised, if visualization is difficult or if a diagnosis needs confirmation, nasal endoscopes can be used to visualize the entire nose better [1].

The oral cavity
The oral cavity should be examined with mirror-directed light so that both hands can be used to manipulate the tongue and other mucosal surfaces. Tongue blades can depress the tongue to see the oropharynx, tonsils and tongue base. Keeping the tongue blades just anterior to the junction of the anterior two-thirds and posterior one-third of the tongue, and asking the patient to breathe gently, will minimize the gagging reflex. With the tongue compressed, a nasopharyngeal mirror can be used to assess the nasopharynx.

The larynx
The larynx should be initially visualized with a laryngeal mirror. The tongue is grasped and gently pulled forward. The mirror is inserted to a point just anterior to the palate and light directed to allow visualization of the pharynx and larynx. It is important not to focus on the vocal folds only, as other important findings related to the base of tongue, posterior pharyngeal walls, pyriform sinus, epiglottis, and vallecula may be missed. To supplement the mirror view, to visualize the larynx during running speech, or if visualization is limited, a flexible laryngoscope can be passed. Usually this is passed through the nose after decongestion and occasionally after application of a topical anaesthetic. Not only is this

instrument valuable in larynx assessment, but also it can be used to visualize the nasopharynx better and can be used for functional assessment of swallowing (fibre-optic endoscopic examination of swallowing; FEES) [2] or even for voice modification or biofeedback training. Video images can be obtained to follow the progress of treatment, for documentation and in discussions with the patient, family or referring physician [3]. To augment further the examination of the larynx, videostroboscopy of the larynx can be performed to assess vocal fold vibration.

The neck

The neck should be palpated for any masses, neck muscular problems or asymmetry. The thyroid is then palpated at rest and during swallowing. Pulsating masses can be auscultated to help identify a vascular lesion. Fine-needle aspiration is a useful tool in obtaining a pathological diagnosis and has obviated the need in many cases for open biopsy. A neurological assessment of the cranial nerves is part of the routine examination, while selective assessments of balance function should be performed if indicated.

General tests

Computed tomography (CT) and magnetic resonance imaging (MRI) scanning are very useful in assessing head and neck masses and ruling out intracranial or skull base disease. CT scans are particularly useful in evaluating sinus disease. A chest radiograph is helpful in patients with head and neck tumours, cough or haemoptysis. Swallowing and gastro-oesophageal reflux assessment may be considered in patients with swallowing complaints. Other medical evaluations will be determined by the suspicions of disease.

Disorders of the ear

Cerumen impaction

Cerumen (ear wax) is produced by the cerumen glands of the external auditory ear canal. Occasionally, cerumen production is excessive or may be drier than normal, resulting in accumulation and cerumen impaction. More often, cerumen impaction occurs as individuals try to clean their ears with cotton-tip applicators or other devices, forcing the cerumen further down the ear canal and preventing self-cleaning. A partial or complete obstruction of the canal can occur with an associated loss of hearing.

The best treatment of cerumen impaction is prevention, by avoiding forcing the cerumen back down the ear canal. The old adage of 'placing nothing smaller than an elbow in the canal' holds true. If a patient is prone to recurrent impaction, occasional use of hydrogen peroxide will help break up the cerumen and, in most cases, over-the-counter cerumen-softening agents are safe. If a patient has a history of recurrent external otitis infections, or has had previous ear surgery or a known or suspected tympanic membrane perforation, these agents should not be used nor should the ears be irrigated; rather, the cerumen should be removed directly by a physician.

External otitis (swimmer's ear)

The lateral part of the external auditory canal is cartilage covered by skin, with sweat and ceromucinous glands and hair follicles. The medial one-third of the canal is bone, with tight adherence of the overlying skin and few glandular structures. Infection or inflammation can occur as a result of chronic dermatitis, loss of cerumen, or prolonged moisture of the canal such as occurs with swimming or in a humid environment. The canal will be swollen and tender and the patient may experience decreased hearing. Tenderness of the pina may help to differentiate this condition from otitis media. The treatment of external otitis is by removal of any debris in the canal and the instillation of antibiotic ear drops for 7–10 days. Acetic acid solutions also work well in preventing bacterial growth by decreasing the pH of the canal. Steroids help rapidly to decrease swelling and discomfort, and dry-ear precautions should be employed until the inflammation has resolved.

Otitis media

Otitis media is an infection of the middle ear. It is typically caused by bacteria, most commonly *Streptococcus pneumoniae*, *Haemophilus influenzae* and *Moraxella catarrhalis*. Although otitis media is uncommon in adults, it can occur particularly in those who have problems with eustachian tube dysfunction or in immunocompromised individuals. The patient will typically notice decreased hearing and pain in the ear and the characteristic signs of a bulging, erythematous tympanic membrane will be seen. Antibiotics and ear inflation (auto-insufflation) by the patient will resolve the infection in the course of a few days, although a serous otitis may persist for a couple of months following resolution.

Serous otitis media occurs secondary to dysfunction of the eustachian tube. It frequently occurs following an upper respiratory infection or after rapid changes in pressure that occur with flying or scuba diving. It generally resolves on its own, although a short course of nasal decongestants (for no longer than 3–4 days) and auto-insufflation by the patient will hasten recovery. Serous otitis media without a definitive precipitating episode in an adult should prompt nasopharyngeal examination to rule out a nasopharyngeal tumour. Since the incidence of nasopharyngeal cancer is much greater in men of Asian descent, the nasopharynx should be evaluated for either a serous otitis or acute otitis media.

Hearing loss

Hearing loss may occur either as a result of impedance of transmission of sound across the middle ear (conductive hearing loss) or secondary to neurosensory loss involving the cochlea or auditory nerve (sensorineural hearing loss). Conductive loss is usually due to a temporary or reversible problem such as cerumen impaction or middle ear effusion. There may also be alteration or fixation of the bones of the middle ear, or ossicular chain; this can occur secondary to trauma or chronic infection. Otosclerosis is a familial change in the character of the bone of the middle ear, resulting in ossicular fixation, particularly of the stapes. Individuals usually present with a unilateral, progressive hearing loss, classically beginning in early adulthood; there is often a strong family history. A normal ear examination and a conductive hearing loss identified by audiogram supports the diagnosis. Surgery on the stapes typically results in return of hearing to a level similar to that of the better-hearing ear. Otosclerosis can be bilateral and, in very aggressive cases, can be associated with a sensorineural hearing loss.

The most common cause of sensorineural hearing loss is an age-related change in hearing, or presbycusis. Generally, this type of loss is slowly progressive, with a loss in the higher frequencies occurring initially. With time and advancing age, the hearing change may progress to involve lower frequencies. As no treatment is available for presbycusis, rehabilitation with assistive listening devices and hearing aids is recommended.

Noise-induced hearing loss typically occurs following prolonged exposure to high-decibel sounds. Treatment is largely preventative, with appropriate hearing protection based on standards related to the intensity and duration of the noise exposure. If the hearing loss is significant enough to affect communication, hearing augmentation is recommended.

Vertigo

Vertigo is a symptom that is associated with a sense of movement, classically a sense of rotation or spinning. In general, true spinning vertigo is related to dysfunction of the labyrinth, or is otological in aetiology. Dizziness, on the other hand, is a non-specific term to describe a symptom that may be due to a variety of disorders including hypotension, neurological disease, or generalized changes in balance function that occur with age. It is important to take a thorough history when trying to identify the cause of dizziness.

The most common cause of true spinning vertigo, other than the self-limited vertigo associated with the use of alcohol, is benign paroxysmal positional vertigo (BPPV). This can be diagnosed through its characteristic pattern. Acute labyrinthitis is an acute inflammation of the labyrinth and is generally considered to be of viral aetiology. Patients present with a relatively sudden onset of vertigo, which tends to be relatively severe, and is associated with nausea and vomiting. Menière's disease is a common cause of intermittent and recurrent episodes of vertigo.

Tinnitus

Tinnitus is defined as noise in the ear. It is more common in older age groups and in those with a known sensorineural hearing loss, particularly noise-induced hearing loss. It can be exacerbated by certain medications, particularly aspirin, and many notice that caffeine and tobacco intensify the symptoms. Treatment begins with elimination of precipitating medications and other agents. As most people notice the tinnitus more in a quiet environment, providing background noise under such conditions helps to buffer the sound.

Oral cavity, oropharynx, nasopharynx

Tonsillar hypertrophy

Tonsillar hypertrophy can be important in patients with snoring or obstructive sleep apnoea syndrome. Chronic tonsillitis causes chronic sore throat, odynophagia and halitosis. Occasionally, cryptic debris can accumulate intermittently, with associated halitosis and, occasionally, pain. Clearing the cryptic debris with a cotton-tip applicator or a water pick may be helpful in maintaining good oral hygiene and minimizing discomfort.

Velopharyngeal insufficiency

Velopharyngeal insufficiency can be the result of lack of innervation to the soft palate via the vagus nerve; this may be seen in cerebral palsy or following poliomyelitis. A prosthesis that lifts the soft palate is often very effective. Bilateral lesions of the vagus nerves are extremely unlikely, whereas resection of a skull base tumour can often result in a unilateral vagal palsy with unilateral weakness of the soft palate. Surgical attachment of the paralysed side to the posterior nasopharyngeal wall can effectively provide symptom relief [4].

Tongue disorders

Most disorders that affect the tongue are related to changes of the mucosa, including hyperkeratosis, dysplasia and atrophy. Most mucosal abnormalities seen are non-specific and of little clinical significance. Many need to be biopsied to rule out carcinoma, but otherwise require no therapy (Figs. 19.1, 19.2). Lack of sense of taste is usually due to a loss of sense of smell, with no actual abnormality of the taste apparatus.

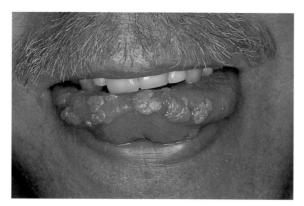

Figure 19.1. *Multiple warts on the tongue.*

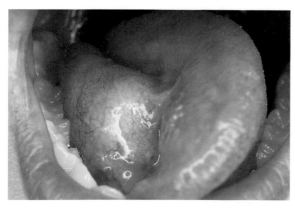

Figure 19.2. *Rannula.*

Decreased taste and/or numbness in a specific part of the tongue should alert the clinician to the possibility of a lesion of the nerve supplying sensation to that portion of the tongue. Interruption of the motor innervation to the tongue is usually the result of stroke or other significant intracranial event, or of surgical trauma in the neck or floor of the mouth. Rarely, a malignant neoplasm of the base of skull or submandibular gland will present with a unilateral tongue palsy.

Salivary gland disorders

Dry mouth (xerostomia) results when the salivary glands cease to function properly. A chronically dry mouth is very uncomfortable, makes eating more difficult and can lead to dental disease. Xerostomia can be due to simple problems, such as inadequate water intake and dehydration, or to more complex autoimmune diseases, such as Sjögren's syndrome in which the tissue ceases to function. A common cause of xerostomia is a medication that alters the autonomic input to the glands. Such medications include antihistamines, and antipsychotic and antidepressant drugs. Xerostomia is also a common side effect of radiation therapy to the oral cavity and/or oropharynx. Treatment first involves identifying and treating the aetiology followed by the use of oral lubricants and medications that directly stimulate the salivary glands.

Neoplasms of the head and neck

Head and neck cancers are more common in men than in women, largely because of the greater tobacco and alcohol exposure in men, although increasing usage in women is eroding this difference. Hoarseness lasting for more than a couple of weeks, dysphagia, odynophagia, haemoptysis, throat pain, or a neck mass should prompt a more thorough evaluation to rule out a neoplasm. The most common malignant tumour of the head and neck is squamous cell carcinoma. Thyroid neoplasms, both benign and malignant, typically present with a thyroid mass, which should prompt further investigation.

Tumours may also develop within the salivary glands. If these are benign or malignant but diagnosed early, excision of the gland may effect a cure. Although excision of the submandibular glands is relatively straightforward, it is much more complex for the parotid glands. Any surgery of the parotid gland must begin with identification and careful dissection of the facial nerve to avoid inadvertent injury, which could result in unilateral complete facial paralysis with inability to close the eye and the lips, and obvious cosmetic deformity.

Sleep disorders

Many conditions can affect sleep. Probably the most common problem is snoring, which represents turbulent airflow during sleep and affects approximately 50% of men and 30% of women. It is more common as people age, and is also more common in those who are overweight. Snoring tends to increase after alcohol intake and when lying flat on the back. Since snoring is a sign of obstruction, it may affect the ability to sleep.

Although snoring is often perceived as a problem for only the snorer's bed partner, it may be a sign of the more serious condition known as obstructive sleep apnoea syndrome (OSAS), in which breathing stops for periods of time during sleep (apnoea). Patients with OSAS commonly complain of excessive daytime sleepiness, headaches and chronic fatigue. The condition can lead to high blood pressure, heart rhythm problems, heart failure, sudden death and automobile accidents due to falling asleep while driving [5]. There are various treatments for sleep apnoea: in those patients who are overweight, weight loss is extremely important and occasionally is enough to relieve the patient of these symptoms [5]; exercise and regimented sleep–wake cycles are also helpful. The main treatment goal is to keep the airway open while the patient is sleeping. This can be done with a nasal constant positive airway pressure (CPAP) device, in which the subject is fitted with a mask over the nose providing a constant flow of air through the nose to prevent collapse of the throat while inhaling. Although it is particularly effective, CPAP is sometimes poorly tolerated. Other options include oral airways, which are devices placed in the mouth that hold the tongue and jaw forward to keep the tongue from falling back and obstructing the airway. Nasal airway devices may be helpful in some patients. Such devices are not particularly comfortable or well tolerated and are often abandoned by the patient who continues to suffer from the effects of sleep apnoea.

Surgical procedures may permanently open the breathing passages without the use of devices. For extremely severe sleep apnoea, a tracheotomy is often done. This is the ultimate surgical procedure for this disease and works 100% of the time, but it does require long-term care of the tra-cheostomy tube. Most patients do not require this procedure.

Other surgical procedures are aimed at improving the nasal airway. Several operations have been developed to open the airway at the level of the throat, the most common area that obstructs. The most popular of these is known as uvulopalatopharyngoplasty (UPPP). Here the surgeon removes the tonsils, which are usually contributing to the problem, and excess tissue from the soft palate and pharyngeal walls. UPPP creates more room in the throat and prevents collapse of the tissues while the person is sleeping. A staged, laser-assisted version can now be performed as an outpatient procedure without general anaesthesia. Techniques have also been developed primarily to pull the tongue forward, preventing it from falling back and blocking the airway [5]. Snoring can also be managed with a new technique called somnoplasty.

Nasal and sinus disorders

The most common nasal complaint is obstruction. Congenital problems such as choanal atresia and nasopharyngeal disease such as adenoid hypertrophy can cause obstruction, as can acquired obstructing lesions of the nasal cavities. The nasal septum should be a straight, relatively thin, flat, midline structure, but it can become deviated with increasing age, resulting in obstruction (partial or complete) of either one or both sides of the nose. Trauma to the nose can also cause deflection of the nasal septum and/or nasal bones. Benign masses, such as polyps (Fig. 19.3) or papillomas, and malignancies often present as unilateral nasal obstruction. Besides the obvious symptom of impaired nasal breathing,

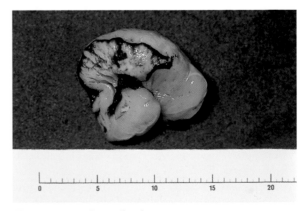

Figure 19.3. *A nasal polyp.*

these patients often complain of an impaired sense of smell, hyponasal speech, dry throat (especially in the morning) and snoring. Tumours may also cause pain and bleeding and, in more advanced cases, can cause anaesthesia of the face or eye symptoms.

Nasal obstruction may improve with medical therapy aimed at reducing swelling of the mucosal lining of the nose with oral decongestants, antihistamines (if allergy is a cause), steroid sprays and humidification. When medical treatment fails, surgery is often curative. Straightening of the septum (septoplasty) and reconstruction of the entire nose (septorhinoplasty) are very effective procedures with few complications. Removal of benign lesions by procedures such as polypectomy is also relatively straightforward, although the polyps have a tendency to recur.

Rhinitis

Allergic rhinitis is a common intermittent cause of nasal obstruction. Other symptoms include clear watery rhinorrhoea, sneezing and itchy nose and eyes. These symptoms occur in the presence of specific allergens, which may be present during certain seasons (e.g. pollen, fungi) or in certain locations (e.g. dust mites, animal dander). Avoidance or elimination of the allergens provides definitive treatment. Alternatively, antihistamines, steroid nasal sprays and sodium cromoglycate nasal sprays may be necessary. Desensitization injections, commonly known as 'allergy shots', frequently succeed in reducing sensitivity to the allergens.

Rhinosinusitis

Rhinosinusitis is an infection of one or more of the eight paranasal sinus cavities. It usually follows a viral upper respiratory infection or an exacerbation of allergic rhinitis. These conditions cause swelling of the nasal mucosa, including the mucosa at the naturally small openings of the sinuses. Anatomical abnormalities and polyps may also block the sinus ostia. Blockage of these openings creates a closed cavity, which is an excellent environment for the colonization and growth of bacteria. Symptoms of acute rhinosinusitis include purulent nasal discharge, nasal obstruction, facial pain and pressure, fever and occasionally headache. Treatment is aimed at opening the closed sinus cavities and eradicating the bacteria. Oral and topical nasal spray decongestants, saline nasal rinses, analgesics, rest and antibiotics are crucial. Most acute episodes of rhinosinusitis in immunocompetent individuals clear with one course of medical therapy.

Chronic rhinosinusitis differs completely from the acute disease, although acute exacerbations may occur in a patient with chronic disease. The common symptoms of chronic rhinosinusitis include chronic nasal and postnasal discharge (which is usually thick mucoid material), varying degrees of nasal obstruction, pressure or a heavy feeling in the face and head. Facial pain and headaches are rarely seen in chronic rhinosinusitis and fever is also uncommon. Patients are treated in a similar manner to those with acute rhinosinusitis, but for longer. Nasal endoscopy helps to determine whether small polyps (Fig. 19.4) or other lesions are obstructing the sinus ostia. A CT scan is the test of choice for assessing location and extent of disease. A patient who has sufficiently severe symptoms and in whom medical therapy fails is a candidate for surgery. A relatively new technique known as endoscopic sinus surgery (ESS) has greatly decreased the morbidity associated with sinus surgery and is the preferred technique [6]. With the increased ability to see the anatomy during surgery, more precise and more thorough removal of diseased tissue can be achieved without the need for external incisions; success rates are approximately 85% [6]. Nasal polyps are often seen in patients with chronic sinusitis; they are removed during ESS and are thought to recur less often after this procedure than after a simple polypectomy.

Facial pain

Facial pain can result from many different disease processes and the most common causes include trauma, sinusitis and dental disease. The history will provide the diagnosis, which is usually confirmed with the physical findings. With appropriate treatment and resolution of the disease, the pain also abates.

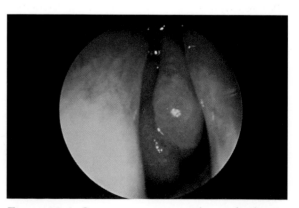

Figure 19.4. *Common appearance of a nasal polyp.*

Laryngeal disorders

The larynx serves to protect the airway from aspiration, provides a valve for generating an effective cough, and is the source of the sound that is shaped by the rest of the vocal tract to produce the voice. Benign laryngeal disorders can affect any or all of these functions. The larynx is protected anteriorly by the thyroid cartilage. The angle of the anterior cartilage tends to be more acute in men (90 degrees) than in women (120 degrees), which makes it more prominent in the neck — hence the term 'Adam's apple'.

Most benign laryngeal disorders cause a change in the voice usually referred to as 'hoarseness'. This term is interpreted as a rough, raspy voice, often with lowering of the pitch. Pain in the region of the larynx, shortness of breath and dysphagia may also be associated with benign laryngeal disorders.

Epiglottitis

Epiglottitis or supraglottitis is an acute infection of the epiglottis and aryepiglottic folds usually caused by *Haemophilus influenzae* type B (Hib). Historically, it was most common in children, aged 2–4 years; however, since the introduction of a Hib vaccine, the incidence in children has declined [7]. Epiglottitis can also occur in adults and, on occasion, can lead to airway obstruction. As the aetiology of epiglottitis in adults is often viral, the Hib vaccine is not expected to reduce the incidence.

Laryngitis

The most common disease of the larynx is laryngitis, an inflammatory condition with several different aetiologies. The most common form of laryngitis is a viral infection and is usually associated with an upper respiratory tract infection. Physical findings include erythema of the vocal folds and arytenoid mucosa, excess mucus and sometimes oedema of the vocal folds. Hydration, humidification, analgesic/anti-inflammatory medications, mucolytics, modified voice use and avoidance of irritants such as cigarette smoke are the mainstays of treatment while the viral illness runs its course; in fact, these treatments will help in any laryngeal disorder. Laryngitis is also caused by gastropharyngeal reflux disease (GPRD) and by exposure to inhaled irritants such as smoke, steam, caustic gases and other noxious substances [8].

Benign laryngeal masses, nodules, polyps and cysts

Any lesion that changes the mass of one or both vocal folds (Figs 19.5, 19.6) or prevents the vocal folds from closing completely during the glottic cycle will cause dysphonia. The common benign lesions of the vocal folds include vocal fold nodules, polyps and cysts; a less common lesion is sulcus vocalis. Each of these has a different aetiology and treatment. Often, the diagnosis of a vocal fold lesion is obvious on indirect or fibreoptic laryngoscopy. Videostroboscopy is of help in differentiating between the different masses [9,10].

Benign neoplasms

The most common benign neoplasm of the vocal fold, by far, is the squamous papilloma [11]. Dysphonia is the first symptom, but neglected or aggressive disease can progress to airway obstruction and even death. The aetiology seems to be human papillomavirus infection, but an infecting

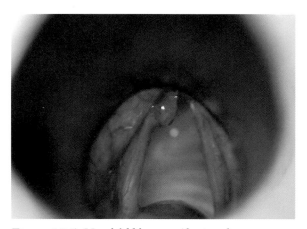

Figure 19.5. *Vocal fold haemmorhagic polyp.*

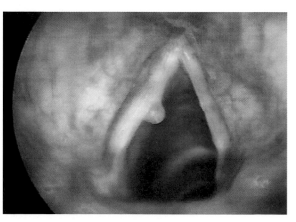

Figure 19.6. *Vocal fold laryngeal polyp.*

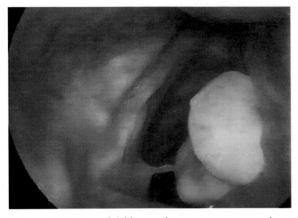

Figure 19.7. *Vocal fold granuloma originating on the vocal process of the right arytenoid cartilage. Note the bilobate appearance where the left vocal fold strikes the granuloma.*

source is usually not apparent. Treatment is microdissection or carbon dioxide laser ablation of the papillomata to restore the airway and normal contours of the vocal folds to improve the voice. The disease is extremely unpredictable and may recur within a month or disappear permanently after only one treatment. Because of this uncertain prognosis, surgical excision must be conservative and preserve all normal anatomy, despite often very extensive disease that obscures all normal landmarks.

Granulomata (Fig. 19.7) are not considered to be true neoplasms and consist of masses of granulation tissue. They commonly occur on the vocal process of the arytenoid cartilage as a result of some irritation, such as endotracheal intubation, frequent coughing and throat clearing, vocal abuse with a hard glottal attack or GPRD [12]. Treatment options include antireflux measures, voice therapy, steroids, surgical excision and Botulinum toxin injection (to decrease the force of arytenoid contact). Granulomas have a tendency to recur after excision if the inciting aetiology, such as GPRD, is not eliminated and this is best addressed prior to surgery.

Gastro-oesophageal and pharyngeal reflux disease

Gastro-oesophageal reflux disease (GERD) and GPRD can be either causative or a cofactor in many diseases and disorders of the oesophagus, pharynx, larynx and upper respiratory tract. Recent studies have shown that reflux is a proba-

ble cause of unexplained cough, globus sensation, hoarseness and chronic throat clearing [13]. Furthermore, GPRD is often confused with sinus disease in that patients complain of thick mucus sticking in the throat and attribute such symptoms to posterior nasal drainage from sinus disease, even if they have no other nasal or sinus symptoms. The throat clearing can become habitual and the symptoms perpetuate.

The typical patient with GPRD often presents with a constellation of symptoms that differ from those with GERD: where GERD patients often complain of dyspepsia and heartburn, those with GPRD will usually have non-specific symptoms, such as mild hoarseness usually worse in the morning, a foreign body or 'globus' sensation, nocturnal cough, or the chronic need to clear the throat. The diagnosis in such patients is usually made by history suggestive of reflux. The physical examination may reveal some thickening or oedema of the posterior commissure or arytenoids, and occasionally will reveal erythema or cherry-red arytenoids. With advanced or prolonged reflux, contact ulcers, granulomas (Fig. 19.7), leukoplakia, evidence of chronic inflammation, or diffuse oedema can be seen. There has been some suggestion that reflux may even be a factor or cofactor in the development of laryngeal cancer.

The treatment of GPRD is dependent on the severity of symptoms and the certainty of the diagnosis. In most cases, diet and lifestyle are the major causes of GERD and GPRD, and dietary and lifestyle modifications will be adequate to alleviate the symptoms: smaller meals; a low-fat diet; avoidance of alcohol, tobacco and caffeine, not eating for 3–4 hours before bedtime, weight control; and elevation of the bedhead will control the symptoms in most patients. With severe reflux and hiatus hernia, avoidance of heavy lifting, stooping or tight clothing may be recommended. If these conservative measures are unsuccessful, a trial of antacids, especially at bedtime, may be suggested. If unsuccessful, a trial of a more aggressive pharmacological treatment can be considered; objective testing may be conducted if the diagnosis is uncertain.

AIDS and otolaryngology

Acquired immunodeficiency syndrome (AIDS) has had a profound impact on otolaryngology, as it has on all areas of medicine. Many patients will experience their first symptoms of AIDS in the head and neck. Although certain infectious processes are much more common in AIDS patients, all common infections may occur, including sinusitis, pharyngitis, tonsillitis, and otitis media and externa. These frequently seen conditions, however, will often fail to respond to the usual course of treatment, requiring repeated courses of antibiotics and perhaps surgery when complications occur. Resistance to treatment should alert the clinician to a possible immuno-deficiency.

Candida infections of the oral cavity, pharynx, larynx and oesophagus are more common in patients with AIDS. Herpes simplex and zoster infections are also more frequent and more severe. Giant herpetic ulcers may affect the mouth, nose or face; other ulcers of the oral cavity, specifically aphthous ulcers, may develop into giant ulcers and are extremely painful and difficult to treat. Hairy leukoplakia (Fig. 19.8) is a benign and painless condition that is also associated with HIV infection.

Nasopharyngeal lymphoid proliferation may present with nasal obstruction, snoring and serous otitis media with hearing loss. The findings of apparent adenoid hypertrophy in an adult with HIV infection risk factors should prompt the appropriate tests. Kaposi's sarcoma is a previously rare neoplasm and is the most common neoplastic process in AIDS patients: these lesions may be in the skin, lymph nodes or any mucosal surface of the head and neck.

The most common neck mass in patients infected with HIV is the enlarged lymph node. If one of these enlarged nodes becomes significantly larger than the rest, a diagnosis of lymphoma, which is associated with AIDS, must be considered. Benign lympho-epithelial lesions of the parotid glands have been noted in patients who are HIV seropositive. These lesions are typically cystic and bilateral, and can grow quite large. Diagnosis is based on the clinical presentation and fine-needle biopsy to rule out other neoplasms.

Excision, which involves superficial or total parotidectomy with facial nerve dissection, is reserved for neoplasms; benign lympho-epithelial lesions of the parotid glands should be followed for repeated aspirations of fluid, as needed for comfort, or for sudden changes in size, which may indicate the development of a lymphoma. In 50% of AIDS patients presentation will be with an opportunistic pulmonary infection such as *Pneumocystis carinii* pneumonia. Cough is the most common symptom of these infectious processes.

References

1. Benninger MS. Nasal endoscopy: its role in office diagnosis. *Am J Rhinol* 1997; 11: 177–180
2. Langmore SE, Schatz MA, Olsen N. Fiberoptic endoscopic examination of swallowing safety: a new procedure. *Dysphagia* 1988, 2: 216–219
3. Benninger MS. The medical examination. In: Benninger MS, Jacobson B, Johnson A (eds) Performing arts medicine, the care and prevention of professional voice disorders. New York: Thieme Medical, 1994: 86–96
4. Netterville JL, Vrabec JT. Unilateral palatal adhesion for paralysis after high vagal injury. *Arch Otolaryngol Head Neck Surg* 1994; 120: 218–221
5. Goode RL. Sleep disorders. In: Cummings CW (ed) Otolaryngology, head and neck surgery. St Louis: Mosby Year Book, 1986; 78: 1449–1457
6. Benninger MS, Mickelson SA, Yaremchuk K. Functional endoscopic sinus surgery: morbidity and early results. *Henry Ford Hospital Med J* 1990; 38: 5–8
7. Frantz TD, Rasgon BM. Acute epiglottitis: changing epidemiologic patterns. *Otolaryngol Head Neck Surg* 1993; 109: 457–460
8. Koufman JA, Wiener GJ, Wu WC, Castell DO. Reflux laryngitis and its sequelae: the diagnostic role of ambulatory 24-hour pH monitoring. *J Voice* 1988; 2: 78–89
9. Woo P, Colton R, Casper J, Brewer D. Diagnostic value of stroboscopic examination in hoarse patients. *J Voice* 1991; 5: 231–238
10. Sataloff RT, Spiegel JR, Hawkshaw MJ. Strobovideolaryngoscopy: results and clinical value. *Ann Otol Rhinol Laryngol* 1991; 100: 725–728
11. Jones SR, Myers EN, Barnes L. Benign neoplasms of the larynx. *Otolaryngol Clin North Am* 1984; 17: 1–178
12. Olson NR. Laryngopharyngeal manifestations of gastroesophageal reflux disease. *Otolaryngol Clin North Am* 1991; 24: 1201–1213
13. Koufman JA. The otolaryngologic manifestations of gastroesophageal reflux (GERD): a clinical investigation of 225 patients using ambulatory pH monitoring and an experimental investigation of the role of acid and pepsin in the development of laryngeal injury. *Laryngoscope* 1991; 53(Suppl): 71–78

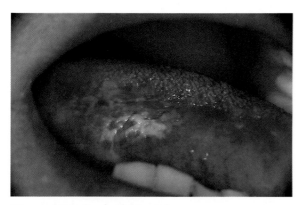

Figure 19.8. *Leukoplakia of the tongue.*

CHAPTER 20

Setting up a Well Man clinic in primary care

M. G. Kirby

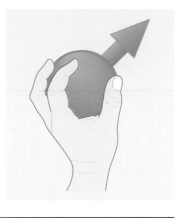

Introduction

Primary health care in the UK and around the world is undergoing a number of fundamental changes. There is increasing recognition of the importance of lifestyle and environmental factors in staying healthy and maintaining quality of life, with the objective of 'Adding life to years, not just years to life'. The World Health Organization/ United Nations International Children's Emergency Fund Alma-Ata Declaration of 1978, which was subsequently reflected in the report by the UK Department of Health, *The Health of the Nation* [1], has led to an increasing interest in health promotion and disease prevention.

The Department of Health set out the framework for a new health strategy for the UK in a Green Paper, *Our Healthier Nation* [2], in 1998. Its twin aims were to improve the health of the nation as a whole by increasing the length of people's lives and the number of years people spend free of illness, and to improve the health of the worst-off in society and narrow the health gap. It was recognized that there are major opportunities to improve people's health: almost 90 000 people die in the UK every year before the age of 65; of these, nearly 32 000 die of cancer and 25 000 die of heart disease, stroke and related illnesses. Many of these deaths could be prevented by changes in lifestyle, and health-promotion activity is seen as a catalyst for this change.

There are sound economic reasons for improving the health of the nation. A total of 187 million working days are estimated to be lost every year owing to sickness, equating to a £12 billion tax on business. The treatment of ill-health is also costly: for example, it has been estimated that the annual cost to the National Health Service (NHS) of treating heart disease, stroke and related illnesses is £3.8 billion. Major advances in information technology have facilitated audit and recall procedures and, each year, general practi-

tioners (GPs) are expected to be more accountable and to provide value for money.

The NHS reforms of the 1990s resulted in major changes to health promotion in general practice. Prior to 1990 the area was entirely under the jurisdiction of individual practices and formed part of the General Medical Services. Since 1990, there has been considerable health promotion activity in general practice in the UK; however, unfortunately, this has been confused by rapid changes in the rules of health promotion, as well as by regional variation in interpretation. Existing payments to primary care practitioners were redistributed and this led to uncontrolled and unevaluated health-promotion activity. Professional concern and uncontrolled costs led to a change in the banding system, in which there was an attempt to address smoking, hypertension and cardiovascular disease on a national basis. This was subsequently replaced in October 1996 by Health Promotion Committees (HPCs), whose function is to advise health authorities as to the acceptability of health-promotion programmes submitted to them by the Primary Health Care Team (PHCT).

The HPCs take into account four main criteria:

1. Current authoritative medical opinion as to the effectiveness of the programme;
2. Health-of-the-nation strategies, priorities and objectives;
3. Local strategies, priorities and objectives;
4. Benefit to patients.

As a result of this, health promotion has become far simpler, more flexible and professionally led. All primary-care practitioners are eligible to be paid for undertaking health-promotion activity and for chronic disease management of asthma, diabetes or both, and practices should describe such activities on an annual basis. A description of the health-promotion programmes must be submitted by 31 December each year and, once approved, programmes stay eligible for payment if the health authority is satisfied that they have been completed as approved, subject to minor variations. In the UK, the annual payment for a health-promotion programme for a GP with an average list size (1884 patients) is currently £2340; this is adjusted pro rata for other list sizes.

Aims of *The Health of the Nation*

The key health areas that have been targeted for improvement are shown in Table 20.1 [1] and the criteria employed in their selection in Table 20.2. This concept has been a tremendous step forward for health care in the UK: for the first time there has been a coherent structure through which prevention could be delivered to the public, drawing on the huge potential of health professionals throughout the country.

Evaluation of the effects of this initiative and the impact on public health will be difficult to establish. However, statistics provided by the Office of Population Censuses and Surveys (OPCS) have indicated little change [3]. This confirms a health-behaviour survey carried out as part of the health-of-the-nation strategy, which indicated little change in the trend of key life-style risks among the population. Ultimately, it will probably be impossible to sift out the effects of the Health of the Nation programme from other social influences that impact on health and quality of life, such as demographic shifts, alterations in the labour market and the distribution of wealth among our population. Nevertheless, the 1998 Green Paper, *Our Healthier Nation*, set out clear targets for improvements in four priority areas by the year 2010 (Table 20.3) [2].

Well Man clinics

Male morbidity and mortality are both greater than those of females in all five key areas shown in Table 20.1 and, as a result of this, Well Man clinics qualify under all five of the HPC criteria stated in Table 20.2. Primary care practitioners may consider that developing a more systematic approach towards the organization of these services for men, including the development of Well Man clinics, could be advantageous in a number of ways (Table 20.4). These objectives can be achieved by introducing a systematic, protocol-led approach to selective disease groups and/or health screening. This can be accomplished by incorporating some (or all) of the following specific tasks into the clinic plan and by addressing those diseases that target men exclusively or preferentially:

- Health information: providing detailed, accurate current health information;
- Health screening: systematically searching for diseases where early detection is important;
- Treatment: monitoring and adjusting for chronic conditions;
- Surveillance: monitoring borderline abnormalities.

Significant health areas for men

Ischaemic heart disease and atherosclerosis

The UK has the second-highest male cardiovascular mortality rate after Finland. Coronary heart disease (CHD) is the single largest cause of death

---

Table 20.1. The Health of the Nation *improvement targets prioritized by key health areas [1]*

- Heart disease and stroke
- Cancers
- Mental illness, depression, anxiety and related consequences, such as suicide
- Sexual health, particularly containment of HIV/AIDS
- Accidents

Table 20.2. *Selection criteria for key areas*

- Should be a significant source of ill-health, disability and premature death
- Should offer scope for improvement
- Should have identifiable risk factors that could be addressed through health promotion
- Should lead to a measurable improvement following health promotion
- Should allow the setting of targets for improvement

Table 20.3. *Healthcare targets set by the 1998 Green Paper 'Our Healthier Nation'*

Healthcare area	Target
▨ Heart disease and stroke	▨ To reduce the death rate from heart disease and stroke, and related illness, among people aged under 65 years by at least one-third
▨ Accidents	▨ To reduce accidents by at least one-fifth
▨ Cancer	▨ To reduce the death rate from cancer amongst people aged under 65 years by at least one-fifth
▨ Mental health	▨ To reduce the death rate from suicide and undetermined injury by at least one-sixth.

Table 20.4. *Benefits of developing a Well Man clinic*

- ▨ Quality of care
- ▨ Health-promotion payments
- ▨ Healthier patients
- ▨ Team building
- ▨ Audit
- ▨ Patient demand
- ▨ Health of the Nation targets
- ▨ Proven clinical effectiveness
- ▨ More effective use of resources
- ▨ Greater utilization of data collected
- ▨ Sensitive to local health care need
- ▨ Optimized purchasing decisions

and the main cause of premature death in both men and women, accounting for 24% of deaths in England in 1994. In the same year, stroke accounted for 11% of all deaths. The opportunity to address lifestyle and risk factors provides scope for preventing illness, disability and death from these conditions. The OPCS *Health Survey for England 1993* showed that only 10% of the population are free from the major risk factors for CHD [4]. Asians residing in England have a particularly high risk of CHD and West Indians a particularly high risk of stroke. A number of other interesting statistics were revealed by the 1993 survey:

- ▨ Of the total male population, 12% are hypertensive and untreated;
- ▨ More than two-thirds of adults have a blood cholesterol level above 5.2 mmol/l;
- ▨ Insufficient physical activity is taken by 80% of adults;
- ▨ A total of 42% of men are overweight (Body Mass Index 25–30);
- ▨ Insufficient exercise is taken by 70% of men, and 61% of adult males who take little or no exercise consider themselves to be very or fairly fit.

Other statistics to be considered include the fact that up to 18% of CHD deaths and 11% of stroke deaths are associated with smoking [5] and 28% of adults in England are regular cigarette smokers [6].

Physical inactivity has been shown to double the risk of CHD [7] and triple the risk of stroke [8]. Conversely, studies suggest causal associations between regular physical activity and reduced rates of CHD, hypertension, non-insulin-dependent diabetes, osteoporosis, colon cancer, anxiety and depression [9]. Some specific benefits of exercise in middle-aged and elderly patients are shown in Table 20.5 [10]. Clearly, the link between exercise and health status is not a new finding; according to the observations of the 18th century Scottish physician, Dr William Buchan:

'Of all the causes that conspire to render the life of man short and miserable, none have greater influence than the want of exercise.'

Health-education campaigns on physical fitness have increased the general population's knowledge and awareness of the benefits of regular exercise. Because no consistent specific recommendations exist for exercise programmes, each person should tailor their regimen to their individ-

Table 20.5. *Benefits of exercise in middle-aged and elderly patients*

Type of exercise	Benefit
Combined weight training, walking	Increased endurance and strength
Tai chi, endurance training, leg strengthening	Reduced risk of fall
Tai chi, endurance, weights	Improved gait and balance
Aerobics (walking, jogging, bicycling)	Lower systolic and diastolic blood pressure
Endurance training, aerobics	Increased glucose tolerance/decreased insulin resistance
Endurance training, aerobics	Increased HDL
	Reduced risk of:
Endurance training, aerobics	CHD
Endurance training, aerobics	Type II diabetes
Physical activity	Colorectal cancer
Weight training	Increased bone density
Weight training, endurance	Positive effect on anxiety, depression and sleep
Endurance, aerobics	Decreased CHD and all-cause mortality

HDL, high-density lipoprotein; CHD, coronary heart disease.

(Adapted from ref. 10 with permission.)

ual baseline fitness level, physical capacity and any coexisting disability. Types of moderate physical activity that can be undertaken by middle-aged patients are listed in Table 20.6 [10]. The GP can assist by defining the individual's perception of the subject and identifying any barriers to the use of regular exercise. Most adults do not need medical testing, but men over 40 and women over 50 with known CHD or multiple risk factors of CHD should seek medical advice before starting exercise programmes.

Another risk factor for cardiovascular disease is increased waist circumference. Waist measurement increases with overweight and central fat distribution, both of which are related to preventable ill-health. In a study by Han and associates, two action levels of waist circumference were determined to identify men whose health risks were increasing (action level 1: 94 cm) or were high (action level 2: 102 cm) [11]. Results showed that, compared with men with waist circumferences below action level 1, those with waist circumferences between action level 1 and 2 were 1.5–2 times as likely to have one or more major cardiovascular risk factors (Fig. 20.1). Men with a waist circumference above action level 2 were 2.5–4.5 times as likely to have one or more major cardiovascular risk factors (Fig. 20.1). The authors conclude that a waist circumference above 94 cm should be a signal to avoid weight gain or to lose weight, to maintain physical activity and to give up smoking in order to reduce the risk of cardiovascular disease. Patients with a waist circumference greater than 102 cm should seek medical advice from a health professional regarding weight management.

Lung disease, cancers and chronic obstructive pulmonary disease (COPD)

Lung cancer is the commonest cause of cancer death in men in the UK. Smoking causes 80% of lung cancer deaths [5], and non-smokers exposed to tobacco smoke most of their lives have a 10–30% greater risk of lung cancer than other non-smokers [12]. Stopping smoking is the most effective way to improve the health of smokers. Men are giving up smoking, but often later in life when they have started to have other symptoms and, therefore, some of the damage has already been done. COPD is caused predominantly by

Table 20.6. *Examples of moderate physical activity suitable for middle-aged patients*

LESS VIGOROUS, MORE TIME

- Washing and waxing a car for 45–60 minutes
- Washing windows/floors for 45–60 minutes
- Playing volleyball for 45 minutes
- Playing touch football for 45 minutes
- Gardening for 35–40 minutes
- Wheeling self in wheelchair for 30–40 minutes
- Walking for 1.75 miles in 35 minutes (20-minute mile)
- Basketball (shooting hoops) for 30 minutes
- Bicycling 5 miles in 30 minutes
- Pushing pushchair 1.5 miles in 30 minutes
- Raking leaves for 30 minutes
- Walking 2 miles in 30 minutes (15-minute mile)
- Water aerobics for 30 minutes
- Swimming laps for 20 minutes
- Wheelchair basketball for 20 minutes
- Basketball (playing a game) for 15–20 minutes
- Bicycling 4 miles in 15 minutes
- Skipping rope for 15 minutes
- Running 1.75 miles in 15 minutes (10-minute mile)
- Shovelling snow for 15 minutes
- Walking up and down stairs for 15 minutes

MORE VIGOROUS, LESS TIME

(From ref. 10 with permission.)

smoking cigarettes and more men die from COPD annually (nearly 30 000) than from lung cancer. The cost of COPD has a huge impact on NHS resources, as an estimated 10% of the adult UK population suffer from the disease; despite this, many do not seek medical advice and only about 25% are diagnosed [13].

Mental health problems and suicide (see Chapter 16)

Mental health causes considerable personal suffering and affects quality of life, leading to significant demands on the NHS and Social Services. In 1992 there were 4000 male suicides [14]. Highest suicide rates are reported in men aged 35–44 years, although there was a 75% increase

in incidence in younger men aged 15–24 years between 1982 and 1992 [15].

Accident prevention

Accidents are the most common cause of death in people under the age of 30. They not only cause considerable short-term illness but also may lead to permanent disability. In 1992 4743 deaths in England were caused by accidental injuries to people aged 15–64 years, over three-quarters of whom were men. The rate of accidental death in men exceeds that in women at all ages. In males, motor-vehicle traffic accidents account for 46% of all accidental deaths. Men are also more likely than women to be involved in sporting accidents [16].

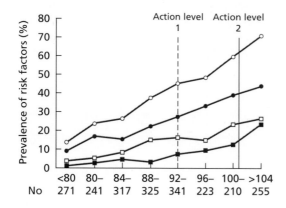

Figure 20.1. *Larger waist circumference identifies men at increased cardiovascular risks. (●) Low high density lipoprotein cholesterol. (□) Hypercholesterolaemia. (■) Hypertension. (○) Any one or more risk factors. (From ref. 11 with permission.)*

Sexually transmitted disease and HIV

Transmission of HIV and sexually transmitted diseases (STDs) can be prevented by sustained changes in sexual behaviour. Ignorance, or perhaps ill-educated risk taking, is rife despite significant advertising campaigns. The correct use of condoms, which gives almost 100% protection, is not widespread enough to prevent an increase in the incidence of HIV and STDs. Over the past decade, HIV infection has emerged as a substantial contributor to male mortality and the majority of HIV infections have been acquired as a result of sex between men. In addition, almost all recipients of contaminated blood products have been males with haemophilia and most injecting drug misusers infected with HIV have been male. Up to the end of 1992, 93% of people with a diagnosis of AIDS and 88% of those infected with HIV were men. Both gonorrhoea and syphilis are also more common in men [17].

Urological disorders

Up to 40% of men aged 65–69 years have clinically detectable benign prostatic hyperplasia (BPH) and the disease becomes progressively more common in the ageing male. Between 1975 and 1990 there was a 62% increase in prostatectomies undertaken in the NHS. Many men present with acute urinary retention (AUR): in 1990, 16% of transurethral resections of the prostate and 35% of retropubic prostatectomies were performed as emergency operations due to AUR [18]. The Department of Health identified BPH as a priority area for research funding during 1993–1994. Prostate cancer is the second-commonest cause of cancer death in men, resulting in nearly 10 000 deaths in the UK each year, and the incidence has risen over the past decade. In the UK, more than 50% of men present with metastatic disease [19] and early diagnosis is essential if a cure is to be achieved.

Testicular tumours have a peak incidence at around the age of 30 years and are the most common tumours in men aged 24–34 years. Early diagnosis is essential and, with modern treatment regimens, mortality continues to fall, even though the incidence of these tumours has increased over the past decade [20].

Alcohol problems

The use of alcohol and subsequent intoxication tend to be associated with loss of inhibition, risk-taking behaviours and increased aggression. The regular consumption by men of four or more units per day is not advisable because of the progressive health risk it carries; however 6% of men drink in excess of 50 units a week.

Drug and substance abuse

Three-quarters of the opioid addicts (most of whom are heroin users) that are notified to the Government Home Office are men [21]. In 1998, 50% of drug offenders in the UK were aged 21–29 years and 88% of these were men [21].

Malignant disease

Cancer incidence is higher amongst men than women, and overall accounted for approximately 26% of deaths in the UK in 1992 and has now overtaken heart disease as the leading cause of mortality: in 1996, there were 156 890 deaths from cancer and 148 186 deaths from heart disease. Many of these deaths are preventable by reducing risk factors and by early detection; for example, 88% of all skin cancers are avoidable [22].

Skin disease

From the age of 20 to 39 years, malignant melanoma accounts for 8% of cancer incidence and 4% of cancer deaths [23]. However, the burden of non-melanotic skin cancer is also considerable: over 31 500 new cases were registered in the UK in 1989 [24].

Diet

Overweight and obesity are ever-increasing problems in the Western world. Between 1980 and 1996 in Great Britain, obesity rates amongst men increased from 6% to 16% [25]. There is little doubt that available statistical and epidemiological evidence indicates the importance of dietary habits as a major influence on both carcinogenesis and arterial disease. Decreased incidence rates of both diseases are considered to be attainable by reducing fat intake and increasing fruit and vegetable consumption. The concept of free radicals in relation to their putative role in human disease is important, particularly in relationship to antioxidants such as vitamins A, C and E, which are constituents of a healthy diet. There is currently no evidence to indicate that taking vitamins as supplements or alternatives to a diet rich in fruit and vegetables will provide extra protection. Eating five portions of fruit and vegetables a day could lead to a 20–30% reduction in death due to heart disease. In addition, it does not matter how the fruit and vegetables are eaten: raw or cooked, fresh or frozen, tinned or dried — all are beneficial. There is a wide variation in fruit and vegetable consumption within the UK: in Scotland and northern England the consumption is less than two portions a day, whereas up to three portions are eaten in southwest and south-east England. The consumption in the UK is about one-half of that in Italy and Spain and one-third of that in Greece, where the incidence of heart disease is 50% less than in the UK.

Is health promotion good value?

Evidence suggests that health promotion is a cost-effective method for improving patients' health. The British Family Heart Study was designed to determine the cost effectiveness of a cardiovascular screening and intervention programme led by practice nurses using a family-centred approach, with follow-up according to degree of risk of cardiovascular disease. The costs of the programme were determined at £5.08–5.78 per patient per 1% reduction in coronary risk [26]. The OXCHECK Study was designed to determine the cost effectiveness of health checks done by nurses in primary care (cardiovascular risk factor screening and intervention programme). The costs of this study were set at £1.46–2.25 per patient per 1% reduction in coronary risk [27]. The Action Heart Intervention Study in the Rotherham area compared changes in lifestyle in a community where health promotion was used with those in another similar community where it was not used [28]. This 4-year health-promotion effort probably reduced smoking by 6.9% and increased the consumption of low-fat milk. The cost effectiveness of this study, calculated at £31 per life year gained,

was good value when compared with health-care interventions for other diseases and health checks such as OXCHECK, the British Family Heart Study and the use of statin lipid-lowering treatment in primary and secondary prevention.

Well Man clinic: financial considerations

A detailed calculation of the impact of running a Well Man clinic on the practice accounts will include costs that are both obvious and hidden. Individual practices will need to decide at partnership level how the activity will be funded and whether it is cost effective. The individual costs that should be considered include the following:

- Staff costs;
- Overheads: such as heat, light, photocopying, correspondence, telephone, etc.;
- Computer costs;
- Medical, e.g. urine dipsticks and pathology costs;
- Equipment, e.g. weighing scales, vitalograph, urinary flow meter;
- Hidden costs, such as increased prescribing costs driven by case finding, referral costs for investigation and treatment and increased attendance at follow-up clinics.

A source of income for running such clinics obviously needs consideration and this potentially can be derived from health authority fees, item-of-service fees, sponsorship, commissioning, Medical Audit Advisory Group support and patient charges (i.e. private clinic).

Professional roles

Teamwork has been the strength of British primary care for some years and the co-ordinated activity needed by the present-day health care system requires a number of different skills that can function efficiently only in the team setting. Teamwork is the key to efficient health promotion and prevention of illness. The doctor, of course, bears a heavy responsibility for the outcome of these activities and leadership is essential. Typically, the team would include the following members:

- Doctor: the buck stops here;
- Team leader: financial and medical responsibility;

- Practice nurse or health visitor: day-to-day clinic work; consults with patients and refers medical questions to GP for decision;
- Receptionist: makes appointments, handles mail and telephone calls;
- Audit assistant: audit of clinic attendance, outcome, etc.

Factors affecting the establishment of a good team and how to assess the quality of the team-work produced are detailed in Table 20.7 [29].

How to proceed

The six essential steps to developing an efficient Well Man clinic are detailed below.

1. Develop effective teamwork

This involves shared goals and understanding of each others' roles. One way of developing effective procedures and inter-personal relationships is to use a SWOT analysis: the group meets to discuss and agree the current strengths (S), weaknesses (W), opportunities (O) and threats (T) in setting up a Well Man clinic. Examples of factors relevant to each area are shown in Table 20.8.

2. Focus on men's health

It is important for members of the team to have a shared understanding of men's health. This may be promoted initially with the use of a brainstorming session at which key areas of men's health are discussed. In this way, it is possible to raise awareness of the diseases from which men suffer, and a protocol can be constructed and an action plan developed.

3. Arrange meeting to discuss practicalities

The practicalities that need to be discussed include the following:

1. Agree the partner or colleague for the project;
2. Define practice priorities in terms of which services need to be provided and which disease areas are important;
3. Arrange literature search and future meeting to present results of this;
4. Establish who will do what, where and when;
5. Agree timing of clinics and provisional start date;
6. Define patient target group, e.g. for men aged 45–60;
7. Estimate numbers of patients attending the clinic;

Table 20.7. *Factors affecting the establishment of a successful Well Man clinic team [29]*

Leadership qualities

1. Inspires trust
2. Selects good staff
3. Has infectious enthusiasm
4. Is a good listener
5. Runs effective meetings
6. Good presenter
7. Accepts responsibility
8. Can tolerate uncertainties
9. Responds positively to conflict and failure
10. Has a good sense of humour
11. Maintains good morale

Factors helpful to team morale

1. Small organization that communicates well
2. High quality and level of training of staff
3. High motivation and dedication
4. Clear sense of direction and goals shared by all
5. Organizational stability and low staff turnover
6. Sensitive to patients' needs
7. Quality assurance with results shared with all concerned
8. Regular reports of progress towards goals and targets
9. An open style of organization and leadership
10. Adaptability to change
11. Able to contain conflict where used constructively

How to measure the quality of team work

1. The views and judgement of people concerned, such as patients, staff, authorities, other professional teams, using appropriate criteria
2. The innovativeness of the team
3. Team vision and shared objectives
4. Participative safety, implying that the team is seen by members as supportive and that information is safe within the team
5. Commitment to excellence and a shared concern for quality of team and individual performance
6. Audit activity
7. Re-audit to assess change

Table 20.8. *SWOT analysis in the development of a Well Man clinic*

Strengths (S)	Weaknesses (W)
▧ Committed team	▧ Premises in poor repair
▧ Clear protocol	▧ Inadequate space
▧ Sound knowledge base	▧ Nurse needs computer terminal
▧ Convenient appointment times	▧ None of the present team has experience in sexual health
▧ Health Authority support	▧ Staff already have time pressures
▧ Health Promotion Committee approval	▧ Generates more work
▧ Patients appreciate	▧ Time not convenient
▧ Variety of work	

Opportunities (O)	Threats (T)
▧ Learning	▧ Lack of motivation
▧ Disease prevention	▧ Falling practice size
▧ Healthier, happier patients	▧ Staff member leaving
▧ Financial support	▧ Future funding uncertain
▧ Increased quality of care	▧ Political change in the NHS
▧ New practice partner enthusiastic	▧ Time pressures
▧ Practice staff enthusiastic	▧ Financial shortage
	▧ Cost of training

8. Define length of appointments;
9. Clarify how staff can get access to a doctor if questions arise during consultation or prescriptions are needed;
10. Inform patients about the clinic:
    - ▧ Practice notice-board
    - ▧ Practice leaflet
    - ▧ Opportunities during consultation
    - ▧ Computer searches
    - ▧ Disease indexes
    - ▧ Local newspaper publicity;
11. Make arrangements for appointments and recall, systematic or opportunistic; make a decision regarding whether non-attenders will be reappointed;
12. Are there any cultural or language implications?
13. Specific approach to men with learning difficulties?
    - ▧ The disabled or housebound;
14. Get approval from the HPC;
15. Develop an audit trail.

4. Arrange follow-up meetings

Such clinic arrangements should be flexible and planning should be seen as a learning process. The team members should be encouraged to be innovative and to acknowledge mistakes made and lessons learned. In this way, the team's knowledge base will be increased and confidence in managing men's health problems will be increased.

5. Audit

Audit activity needs to be simple and focused on specific terms of reference. It is a means of making sure that the best possible care is being provided to the patients. Feedback and re-audit are necessary in order to ensure that any agreed recommendations are implemented and effective. For an effective audit, a positive approach is essential: 'Am I (or are we) doing well'; 'can I (or can we) do better?' Audit should involve staff, not just the doctors, and is a collective way of improving patient care. Staff performing the audit should be team members and attend meetings to discuss the results. Remember to have a clear purpose in mind and ask simple questions: 'keep it short and simple' (KISS) [30].

6. Protocols

A clinic can function effectively only if there is a clear understanding of agreed procedures and guidelines. It is important to define clearly what information is to be recorded and where; this keeps the clinic focused and the staff interested and motivated, and facilitates audit and report. Such a protocol will allow the prompt recognition of trends and allows the staff to attach value to what they are doing. It is important to ensure that, at each attendance, the minimum data set per patient is recorded and that, at regular defined intervals, a collation of these data occurs by a defined individual and the audit cycle is completed.

A sample protocol for a Well Man clinic is shown in Table 20.9.

Table 20.9. *Sample protocol for a Well Man clinic*

Personal data

Name

Date of birth

Address

Occupation

Marital status

Employment situation

Smoking status

Average alcohol consumption

Sexual orientation (if relevant)

Enquire about skin health and discuss avoidance of sunburn

Health problems

Current and significant past

Therapy history

Current medication

Prescription and self-medication

Family history

▢ Heart disease	▢ High blood pressure	▢ Stroke
▢ Prostate cancer	▢ Hypothyroidism	▢ Diabetes
▢ Other forms of cancer	▢ Gout	▢ Epilepsy

Cholesterol

▢ Ever tested?	▢ Needs testing?

Stress

Enquire about level of stress and consider the use of a rating scale [31]. Reinforce advice regarding safe limits of alcohol

Depression

Enquire about depression and consider use of a rating scale [31]

Accidents

Eyesight check, take care with prescribed drugs when driving; don't drink and drive; all drugs at home to be kept under lock and key

Sexual health

Discuss safe sex methods and precautions against sexually transmitted diseases; advise use of condoms and reduction of numbers of sexual partners

Table 20.9. *cont.*

Exercise history

How much and how often, daily exercise where possible, but at least 20 minutes three times a week

Steps to ensure safe exercise

- Wear suitable footwear, preferably with ankle support and designed for walking or jogging
- Consider the use of shock-absorbing inserts if there is arthritis pain in knees or hips
- Drink plenty of water before and after exercise
- Wear clothing that allows ease of movement and evaporation of water
- Avoid exercising outdoors in very warm or very cold weather
- Stop exercising immediately if the following symptoms occur: chest pain, shortness of breath, dizziness, light-headedness or palpitations
- Do not exercise if suffering from any infectious condition, such as a cold or influenza
- Consider supervised training in a gymnasium

Exercise with a partner if possible

Prostate health

Ask the following questions:

- Are you bothered by urinary function?
- Do you get up at night to pass water?
- Have you noticed a deterioration in your urinary stream?

An affirmative answer should lead to the use of the International Prostate Symptom Score and Quality of Life Assessment

Testicular health

Offer a leaflet on self-examination

Osteoporosis risk

Provide check-list for risk factors for osteoporosis in men and consider use of DXA scan to evaluate if positive

Risk factors

Previous fracture	Hypogonadism	Steroid use
Alcohol excess	Heavy smoking	COPD
Intestinal disease	Gastric surgery	Coeliac disease
Thyroid disease	Hypercalciuria	Ankylosing spondylitis
Low calcium intake	Family history of fractures caused by osteoporosis	
Anti-convulsant therapy	Anorexia nervosa	

Examination

- Height/weight: calculate and explain the BMI
- Measure waist circumference: larger waist circumference identifies people at increased cardiovascular risk (Fig. 20.1) [11]
- Blood pressure: < 140/85 mmHg, reassure and recommend a further check, not longer than 5 years; 140/85–150/90 mmHg, recommend annual review; unless patient is diabetic or has other cardiovascular risk factors ≥ 150/90 mmHg, repeat three times over the next 4 weeks and then review with the GP
- Rectal examination where appropriate

Investigations

- Urinalysis: dipstick test for blood, glucose and protein; if abnormal, send MSU to laboratory; ensure the patient has instructions for collection of MSU and refer patient to GP for advice
- Peak expiratory flow rate

Table 20.9. *cont.*

Investigations cont.

    Consider use of vitalograph if early COPD suspected

Blood tests

    Blood cholesterol: where indicated according to other cardiovascular risk factors

    HIV and PSA test should not be requested without suitable pretest counselling

Review all data collected

Give advice and appropriate leaflets on smoking, diet and weight control, exercise, lifestyle, avoidance of sunburn, sexual health, family history of coronary heart disease, any previous cardiovascular events, prostate health, testicular health and bone health

Immunizations

Ensure the patient is fully immunized according to approved guidelines

Follow-up

If no problems detected, offer repeat appointment in 5 years; if any significant abnormality detected, refer to doctor

Audit

Every 6 months audit data will be reviewed, numbers seen and non-attenders, problems detected, outcomes, consider patient satisfaction survey

Complaints

Referral to practice-based complaints procedure at earliest opportunity

Current concerns

Any questions about health that are worrying the patient at this time

Erectile dysfunction

Many primary-care practitioners are considering the advisability of setting up an inhouse service for erectile dysfunction

Patients with a history of heart disease

A focused history and examination in these patients is important because they are at high absolute risk for further problems, with a four- to eight-fold increased risk of recurrence [32]; there is also good evidence of benefit [33], and risk management and treatment are cost effective [34]

This is a special group that needs an additional protocol:

1. History of cardiac event
2. Date of admission to hospital
3. What diagnosis was made?
4. Details of current medication
5. Is the patient compliant with medication?
6. Is blood pressure controlled?
7. Is the patient currently smoking?
8. Hospital follow-up arrangements
9. What tests have been performed:
       Cholesterol
       Has diabetes been excluded?
       ECG
       Exercise treadmill test

Table 20.9. *cont.*

Patients with a history of heart disease cont.

- Echocardiogram

10. Are there any current complaints:
- Chest pain
- Palpitations
- Shortness of breath
- Cough
- Ankle swelling
- Orthopnoea
- Paroxysmal nocturnal dyspnoea

Check patient is on aspirin

Aspirin should be in routine use unless there is a contraindication

ACE inhibitor indicated

Consider the use of ACE inhibition if the patient has a past history of cardiac failure, hypertension, diabetes or microalbuminuria

Investigations

BMI	Blood pressure	Urinalysis
Blood sugar	Blood lipids	ECG
Echocardiogram		

Review of history and examination

Be prepared to give advice with appropriate supportive literature on cardiac symptoms, smoking, alcohol, exercise, cardiac rehabilitation programme, diet and obesity, medication, reinforce importance of regular follow-up. Are the blood lipids in the target area? Is the patient on aspirin? Is an ACE inhibitor indicated? Was the patient prescribed a beta-blocker and has it been continued? Is there any indication for the use of anticoagulation: for example, has the patient ever been, or is he currently, in atrial fibrillation?

ACE, angiotensin-converting enzyme; BMI, body mass index; COPD, chronic obstructive pulmonary disease; DEXA, dual energy X-ray absorptiometry; ECG, electrocardiogram; HIV, human immunodeficiency virus; MSU, midstream urine; PSA, prostate-specific antigen.

Conclusions

Health and lifestyle up to the age of 65 years are likely to be major determinants of the quality of life after that age, and the health of men in the working age group will be a key factor in any nation's economic activity and success. Ill-health and disability can wreak havoc in the family unit, causing much unhappiness. With increased media activity, it is likely that men born after the Second World War will become more health conscious and present for a medical check because they want to remain healthy and not to succumb to premature illness or death.

The 1998 Green Paper acknowledges that loss of good health is no longer about blame, but about opportunity and responsibility. Individuals can find it hard to make a difference, but when they are supported by the Primary Health Care Team (PHCT) and work together with families, local agencies, communities and the government, deep-seated problems can be tackled.

There are many gaps and unanswered questions in the data on preventive health care for men, and physicians must therefore use available recommendations when developing any form of health-improvement programme. Each practice will wish to individualize its programme after assessing the health needs of the local population, deciding on the range and location of health services and determining local targets and standards. Activity will have to be tailored according to resources available, in partnership with government and health authority initiatives. This chapter is designed to provide the building blocks to construct a comprehensive programme for the health of men in primary care.

References

1. Department of Health. The Health of the Nation: a strategy for health in England. London: HMSO, 1992
2. Department of Health. Our Healthier Nation: A Contract for Health. Wetherby: Department of Health, 1998
3. OPCS. *Social Trends* 1997; 27: 1–30
4. OPCS. Health Survey for England 1993. London: HMSO, 1994
5. Health Education Authority. The smoking epidemic. A manifesto for action in England. London, 1992
6. OPCS. The General Household Survey 1992 Report. London: HMSO, 1994
7. Wannamethee G, Shaper AG. Physical activity in stroke in middle aged men. *Br Med J* 1992; 204: 597–601
8. Feingard RH. Physical fitness and blood pressure. *J Hypertens* 1994; 11(Suppl 5): 547–552
9. Pate RR, Pratt M, Blair SN *et al.* Physical activity and public health: a recommendation from The Centers for Disease Control and Prevention and the American College of Sports Medicine. JAMA 1995; 273: 402–407
10. Gunnarsson OT, Judge JO. Exercise at midlife: how and why to prescribe it for sedentary patients. *Geriatrics* 1997; 52: 71–80
11. Han TS, van Leer EM, Seidell JC, Lean ME. Waist circumference action levels in the identification of cardiovascular risk factors: prevalence study in a random sample. *Br Med J* 1995; 311: 1401–1405
12. Independent Scientific Committee on Smoking and Health. Fourth report. London: HMSO, 1998
13. Pearson MJ, Littler J, Davies PDO. An analysis of medical workload by speciality and diagnosis in Merseyside. Evidence of specialist to patient mismatch. *J R Coll Phys Lond* 1994; 28: 230–234
14. Meltzer H, Gill B, Pettigrew M. The prevalence of psychiatric morbidity among adults aged 16 to 64, living in private households in Great Britain. OPCS surveys of psychiatric morbidity in Great Britain. Bulletin 1. London: HMSO, 1994
15. Charlton J, Kelly S, Dunnell K, Evans B. Trends in suicide deaths in England and Wales. *Popul Trends* 1992; 69: 10–16
16. Department of Health. On The State of the Public Health. London: HMSO, 1992: 100
17. Department of Health. On the State of the Public Health. London: HMSO, 1992: 99
18. Donovan J, Frankel S, Nanchahal K *et al.* Prostatectomy for benign prostatic hyperplasia. Epidemiologically based needs assessment: Report 8. London: Department of Health, 1992
19. Schroder FH. Prostate cancer: To screen or not to screen? *Br Med J* 1993; 306: 407–408
20. Department of Health. On the State of the Public Health. London: HMSO, 1992: 96
21. National Audit of Drug Misuse Statistics. Drug misuse in Britain. London: Institute for Studies of Drug Dependence, 1990
22. Sunshine and Skin Cancer: Consensus Statement by the UK Skin Cancer Prevention Work Party, London: British Association of Dermatology, 1994
23. OPCS. Cancer statistics. Registration of cancer diagnosed in 1989 — England and Wales. Series MB1, No 22. London: HMSO, 1994
24. OPCS. Cancer statistics — registrations. Series MB1, No.22. London: HMSO, 1989
25. Kelly S, Dunnell K, Fox J. Health trends over the last 50 years. *Health Trends* 1998; 30: 10–15
26. Wonderling D, McDermott C, Buxton M *et al.* Costs and cost effectiveness of cardiovascular screening and intervention: The British Family Heart Study. *Br Med J* 1996; 312: 1269–1273
27. Langham S, Thorogood M, Normand C *et al.* Costs and cost effectiveness in health checks conducted by nurses in primary care: the OXCHECK Study. *Br Med J* 1996; 312: 1265–1268
28. Baxter T, Milner P, Wilson K *et al.* A cost-effective, community-based heart health promotion project in England: prospective comparative study. *Br Med J* 1997; 315: 582–585
29. Pritchard P, Pritchard J. Teamwork for primary and shared care: a practical workbook (Practical Guide for General Practice 17), 2nd edn. Oxford: Oxford Medical Publications, 1994
30. Samuel O, Sakin P, Sybald B. Counting on quality: A medical audit workbook. London: RCGP, 1993
31. Rating scales for depression and anxiety. *Beaumont psychiatry in practice*. 1993; 2: 17–20
32. Shaper AG, Pocock SJ, Walter M *et al.* Risk factors for ischaemic heart disease: the prospective phase of the British Regional Heart Study. *J Epidemiol Community Health* 1985; 39: 197–209
33. Lancaster T, Sleight P. Secondary prevention of coronary heart disease. In: Lawrence M, Neil A, Fowler G, Mant D (eds) Prevention of cardiovascular disease: an evidence based approach. Oxford: Oxford University Press, 1996
34. Pharoah PDP, Hollingworth W. Cost effectiveness of lowering cholesterol concentration with statins in patients with and without pre-existing coronary heart disease: life table method applied to health authority population. *Br Med J* 1996; 312: 1443–1448

Index

A

abciximab, PTCA patients, 104, 108
abdominal hernias, *see* groin hernias
abscess, prostatic, 20
acaricides, 180
accident prevention, 235
ACE inhibitors, hypertension, 97
Achilles tendon, sports injuries, 203–4, 204
acromioclavicular joint, 204
  degenerative changes, 205
  dislocation, 207
  injuries causing tenderness around, 206
acyclovir, genital herpes, 170
adenoma, colorectal
  to carcinoma sequence, 51, 60
  endoscopy and removal, 54, 55
adenomatous polyposis, familial, 59
adenopathy, STDs, 168
adjuvant therapy, colorectal cancer, 57–8
adolescent suicide, 185
adrenal hydroxylase deficiency, 150, 151
adrenal hypertension, 94
adrenoceptor antagonists, *see* alpha-1-adrenoceptor blockers; beta blockers
affective/mood disorders (incl. depression), suicide risk due to, 188
  identifying, 190–1
  prevention, 193
age
  osteoporosis and, 211
    pathogenesis of age-related bone loss, 212
    treatment of, 217
  prostate cancer and, 118
  suicide and, 185
AIDS, *see* HIV disease
airway, upper, *see* ENT
alcohol consumption, 158
  colorectal cancer and, 53
  suicide and, 188
alendronate, osteoporosis, 217
allergic rhinitis, 226

alpha-1-adrenoceptor blockers/antagonists
  benign prostatic hyperplasia, 14
  hypertension, 97
5-alpha-reductase inhibitors, benign prostatic hyperplasia, 14
alprostadil, *see* prostaglandin E₁
ambulatory BP monitoring, 96
ambulatory surgery, hernia, 49
amoebiasis, 177
AMS penile prostheses
  inflatable, 135
  semi-rigid rods, 134
anaemia, colorectal cancer, 54
anal disease, *see* anus; perianal region
androgen(s), in male menopause
  changes in levels, 138–9, 140
  therapeutic use, 141–3
    new systems, 144
androgen ablation, metastatic prostate cancer, 18
androgen receptor and male menopause
  receptor status, 139–40
  selective modulators, 144
anejaculation, *see* ejaculation
angioplasty, coronary, *see* coronary angioplasty
angiotensin II receptor antagonists, hypertension, 97
angiotensin-converting enzyme inhibitors, hypertension, 97
anion-exchange resins in hyperlipidaemia, 92
ankle, sports injuries, 202–4
anti-androgens, metastatic prostate cancer, 18
antibiotics
  H. pylori eradication, *see* *Helicobacter pylori*
  prostatitis, 20, 21
  STDs
    genital ulcers, 170
    urethritis, 177
anticoagulant therapy, post-vascularization
  PTCA, 104
  stents, 108
antidepressants with suicide risk, 193
antihypertensives, 96–7

erectile dysfunction caused by, 128
antioxidant vitamins and prostate cancer, 121
antiplatelet agents, new, post-PTCA, 104
antiprotozoal agents, 177
antiretrovirals, 180–1
antisocial personality and suicide, 189
antisperm antibodies, 140
antivirals
  HIV, 180–1
  HSV, 170
anus, *see also* perianal region
  STDs affecting, 167
    examination, 164
    trauma in gay men, 162
anxiety disorders and suicide, 188
aortic coarctation and hypertension, 95
apnoea, obstructive sleep, 225
apolipoprotein E, 90, 91
apomorphine, 131
arterial supply, penis, 6, 125–6
  revascularization in erectile dysfunction, 133
ASPIRE, 92
aspirin
  coronary revascularization
    with balloon angioplasty, 104
    with stents, 108
  hyperlipidaemia, 92
assisted reproductive techniques, 153–4
atherectomy, *see* coronary atherectomy
atherosclerosis, 232–4, *see also* ischaemic heart disease
athletes, *see* sports
audit, Well Man clinic, 239
autonomic nerves, penis, 7, 126
avulsion injury/fracture
  finger, 210
  pelvis/hip/thigh, 199
azoöspermia, 152
  fructose testing, 149

B

bacterial prostatitis, 18–19, 20–2
  acute, 20

chronic, 20–2
bacterial STDs, 161
balloon dilatation
    coronary angioplasty, coronary
        vessels, *see* coronary
        angioplasty
    coronary stent, 108
barium enema, colorectal cancer, 55
basal cell carcinoma, genital, 87
Bassini–Shouldice operation, 47, 48
beta blockers, hypertension, 96–7
biopsy of testis in infertility, 151
biphosphonates, osteoporosis, 217
bladder cancer and smoking, 68–9
bleeding/haemorrhage
    bowel cancer, from rectum, 54
    peptic ulcer, 39
blood pressure
    measurement, 96
    raised, *see* hypertension
    twenty four-hour
        ambulatory monitoring, 96
        variations, 94
blood vessels
    in hypertension, 95
    penile, 6–7, 125–6
bone
    fracture, *see* fractures
    loss, 212
    mass/density
        development, 212
        measurement, 215
        reduced, *see* osteoporosis
bowel
    cancer, *see* colorectal cancer
    gay (syndrome), 176
    strangulation/obstruction by
        hernia, 46
bowel habit, colorectal cancer, 54
bowenoid papulosis, 82
Bowen's disease, 81, 82
brain, hypertension effects, 95
Buck's fascia, 5, 125

C

caffeine and colorectal cancer, 53
calcium antagonists, hypertension,
    97
calcium supplements, osteoporosis,
    216, 217
calculi, prostatic, 19
Calymmatobacterium granulomatis, see
    granuloma inguinale
cancer, 2, 236, *see also* premalignant
    lesions *and specific*
    organs/tissues
    dietary prevention, 73
    metastatic, *see* metastases
    smoking and, *see* smoking
car accidents, 157

carcinoembryonic antigen, colorectal
    cancer, 57
carcinoma, progression from
        colorectal adenoma to, 51, 60,
        see also specific types of
        carcinoma and specific cancers
carcinoma in situ, penile, 81–2
cardiovascular (incl. heart) disease,
        1–2, 89–115, 232–4, *see also*
        ischaemic heart disease
    diet and, 234, 237
    history of, in Well Man clinic
        protocol, 242
    smoking and, 69
CAVEAT trial, 109–10, 110
cavernosometry, 130
cavernous artery, 6, 125
cavernous body of penis, *see* corpus
        cavernosa
cavernous nerves, 7
cerebrovascular effects of
        hypertension, 95
cerumen impaction, 222
cervical mucus, sperm penetration
        tests, 150
chancre, 167
chancroid (*Haemophilus ducreyi*), 79,
        167, 168
    diagnosis, 169
    treatment, 170
chemotherapy
    colorectal cancer, adjuvant, 57, 58
    erythroplasia of Queyrat, 81
    testicular cancer
        avoiding, 28
        non-seminomatous germ cell
            tumour, 28, 28–9
        seminoma, metastatic, 28
childhood disease causing infertility,
        148
Chlamydia trachomatis
    lymphogranuloma venereum with,
        see lymphogranuloma
        venereum
    N. gonorrhoeae and, co-existing,
        172
    urethritis, 172
    treatment, 173
cholesterol levels, 89
    drugs lowering, 91–2
chronic obstructive pulmonary
        disease, 234–5
cigarettes, tar/nicotine content, *see*
        also smoking
    lung cancer occurrence and, 65
    reducing, 65, 73
cimetidine, peptic ulcer, 38
CMV, 179, 180
colitis, *see* proctocolitis; ulcerative
        colitis

Colle's fascia, 5
colonoscopy, colorectal cancer, 54
    in follow-up, 57
colorectal (incl. colon) cancer, 2,
        51–61
    clinical presentation, 54
    epidemiology, 51–2
    hereditary non-polyposis, 60
    high-risk groups, 59–60
    investigations, 54–5
    pathogenesis, 51
    predisposition and aetiology, 51–4,
        59–60
    preoperative staging, 55
    prevention, 58–9
    prognosis, 58
    screening, 59
    surgery, 55–6
        adjuvant therapy, 57–8
        follow-up, 56–7
compulsive personality and suicide,
        189
condom, correct use, 182
conductive hearing loss, 223
condyloma acuminatum, *see* HPV
condyloma latum, 174–5
coracoclavicular ligament, 204
    injuries, 205
coronary angioplasty
    laser, 113
    percutaneous transluminal
        (PTCA), 101–8, 113–14
        acute complications, 101–7
        acute results, 101
        directional atherectomy vs, 106,
            109
        late results/complications, 107–8
        limitations, 108
coronary artery bypass graft,
        emergency, failed angioplasty,
        105
coronary artery disease, *see* ischaemic
        heart disease
coronary atherectomy, 109–13
    directional, 109–10
        indications/contraindications,
            111
        post-PTCA, 105
        PTCA compared with, 106,
            109
    extraction, 111–13
    rotational, 110–11
coronary dissection in PTCA, 103
coronary heart disease, *see* ischaemic
        heart disease
coronary stent, 108–9
    design, 108
    post-PTCA, 105
coronary thrombus in PTCA,
        103–4

corpus cavernosa, *see also* cavernosometry; intracavernosal PGE₁ injections
circulation, 6
in erection, 8, 126
corpus spongiosum, 5, 125
corticosteroid-induced osteoporosis, 216–17
cost considerations, Well Man clinic, 237
Cowper's glands, 8
creatine kinase levels and post-PTCA MI, 105–6
Crohn's disease and cancer, 60
cruciate ligament injuries, anterior and posterior, 199, 200, 201
cryotherapy, viral warts, 175
cutaneous lesions, *see* skin lesions
cyclic GMP phosphodiesterase 5 inhibitors, 9, 131
cyst(s)
epididymal, 77
laryngeal, 227
cytomegalovirus (CMV), 179, 180

D

day-case surgery, hernia, 49
deafness, 223
deaths/mortalities (causes), 1, 156, *see also* suicide
accidental, 235
colorectal cancer, 52
hernia operations, 50
lifestyle factors, 2
prostate cancer, 118
fruit and vegetable intake and, 121
PTCA patients, 105
smoking-related, 63–75
Europe, 70–2
non-cancer, 69, 70
dehydroepiandrosterone (DHEA) and DHEA sulphate, male menopause and, 139
depot testosterone, male menopause treatment, 141
depression, *see* affective disorders
dermatological disorders, *see* skin lesions
detumescence, 9
diabetes
erectile dysfunction and, 130
hypertension and, 93–4
diet, 236–7
in cancer aetiology
colorectal cancer, 52–3
prostate cancer, 119–21, 121–2
in cancer prevention, 73
colorectal cancer, 58–9

prostate cancer, 121
as lipid lowering strategy, 91
in osteoporosis prevention, 217
digital rectal examination of prostate
benign prostatic hyperplasia, 14
infertility and, 149
dihydrotestosterone, 139, 141
benign prostatic hyperplasia and, 12
diltiazem, hypertension, 97
diuretics, hypertension, 96
donovaniasis, *see* granuloma inguinale
dorsal artery of penis, 6, 125
revascularization procedures, 133–4
doxazosin, benign prostatic hyperplasia, 14
driving accidents, 157
drugs, *see also specific (types of) drugs*
adverse reactions
erectile dysfunction, 127, 128
genital area, 165–6
diagnostic studies in erectile dysfunction, 129–30
misuse, *see* substance abuse
therapeutic use
erectile dysfunction, 130–3
hyperlipidaemia, 91–2
hypertension, 96–7
oligospermia (idiopathic), 153
peptic ulcer, 38–9
prostate cancer, metastatic, 18
prostatic hyperplasia (benign), 14–15
suicidal patients, 193
warts, 175
dry mouth, 224
dual energy X-ray absorptiometry, 215
Dukes' classification, colorectal cancer, 59
duodenal ulcers, *see* peptic ulcers

E

ear, *see also* ENT
disorders, 222–3
examination, 221
ear wax, impaction, 222
EBV, 179
economics, Well Man clinic, 237
ectoparasitic STDs, 161, 177–8
treatment, 180
education, health, *see* health promotion
ejaculation, 9–10, 148
failure/loss (anejaculation), 152
testicular cancer treatment-related, 29
retrograde, 151

ejaculatory duct obstruction, 149, 152
elbow, sports injuries, 207–9
elderly
exercise benefits, 233
suicide, 185–6
emission of semen, 9, 148
endocrine causes
hypertension, 94
infertility, 151
screening, 140, 150
menopause (male), 138–40
screening, 140–1
osteoporosis, 212
treatment, 216
endocrine therapy, *see also* hormone replacement therapy
erectile dysfunction, 130–1
metastatic prostate cancer, 18
endodermal sinus (yolk sac) tumour of testes, 79
endoscopy
colorectal cancer, 54
peptic ulcers, 36–7
sinus surgery, 226
ENT (ear, nose and throat)
history-taking, 221
physical examination, 221–2
Entamoeba histolytica, 177
enteritis and STD, 176–7
environmental factors, hypertension, 94
epicondylitis
lateral, 207, 208
medial, 207, 208
epidermoid cell carcinoma, *see* squamous cell carcinoma
epididymis
cyst, 77
obstruction, 152
epididymo-orchitis, 78
epigastric artery, inferior, in erectile dysfunction revascularization treatment, 133
epiglottis, 227
Epstein–Barr virus, 179
erectile function
anatomical aspects, 5–7, 125–6
disorders (impotence), 3, 125–36
diagnosis, 127–30
management, 3, 130–6
physiology, 8–9, 126–7
erythroplasia of Queyrat, 81
Escherichia coli, urinary tract infection, 19
ethnicity/race
colorectal cancer and, 51–2
suicide and, 186
etidronate, osteoporosis, 216, 217
Europe, smoking-related deaths, 70–2

evidence-based guidelines
    hyperlipidaemia, 92–3
    male menopause, 143–4
    osteoporosis, 218
exercise (or its lack), 233–4, *see also*
    sports
    benefits, 233–4, 235
    colorectal cancer and, 53
    coronary heart disease and,
      233–4
    history (in Well Man clinic
      protocol), 241
extraction atherectomy, 111–13
eye, hypertensive disease, 96

F

facial pain, 226
falls, osteoporotic fractures, 217
familial adenomatous polyposis, 59
family history
    suicide, 188
    in Well Man clinic protocol, 240
family screening, lipid levels, 91
fascia, penile, 5, 125
fat, dietary, *see also* lipid levels
    in hyperlipidaemia, reducing
      intake, 91
    in prostate cancer aetiology,
      119–21
feet, sports injuries, 202–4
femoral bone fracture
    neck, in osteoporotic, 214–15
    sport-related, 197
femoral hernias, *see also* groin hernias
    aetiology, 44–5
    epidemiology, 43
fertility, diminished/absent, *see*
    infertility
financial considerations, Well Man
    clinic, 237
firearm suicide, 186
flexor tendon injuries, hand, 209
follicle-stimulating hormone (FSH),
    8, 147–8
foot, sports injuries, 202–4
fractures
    osteoporotic, 214–15
      falls and, 217
    sport-related, *see* sports
French operation, 47
fructose testing, semen, 149
fruit intake
    cancer prevention and, 73
      prostate, 121
    heart disease prevention and, 237
fundiform ligament, 5

G

gastric acid, 33
gastric cancer and smoking, 67

gastric outflow obstruction, peptic
    disease, 40
gastric ulcers, *see* peptic ulcers
gastro-oesophageal/pharyngeal reflux
    disease, 228
gastroscopy, peptic ulcers, 36–7
gay men/homosexuals
    anorectal trauma, 162
    bowel disease, 176–7
    STDs, 162, 162–3
gender and colorectal cancer,
    51–2
genetic disease
    colorectal cancer as, 51, 60–1
    infertility in, 148
genetic factors
    hypertension, 93–4
    peptic ulcer, 33
    prostate cancer, 16
    suicide, 188
genitalia, *see* reproductive tract
germ cell tumours of testes, 78–9
    histological types, 26–7
Giardia lamblia, 177
glandular fever (infectious
    mononucleosis), 179
glenohumeral joint, 204–5
    degenerative changes, 205
    dislocation, 206–7
glyceryl trinitrate (nitroglycerine),
    intracoronary, PTCA patients,
    104
glycoprotein IIb/IIIa receptor
    (platelet) blocker, PTCA
    patients, 104, 108
cGMP phosphodiesterase 5
    inhibitors, 9, 131
golfer's elbow, 207, 208
gonadotrophin-releasing hormone,
    see luteinizing hormone-
    releasing hormone; luteinizing
    hormone-releasing hormone
    analogues
gonorrhoea, 171, 172–3
    C. trachomatis and, coexisting,
      172
    diagnosis, 171
    treatment, 173
granuloma, laryngeal, 228
granuloma inguinale (donovaniasis;
    C. granulomatis), 164, 167
    treatment, 170
groin hernias, 43–50
    anatomy and aetiology, 43–5
    diagnosis, 45–6
    embryology, 45
    epidemiology, 43
    treatment, 46–50, 77
      complications, 49–50
guns and suicide, 186

H

H_2-receptor antagonists, peptic ulcer,
    38
Haemophilus ducreyi, *see* chancroid
Haemophilus influenzae type B and
    epiglottis, 227
haemorrhage, peptic ulcer, 39
hairy leukoplakia, 229
hand, sports injuries, 209–10
head and neck, 221–9
    history taking, 221
    neoplasms, 224–5
    physical examination, 221–2
health, risk-taking, 155–60
health care personnel, Well Man
    clinic, 237–8
Health of the Nation, 231
    aims, 231
health promotion (incl. education),
    159–60
    programmes in primary care,
      231
    sexual health, 181
    value, 237
hearing loss, 223
heart
    disease, *see* cardiovascular disease;
      ischaemic heart disease
    hypertension effects, 95
Helicobacter pylori infection, 34–6
    eradication (antibiotics), 36, 38
      confirmation, 35
      recurrence rates, 34
    genetic factors for occurrence, 33
hemi-zona assay, 150
hepatic metastases, colorectal cancer,
    scanning, 57
hepatitis, viral, 179–80
heredity, *see* genetic disease; genetic
    factors
hernias, *see* groin hernias
herpes simplex virus (HSV)
    genital, 79, 164
    other areas, 167
high-density lipoprotein, 89, 90, 91
hip
    osteoporotic fractures, 217
    sports injuries, 197–9
histamine H_2-receptor antagonists,
    peptic ulcer, 38
HIV disease/AIDS, 158–9, 180–1,
    236
    cutaneous lesions, 178
      genital, 80, 174
    otolaryngology, 228–9
    risk-taking behaviour, 158–9, 181
    treatment, 180–1
HMG CoA reductase inhibitors, *see*
    statins

homosexuals, *see* gay men
hormone(s)
　causing disease, *see* endocrine
　　causes
　therapeutic use, *see* endocrine
　　therapy; hormone replacement
　　therapy
hormone replacement therapy
　(HRT)
　female menopause, 137, 144
　male menopause, 141–4
　　efficacy, 141–2
　　future directions, 143–4
　　safety issues, 142–3
HPV (human papilloma virus)
　bowenoid papulosis, 82, 84
　genital warts (condyloma
　　acuminata; genital warts), 80,
　　173–4, 174–6
　　treatment, 175
　tongue lesions, 224
HSV, *see* herpes simplex virus
human immunodeficiency virus
　disease, genital cutaneous
　　lesions, 80
human papilloma virus, *see* HPV
hydrocele, 77
　encysted, of cord, 79
hydroxymethylglutaryl CoA
　reductase inhibitors, *see* statins
5–hydroxytryptamine, *see* serotonin
hyperinsulinism and hypertension,
　93–4
hyperlipidaemia (lipaemia), 89–93
　aetiology, 89–90
　female:male ratio, 89
　investigation, 90–1
　shared care and evidence-based
　　guidelines, 92–3
　treatment, 91–2
hyperprolactinaemia
　infertility and, 150
　osteoporosis and, 216
hypertension, 93–8
　essential, aetiology, 93–4
　female:male ratio, 93
　investigation, 96
　pathological effects, 95–6
　prevention, 97
　secondary, aetiology, 94–5
　treatment, 96–7
　　drug, *see* antihypertensives
hypogonadism, 8
　bone loss/osteoporosis in, 213, 214
　　treatment, 216
　hypogonadotrophic, 151
　　testosterone replacement, 130–1,
　　142

imaging, *see* radiology
implants, penile, 134–6
impotence, *see* erectile function
in vitro fertilization, 153
infections
　ear
　　external, 222
　　internal, 222–3
　genital, *see also* sexually-
　　transmitted disease
　　external, 79–80
　　internal, 151
　HIV/AIDS-related opportunistic,
　　80, 174, 229
　infertility caused by, 148, 151
　laryngeal, 227
　paranasal sinus, 225
　with penile prostheses, 135–6
　prostate, *see* bacterial prostatitis
infertility, 147–55
　assisted reproductive techniques,
　　153–4
　clinical evaluation, 148–9
　diagnosis/investigations, 149–50
　　laboratory tests, 149–50
　in testicular cancer, treatment-
　　related, 29
inflammatory bowel disease and
　cancer, 60
inflatable penile prosthesis, 134–5
inguinal hernias, *see also* groin
　hernias
　aetiology, 44
　direct, 44, 46
　epidemiology, 43
　indirect, 44, 46–7
　surgery, 46–7
　　inguinoscrotal hernia, 77
inheritance, *see* genetic disease;
　genetic factors
injury/trauma, *see also* accident
　prevention
　anorectal, gay men, 162
　genital (sexual activity), 80, 165
　road traffic accidents, 157
innervation, penis, 7, 126
insemination, intra-uterine, 153
insulin levels/resistance and
　hypertension, 93–4
interviewing/questioning
　STDs, 163–4
　suicide risk, 190–2
intestine, *see* bowel
intracavernosal PGE$_1$ injections
　diagnostic, 129
　therapeutic, 131–2
intracytoplasmic sperm injection,
　153

intra-epithelial neoplasia, prostatic,
　15
intra-urethral PGE$_1$ delivery, 133
intra-uterine insemination, 153
ischaemia, myocardial, with PTCA,
　103
ischaemic heart disease (coronary
　disease), 89–115, 232–4
　history (in Well Man clinic
　　protocol), 242
　lifestyle and, 159
　　diet, 234, 237
　　smoking, 69
　lipids and, *see* hyperlipidaemia
　revascularization surgery, 101–5
Isospora belli, 177

K

Kallman's syndrome, 151
kidney
　cancer, smoking and, 69
　hypertension affecting, 95–6
　hypertension caused by, 94
knee, sports injuries, 199–202

L

labyrinthine disorders, 223
laparoscopic surgery, hernia, 49
larynx, 227–8
　cancer, smoking and, 67
　examination, 221–2
laser coronary angioplasty, 113
leg, sports injuries, 202–4
leukaemia and smoking, 69
leukoplakia
　glans penis, 84–5
　tongue, 229
lice, pubic, 177–8, 180
Lichtenstein operation, 47, 48
lifestyle, 2
　and heart disease, *see* ischaemic
　　heart disease
　risk-taking, 155–60
ligaments
　ankle, 202
　　sports injuries, 202, 203
　elbow, 207
　　sports injuries, 208
　knee, 199
　　sports injuries, 199, 200, 201
　shoulder, 204
　　sports injuries, 205
lindane, 180
lingual disease, *see* tongue
lip cancer and tobacco, 66
lipid levels
　drugs lowering, 91–2
　raised, *see* hyperlipidaemia
　recommended, 89

lipoprotein, 89–90
  high-density, 89, 90, 91
  low-density, 90, 91
  very-low-density, 90
lipoprotein(a), 90, 91
Littré's glands, 8
liver metastases, colorectal cancer,
    scanning, 57
louse, pubic, 177–8, 180
low-density lipoprotein, 90, 91
lubricants with condoms, 182
lung
  cancer (smoking-related), 2, 68
    historical epidemiology, 63–5
  chronic obstructive disease, 234–5
luteinizing hormone (LH), 8, 147–8
  and male menopause, 139
luteinizing hormone-releasing
    hormone (gonadotrophin-
    releasing hormone; GnRH;
    LHRH), 8, 147
luteinizing hormone-releasing
    hormone analogues in prostate
    cancer, 18
  osteoporosis associated with,
    213–14
lymphadenectomy, para-aortic,
    testicular cancer, 29
lymphadenopathy
  HIV disease, 229
  STDs, 168
lymphatics, penis, 7
lymphoepithelial lesions of parotid,
    benign, 229
lymphogranuloma venereum (in
    C. trachomatis infection), 79,
    164–5, 168
  diagnosis, 169
  treatment, 170
lymphoma in AIDS, 229

M

malignancy, see cancer
mallet finger, 210
meat, dietary, and prostate cancer,
    119, 120, 122
media, male images, 159–60
medicated urethral system for
    erection, 133
melanoma, penile, 87
menopause
  female, 137
    HRT, 137, 144
  male, 137–46
    aetiology, 138–40
    definition and size of problem,
      137–8
    investigations, 140–1
    treatment, 141–4

mental health, 157–8
  problems, see
      psychological/psychiatric
      problems
Mentor Alpha-1, 135
Mentor GRF, 135
metastases
  colorectal cancer in liver,
    scanning, 57
  prostate cancer, management, 18
  testicular cancer, management, 28,
    28–9
micronutrients prostate cancer
    prevention, 121, 122
microsporidiosis, 177
misoprostol, peptic ulcer, 39
molluscum contagiosum, 174
mononucleosis, infectious, 179
mood disorders, see affective
    disorders
mortalities, see deaths
motor vehicle accidents, 157
mouth, see oral cavity
mucous discharge, colorectal cancer,
    54
muscles
  of erectile function, 6
  sports injuries/strains
    knee, 201
    leg/ankle/foot, 203, 204
    pelvis/thigh, 197, 199
MUSE, 133
myocardial infarction after PTCA,
    non-Q wave, 105–6
myocardial ischaemia, see ischaemia;
    ischaemic heart disease

N

nasal/nasal sinus, see nose; paranasal
    sinuses
nasopharynx, 223–5
  examination, 221
nationality and suicide, 186
neck, see head and neck
Neisseria gonorrhoeae, see gonorrhoea
neoplasms, see tumours
nerve supply, penis, 7, 126
neurotransmitters in erection, 9,
    126–7
nicotinates, 92
nicotine content of cigarettes, see
    cigarettes
nitric oxide and erection, 9, 126, 127
nitroglycerine, intracoronary, PTCA
    patients, 104
nocturnal penile tumescence
    monitoring, 129
nodules, laryngeal, 227
noise-induced hearing loss, 223

non-gonococcal urethritis, 171, 172
  treatment, 173
non-polyposis colorectal cancer,
    hereditary, 60
non-steroidal anti-inflammatory
    drugs in peptic ulcer disease
  as cause, 33–4
  discontinuing, 38
Norwegian scabies, 178
nose, 225–6
  examination, 221
  tumours, 225–6
    malignant, smoking and, 67
Nottingham Health Profile, vertebral
    fractures, 214

O

obesity and overweight, 236
  cardiovascular disease and, 234,
    237
obstructive pulmonary disease,
    chronic, 234–5
obstructive sleep apnoea syndrome,
    225
occupation and colorectal cancer, 53
ocular disease, hypertensive, 96
oesophageal cancer and smoking, 67
oesophageal reflux, 228
oligospermia, idiopathic, 152–3
omeprazole, peptic ulcer, 38
oral cavity (incl. mouth), 223–4
  cancer, tobacco and, 66, 66–7
  examination, 221
  HIV disease-related lesions, 229
  STDs affecting, 167, 171, 175
orchiectomy, 28
organ transplant recipients,
    anogenital lesions, 80
orgasm, 9
oropharynx, 223–5
  examination, 221–2
osteoporosis, 211–19
  fractures, see fractures
  investigations, 215–16
  prevalence, 211–12
  prevention, 217–18
  primary, 213
  risk assessment (Well Man clinic
    protocol), 241
  secondary, 213–14, 216, 216–17
  testosterone in, see testosterone
  treatment, 142, 216–17
    follow-up, 218
    shared care/evidence-based
      guidelines, 218
otitis externa, 222
otitis media, 222–3
otolaryngology, see ENT
otosclerosis, 223

Our Healthier Nation, 231
overweight, *see* obesity

P

Paget's disease, extramammary, 86–7
pain
    facial, 226
    knee, 201
    prostatic area, 22
Palmaz–Schatz stent, 108, 109
pancreatic cancer and smoking, 67–8
papaverine in erectile dysfunction,
    132
    and phentolamine, 132
papilloma, laryngeal squamous,
    227–8
papilloma virus, *see* HPV
papular lesions, STDs, 173–4
papulosis, bowenoid, 82
para-aortic lymphadenectomy,
    testicular cancer, 29
paranasal sinuses, 226–7
    infection, 225
    tumours, 226–7
        malignant, smoking and, 67
parasitic STDs, 161
    ectoparasites, *see* ectoparasitic
        STDs
    treatment, 177, 180
parotid gland
    benign lymphoepithelial lesions,
        229
    tumours, 224–5
patellar tendon/ligament trauma,
    201, 202
patellofemoral joint disorders/pain,
    201
Pediculosis pubis (pubic lice), 177–8,
    180
pelvic sports injuries, 197–9
penile arteries, 6, 125
    revascularization, 133–4
penis
    anatomy, 5–7
    erection, *see* erectile function
    prosthetic implants, 134–6
    STDs affecting, appearances, 80,
        166, 167, 174
    traumatic erosion, 166
pepsin, 33
peptic ulcers (gastroduodenal ulcers),
    33–41
    aetiology, 33–5
    clinical features, 36
    complications, 39–40
    diagnosis, 35–6
    investigations, 36–7
    management, 36, 37–9
    pathogenesis, 35

percutaneous transluminal coronary
    angioplasty, *see* coronary
    angioplasty
perforated peptic ulcer, 39
perianal regions, STDs, 167, 176
    examination for, 164, 165
perineal squamous cell carcinoma, 86
permethrin, 180
personality and suicide, 188–9
pharyngitis following oral sex, 171
pharynx, 66, *see also* nasopharynx;
    oropharynx;
    uvulopalatopharnygoplasty
    cancer, and smoking, 66
    reflux of stomach contents into,
        228
phentolamine in erectile dysfunction
    intracavernosal, with papaverine,
        132
    sublingual, 131
phosphodiesterase 5 inhibitors, 9,
    131
Phthirus (*Pediculus*) *pubis*, 177–8, 180
physical activity, *see* exercise; sports
platelet glycoprotein IIb/IIIa receptor
    blocker, PTCA patients, 104,
    108
polyp(s)
    colorectal
        endoscopy, 54
        surgery, 54, 55
    laryngeal, 227
    nasal, 225, 226
polyposis coli, familial (FAP), 59
premalignant lesions
    genitalia (external), 81–5
    prostate, 15, 117, 119
priapism, 9
    intracavernosal drug-induced,
        131–2, 132
proctitis, 175–6
    herpes, treatment, 170
proctocolitis, 175–6
professional roles, Well Man clinic,
    237–8
prolactin excess, *see*
    hyperprolactinaemia
prostaglandin E_1 (alprostadil) in
    erectile dysfunction
    intracavernosal
        diagnostic, 129
        therapeutic, 131–2, 132
    intra-urethral, 133
prostaglandin E_1 analogue, peptic
    ulcer, 38
prostate, 7, 11–23, 117–23
    anatomy/physiology, 7, 11–12
    assessment (in Well Man clinic
        protocol), 241

benign hyperplasia, 3, 12–15, 236
    clinical effects, 13
    diagnosis, 13–14
    epidemiology, 117, 236
    examination, 14
    history-taking, 14
    risk factors, 13
    special investigations, 14
    testosterone therapy and risk of,
        143
cancer, 2, 15–18, 117–23, 159,
    236
    aetiology/risk factors, 16,
        117–23
    diagnosis, 16–17
    epidemiology, 15, 117, 236
    metastatic disease, 18
    osteoporosis complicating
        treatment, 213–14
    prevention, 121
    testosterone therapy and risk of,
        143
    treatment options, 17–18,
        117–18
digital examination, *see* digital
    rectal examination
in infertility
    palpation, 149
    ultrasound, 151
intraepithelial neoplasia, 15
treatment options, 14–15
prostate-specific antigen (PSA), 12
    measurement, 16–17
        in testosterone-treated patients,
        143
prostatectomy (prostate resection)
    radical, cancer, 17
    transurethral, in benign
        hyperplasia, 15
prostatitis, 18–22
    classification, 19–20
prostatodynia, 22
prosthetic implants, penile, 134–6
proton pump inhibitors, peptic ulcer,
    38
protozoal STDs, 161
    treatment, 177
psychogenic erectile dysfunction
    history-taking, 127
    treatment, 130
psychological/psychiatric problems,
    2, 235
    suicide related to, 187–8, 235
psychosocial factors, suicide, 187
psychotherapy, suicidal patients, 193
psychotropic drug-induced erectile
    dysfunction, 128
Pthirus (*Pediculus*) *pubis*, 177–8, 180
pubic lice, 177–8, 180

pudendal arteries, internal, 6, 125–6
pudendal nerve, 7
pulmonary disease, *see* lung

Q

questioning techniques, *see* interviewing
Queyrat's erythroplasia, 81

R

race, *see* ethnicity
radiology/imaging
  colorectal cancer, 55
  head and neck, 222
  osteoporosis, 215
  sport injuries
    elbow, 209
    knee, 201
    leg/ankle/foot, 204
    pelvis/hip/thigh, 197
    shoulder, 206
    wrist/hand, 209
radiotherapy
  colorectal cancer, adjuvant, 57, 58
  prostate cancer, 17
  testicular cancer, 28
ranitidine, peptic ulcer, 38
rannula, 224
rectum, *see also* digital rectal examination; proctitis; proctocolitis; transrectal ultrasound
  bleeding, in bowel cancer, 54
  cancer, *see also* colorectal cancer
    epidemiology, 52
    postoperative adjuvant therapy, 58
    postoperative complications, 56
    surgery, 55–6
  STDs affecting, 167
  trauma in gay men, 162
5-α-reductase inhibitors, benign prostatic hyperplasia, 14
reflux
  gastro-oesophageal/pharyngeal, 228
  intraprostatic urinary, 19
renal problems, *see* kidney
reproduction, *see* assisted reproductive techniques; infertility; sexual function
reproductive tract/genitalia
  cutaneous lesions (external genitalia), 79–87
    non-infectious ulcers, 165–6
  evaluation in infertility, 149
  external examination with STDs, 164, 165
  infections, *see* infections

resins in hyperlipidaemia, 92
respiratory disorders, *see* ENT; lung
restenosis after coronary revascularization
  with angioplasty, 107–8, 114
  with atherectomy, 110, 111
  with stenting, 109
retinopathy, hypertensive, 96
revascularization, arterial
  coronary, 101–15
  in erectile dysfunction, 133–4
rhinitis, allergic, 226
rhinosinusitis, 226
Rigiscan, 129
risk-taking behaviour, 155–60
  sexual behaviour, 158–9, 181
road traffic accidents, 157
Rotablator, 110, 111
rotational coronary atherectomy, 110–11
rotator cuff changes
  differential diagnosis, 205
  tears, 207
Royal Marsden Hospital testicular cancer staging, 27

S

salivary glands, 224
  lymphoepithelial lesions of parotid, 229
Sarcoptes scabiei, 177–8, 178–9
sartans, hypertension, 97
scabies, 177–8, 178–9
schizophrenia and suicide, 188
screening
  colorectal cancer, 59
  endocrinopathies
    causing infertility, 140, 150
    causing male menopause, 140–1
  lipid levels, 90–1
  prostate cancer, 16–17
scrotum
  anatomy, 7
  masses, 77–9
  varicocele, *see* varicocele
selenium supplementation and prostate cancer prevention, 121, 122
semen/seminal fluid
  analysis, 149–50
    WHO's normal values, 149, 150
  ejaculation, *see* ejaculation
  emission, 9, 148
  intra-uterine insemination, 153
seminal vesicles, 7
seminiferous tubules, 7
seminoma, 27, 79
  treatment, 28

semi-rigid penile prosthesis, 134
sensorineural deafness, 223
serotonin deficiency and suicide, 188
serotonin reuptake inhibitors, selective, suicidal patients, 193
serous otitis media, 222–3
sex hormone-binding globulin and male menopause, 138–9, 139
sexual behaviour
  risk-taking, 158–9, 181
  safe practices, 182
sexual function (incl. reproduction), 5–10, 125–44
  anatomy, 5–8
  disorders, 3, 125–44
  physiology, 8–10, 147–8
sexually-transmitted diseases, 79–80, 161–84, 236
  diagnosis, 169
  examination, 164
  gay men, 162–3
  history-taking, 163–4
  pathogens causing, 161
  prevention, 181–2
  treatment, 169–71, 173, 174, 175, 176–7, 178, 180, 180–1
shared care, guidelines
  hyperlipidaemia, 92–3
  male menopause, 142–3
  osteoporosis, 218
shoulder, sports injuries, 204–7
sinuses, paranasal, *see* paranasal sinuses
skin lesions, 236
  genital, 79–87
  in STDs, examination for, 165
sleep disorders, 225
smoking (and other tobacco use), 63–75, 157
  cancer and, 66–9
    colorectal, 53
    lung, *see* lung
  cessation programmes, 72–3
  fatal non-cancer diseases, 69, 70, 234
    lung, 234–5
  historical epidemiology of disease, 63–5
  non-fatal diseases, 69, 71
snoring, 225
snuff dipping, 67
social factors in death, 156
  suicide, 187, 192
social inequalities, 3
sore throat following oral sex, 171
sperm/spermatozoa, *see also* semen
  absence in semen, *see* azoöspermia
  antibodies to, 140

cervical mucus penetration tests, 150
formation (spermatogenesis), 147–8
arrest, 152
intracytoplasmic injection, 153
reduced numbers in semen (oligospermia), idiopathic, 152–3
tests, 149
functional, 149–50
spermatic cord
anatomy, 7
encysted hydrocele, 79
spermicides, 182
spinal vertebrae, osteoporotic fractures, 214–15
sports
injuries (incl. fractures), 197–210
elbow, 207–9
hand/wrist, 209–10
knee, 199–202
leg/ankle/foot, 202–4
pelvis/hip/thigh, 197–9
shoulder, 204–7
promoting participation in, 159
squamous cell carcinoma (epidermoid cell carcinoma)
penile, 85–6
perineal, 86
squamous cell carcinoma in situ, penile, 81–2
squamous papilloma, laryngeal, 227–8
staffing, Well Man clinic, 237–8
statins (HMG CoA reductase inhibitors), 91–2
fibrates combined with, 92
stent, see coronary stent
steroid-induced osteoporosis, 216–17
stomach, see peptic ulcer and entries under gastric
stones/calculi, prostatic, 19
Stoppa operation, 47
substance and drug abuse, 158, 236
suicide and, 188
suicide, 158, 185–95
attempted, 186–7
previous history, 191
contributing factors, 187–9
mental health problems, 187–8, 235
gesturers, 187
ideators, 187
identification of risk, 190–2
incidence, 185–6
methods, 176
prevention, 192–4
supraglottis, 227

surgery, see also specific procedures
colorectal cancer, see colorectal cancer
colorectal polyp, 54, 55
coronary revascularization, 101–15
erectile dysfunction, 133–6
groin hernia, 46–50
complications, 49–50
inguinoscrotal hernia, 77
nasal, 226
obstructive sleep apnoea syndrome, 225
paranasal sinus, 226
penis
malignant lesions, 85, 86, 86–7
premalignant lesions, 81–2, 82
peptic ulcer, 39
prostate
benign hyperplasia, 14
cancer, 17
scrotal masses
epididymal cyst, 77
hydrocele, 77
inguinoscrotal hernia, 77
testicular cancer, 28, 29
varicocele, 78, 151
Surgitek Uniflate-1000, 135
SWOT analysis, development of Well Man clinic, 238, 239
syphilis (T. pallidum infection), 79, 164
chancre, 167
condylomata lata, 174–5
diagnosis, 169
treatment, 170

T

tar content of cigarettes, see cigarettes
team, Well Man clinic, 237–8
teamwork, Well Man clinic, 238
tendons, sports injuries
hand/wrist, 209
leg/ankle/foot, 203–4, 204
tenesmus, colorectal cancer, 54
tennis elbow, 207, 208
medial, 207, 208
teratoma, testicular (non-seminomatous germ cell tumour), 27, 79
treatment, 28
testicles (testes)
anatomy, 7
relation to groin, 45
biopsy in infertility, 151
development, 45
maldescent, 25

in spermatogenesis, 148
testicular tumour/cancer, 3, 25–31, 78–9, 236
aetiology, 25
diagnosis, 3, 25–6
delayed, 27
early, 27–8
epidemiology, 25, 236
examination, 26
histological classification, 26–7
staging classification, 27
treatment, 27–9
side-effects, 29
testosterone
in erectile dysfunction
evaluation, 128–9
therapeutic use, 130–1
function, 8
in hypogonadotrophic hypogonadism, 130–1, 142
in male menopause
changes in levels, 138–9, 139, 140
measurement of levels, 140–1
therapeutic use, 141–3, 144
in osteoporosis
in pathogenesis, 212
replacement, 142, 216, 217
The Health of the Nation, see Health of the Nation
thiazide diuretics, hypertension, 96
thigh, sports injuries, 197–9
thrombus, coronary, with PTCA, 103–4
thyroid neoplasms, 224
tinnitus, 223
tobacco, see smoking; snuff
tongue disorders, 224
in HIV disease, 229
tonsillar hypertrophy, 223
transdermal delivery of testosterone
in hypogonadotrophic hypogonadism, 131
male menopause, 141
transluminal coronary angioplasty, percutaneous, see coronary angioplasty
transluminal extraction catheter atherectomy, 111–13
transplant recipients, anogenital lesions, 80
transrectal ultrasound
colorectal cancer, 55, 56
prostate in infertility, 151
transurethral prostate resection in benign hyperplasia, 15
trauma, see injury
trazodone, 130, 131

treponemal tests, 169, *see also* syphilis
Trichomonas vaginalis, 171
    treatment, 173
trinitroglycerin, intracoronary,
        PTCA patients, 104
tumescence, penile, 9
    nocturnal, monitoring, 129
tumour(s) (benign/unspecified/in
        general)
    external genitalia, 81
    head/neck, 224–5, 225–6
    laryngeal, 227–8
tumour(s) (malignant), *see* cancer
tumour markers
    colorectal cancer, 57
    testicular cancer, 26
tunica albuginea, 5–6, 125

U
ulcer(s), genital, 164–71
    diagnosis, 169
    treatment, 169–71
ulcerative colitis and cancer, 60
ulnar nerve pathology, 209
ultrasound
    colorectal cancer, 55, 56
    infertility, 151
urea breath test, *H. pylori* infection,
        35
urethra
    examination with STDs, 164
    PGE₁ delivery, 133

urethritis syndrome, 171–3
urinary reflux, intraprostatic, 19
urinary tract, lower
    infections, prostatitis and, 19, 21
    symptoms in benign prostatic
        hyperplasia, 13
urological disorders, 236
uvulopalatopharyngoplasty, 225

V
vacuum erection device, 133
varicoceles, 77–8
    in infertility, 149, 151
    treatment, 151
    ultrasound, 151
vas deferens
    congenital absence, 152
    obstruction, 152
vasculature, *see* blood vessels
vegetable intake
    cancer prevention and, 73
        prostate, 121
    heart disease prevention and, 237
velopharyngeal insufficiency, 224
venereal diseases, *see* sexually-
        transmitted diseases
venous drainage, penis, 6–7, 126
    incompetence, treatment, 134
verapamil, hypertension, 97
verrucous carcinoma, penis, 85
vertebrae, osteoporotic fractures,
        214–15

vertigo, 223
very-low-density lipoprotein, 90
viruses, sexually-transmissible, 161,
        173–6, 179–81
vitamins, antioxidant, prostate
        cancer and, 121
vocal fold lesions, 227

W
waist circumference and
        cardiovascular disease, 234
warts, genital, *see* HPV
wax in ear, impaction, 222
Well Man clinic, 3, 231–44
    benefits, 232, 233
    factors affecting success, 238
    financial considerations, 237
    protocols, 239–43
    staffing, 237–8
wrist, sports injuries, 209–10

X
xerostomia, 224
X-ray absorptiometry, dual energy,
        215

Y
yolk sac tumour of testes, 79

Z
zona pellucida and functional tests of
        sperm, 150